LABORATORY PROCEDURES

for Veterinary Technicians

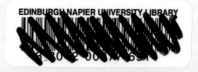

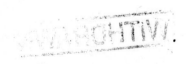

LABORATORY PROCEDURES
for Veterinary Technicians

FIFTH EDITION

Charles M. Hendrix, DVM, PhD
Professor of Parasitology
Department of Pathobiology
Auburn University College of Veterinary Medicine
Auburn, Alabama

Margi Sirois, EdD, MS, RVT
Program Director
Veterinary Technician Program
Penn Foster College
Scottsdale, Arizona

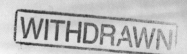

with 420 illustrations, more than 400 in full color

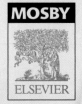

11830 Westline Industrial Drive
St. Louis, Missouri 63146

Notice

Neither the Publisher nor the Authors assume any responsibility for any loss or injury and/or damage to persons or property arising out of or related to any use of the material contained in this book. It is the responsibility of the treating practitioner, relying on independent expertise and knowledge of the patient, to determine the best treatment and method of application for the patient.

The Publisher

Previous editions copyrighted 1985, 1992, 1997, 2002

ISBN: 978-0-323-04572-8

Publishing Director: Linda L. Duncan
Publisher: Penny Rudolph
Managing Editor: Teri Merchant
Publishing Services Manager: Julie Eddy
Associate Project Manager: Laura Kudowitz
Senior Book Designer: Julia Dummitt

Printed in the United States of America

Last digit is the print number: 9 8 7 6 5 4

To my students—past, present, and future

CMH

To my family—especially Dan, Jen, and Daniel

MS

Contributors

Elaine Anthony, MA, CVT
Associate Professor, Veterinary Technology
St. Petersburg College, Pinellas Park, Florida
Nutritional Consultant, Nestle Purina

Eloyes Hill, BS, MT (ASCP)
Instructor, Veterinary Technology Program
Animal and Range Sciences
North Dakota State University, Fargo, North Dakota

Lisa A. Martini-Johnson, DVM
Assistant Professor; Assistant Director
Veterinary Technology Program
Lehigh Carbon and Northampton Community Colleges
Schnecksville, Pennsylvania

Preface

In recent years, the numbers and types of clinical laboratory tests now available for use in the veterinary practice have significantly increased. These technological advances have resulted in improved patient service and higher practice revenue and have greatly expanded the role of the veterinary technician. This book represents an effort to collect the relevant clinical laboratory information needed by the practicing veterinary technician. Veterinary assistant and veterinary technology students will also find this a valuable everyday reference. Principles and procedures for laboratory diagnostics in the areas of clinical chemistry, microbiology, hematology, hemostasis, parasitology, urinalysis, immunology, and cytology are presented. A basic understanding of the anatomy and physiology of common species has been assumed throughout the text but reviews of anatomy and physiology topics are included in some sections.

NEW TO THIS EDITION

This new edition has been significantly updated with expanded information that reflects the latest developments in the veterinary clinical laboratory. Specific features of this new edition include:

- Extensive full-color illustrations including numerous photomicrographs of blood cells, cytology and microbiology samples, and urine sediment
- New sections on laboratory mathematics, hematopoiesis, molecular diagnostics, and the physiologic basis of immunity
- Expanded information on clinical analyzers and quality assurance
- Key points and recommended readings for each chapter

- A glossary of key terms
- Information on professional associations related to veterinary clinical pathology

PROCEDURE BOXES

Step-by-step procedure boxes for all commonly performed hematology, cytology, and parasitology laboratory tests are included in this new edition. The procedure boxes represent those skills that veterinary technician students must perform during their educational program, as well as additional procedures that are commonly performed by veterinary technicians in private veterinary practice. The following procedures are included in specially colored boxes within the chapters:

Chapter 1: The Veterinary Practice Laboratory

- Operating the microscope
- Calibrating the microscope
- Using the refractometer

Chapter 2: Hematology and Hemostasis

- Preparation of wedge film blood smear
- Preparation of coverslip blood smear
- Evaluating bone marrow aspirate

Chapter 3: Clinical Chemistry

- Plasma sample preparation
- Serum sample preparation
- Intravenous glucose tolerance test
- ACTH stimulation test
- Dexamethasone suppression tests
- Protocol for combined dexamethasone suppression and ACTH corticotropin stimulation test

Chapter 4: Diagnostic Microbiology

- Typical sequence of testing of microbiology specimens
- Quadrant streak method for isolating bacteria
- Inoculating agar slant and butt

Chapter 5: Urinalysis

- Routine urinalysis
- Preparing urine sediment for microscopic examination

Chapter 6: Internal Parasites

- Examining tapeworm segments
- Direct smear
- Preparing flotation solutions
- Standard flotation
- Centrifugal flotation
- Fecal sedimentation
- Wisconsin double centrifugation technique
- Modified Wisconsin technique
- Cellophane tape technique
- Baermann technique
- Direct examination of blood
- Thick blood smear
- Buffy coat method
- Modified Knott's technique

Chapter 9: Cytology

- Collecting swab samples
- Collecting a scraping sample
- Collecting a Tzanch sample
- Collecting an imprint sample
- Fine needle biopsy aspiration technique
- Fine needle biopsy nonaspirate technique
- Punch biopsy sample collection
- Preparing a compression smear
- Modified compression smear technique
- Starfish smear technique
- Line smear technique

CONTRIBUTORS

Contributing authors to this edition include experienced veterinary technician educators from AVMA-accredited veterinary technology programs. Their knowledge and commitment to enhancing the learning of these complex subjects are evident in the improved organization of the chapters, as well as the inclusion of many new diagrams and boxes that summarize important test principles.

It is our hope that this text will serve as an every day reference guide for the veterinary technician in the clinical laboratory.

Charles M. Hendrix
Margi Sirois

Acknowledgments

This volume would not have been possible without the hard work of all the contributors to this and the previous editions. We sincerely thank them for their efforts. We are grateful for the expert assistance of our Elsevier editor, Teri Merchant, and appreciate her endless patience and humor. Numerous new illustrations in this edition would not have been possible without the assistance of the doctors and staff at the Gardner Animal Care Center in Gardner, Massachusetts; VCA St. Petersburg Animal Hospital in St. Petersburg, Florida; Oakhurst Veterinary Hospital in Seminole, Florida; and the Florida Veterinary Clinic in St. Petersburg, Florida. Special thanks also to Dr. Barry Mitzner for his assistance with illustrations.

Finally, we are fortunate to have friends, families, students, and colleagues who encourage and inspire us. We are indebted to all of you.

Contents

LABORATORY PROCEDURES

for Veterinary Technicians

CHAPTER 1

The Veterinary Practice Laboratory

Margi Sirois

KEY POINTS

- Proper quality control procedures are essential to the production of diagnostic quality laboratory results.
- A comprehensive laboratory safety program must be implemented in the practice laboratory to ensure the safety of employees.
- The veterinary practice laboratory must have a high-quality binocular microscope that is properly used and maintained.
- Clinical centrifuges are used for preparing samples for analysis.
- The refractometer is used for several types of tests and must be calibrated on a regular basis to ensure diagnostic-quality results.
- Most clinical chemistry analyzers use spectrophotometric methods and test principles based on Beer's law.
- Chemistry assays may use end point or kinetic methods.
- Electrochemical analyzers are primarily used for electrolyte assays.
- Chemistry analyzers have different advantages, benefits, and limitations.
- Cell counters for use in the veterinary practice laboratory may use either impedance or laser-based technology.
- Buffy coat analyzers provide estimates of cell counts.
- A variety of additional supplies and equipment may be needed in the veterinary practice laboratory depending on the specific tests performed.

Veterinarians depend on laboratory results to help establish diagnoses, track the course of diseases, and offer prognoses to clients. The veterinary practice laboratory can also be a significant source of income for the practice. Rapid availability of test results improves patient care and client service. Although some veterinary clinics utilize outside reference laboratories for test results, this may delay implementation of appropriate treatments for patients. Most diagnostic tests can be performed in-house by the well-educated veterinary technician. Veterinary practice laboratories have become increasingly sophisticated. Analytical instruments are affordable and readily available for inclusion in even the smallest veterinary clinic.

ROLE OF THE VETERINARY TECHNICIAN

The veterinary technician/veterinarian team approach works efficiently in a laboratory situation. A veterinarian is trained to interpret test results, whereas a veterinary technician is trained to generate these results. Consistent generation of reliable laboratory results requires an educated veterinary technician. A veterinary technician must understand the value of quality control in the laboratory.

LABORATORY DESIGN

General Considerations

The veterinary clinical laboratory should be located in an area that is separate from other hospital operations (Fig. 1-1). The area must be well lit and large enough to accommodate laboratory equipment, as well as provide a comfortable work area. Countertop space must be sufficient so that sensitive equipment such as chemistry analyzers and cell counters can be physically separated from centrifuges and water baths. Room temperature controls should provide a consistent environment, which in turn provides for optimal quality control. A draft-free area is preferable to one with open

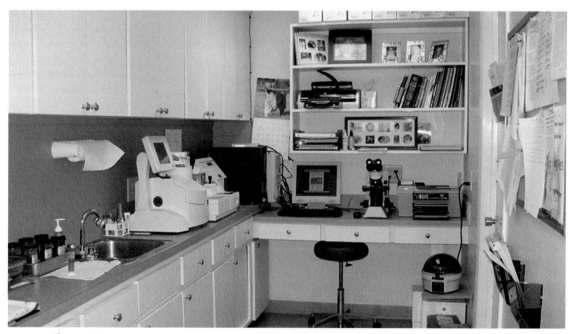

Figure 1-1. The clinical laboratory should be separate from the main traffic flow in the clinic.

windows or with air conditioning or heating ducts blowing air on the area. Drafts can carry dust, which may contaminate specimens and interfere with test results. Although each veterinary practice is unique, every practice laboratory has certain components, including a sink, storage space, electrical supply, and Internet access.

Sink

The laboratory area needs a sink and a source of running water to provide a place to rinse, drain, or stain specimens and reagents and to discard fluids. In every veterinary practice caution should be paramount; handling and disposing of hazardous laboratory materials bear legal and ethical responsibilities that have increased substantially in recent decades. Certain basic laboratory practices are essential for protection of workers and the environment. Some of these practices are simply good laboratory hygiene, whereas federal, state, and local regulations have mandated others. A thorough understanding of the laws is at the foundation of proper laboratory practices regarding hazardous chemicals and specimens. When in doubt, the veterinary technician should never dispose of unknown reagents or chemicals down any sink drain.

Storage Space

Adequate storage space must be available for reagents and supplies to avoid clutter on the laboratory counter space. Drawers and cabinets should be available so that needed supplies and equipment are conveniently located near the site they will be used. Some reagents and specimens must be kept refrigerated or frozen. A refrigerator and freezer should be readily available. A compact countertop refrigerator is sufficient for most practice laboratories. Frost-free freezers remove fluid from frozen samples, making them more concentrated if they are left in the freezer too long. For long-term storage of fluid samples (serum, plasma, etc.), a chest freezer or freezer that is not self-defrosting should be used.

Electrical Supply

Placement of electrical equipment requires careful consideration. Sufficient electrical outlets and circuit breakers must be available. Circuits must not be overloaded with ungrounded three-prong adapters or extension cords. Veterinary technicians should avoid working with fluids around electrical wires or instruments. An uninterruptible power supply may be necessary if sensitive equipment will be used or if the practice is located in an area subject to frequent power outages.

Internet Access

The diagnostic laboratory of the twenty-first century veterinary clinic should have Internet access in the laboratory or at another location within the veterinary clinic. Many reference laboratories use e-mail or fax to report the critical results of submitted diagnostic tests. In a veterinary clinic that has access to a digital camera attachment for the compound microscope, the veterinarian and the veterinary technician should use the Internet as a diagnostic aid. Photographic images such as scanned microscopic images of blood smears and urine sediments may be sent as email attachments to an outside reference laboratory for diagnostic assistance.

The Internet also may be a valuable resource for veterinary medical information. However, information on the Internet may be oversimplified, incomplete, or even inaccurate. The veterinary technician should use Internet sources for additional information along with consultation with the veterinarian. Together, the veterinarian and the technician should examine all Internet resources carefully to determine the quality of the website.

Two basic determinants are used to assess Web site quality. First, high-quality Internet sites are unbiased—the group providing the information should not have a vested interest (such as selling a product) in slanting the information a certain way. Second, sources should be staffed by recognized experts in the field, such as those from a government agency, college or university diagnostic laboratory, or the American Veterinary Medical Association.

Other signs of the quality of a Web site include the following:

- Funding and sponsorship are clearly shown.
- Timeliness (date of posting, revising, and updating) is clear and easy to locate.
- Information about the source (e.g., the organization's mission statement) is clear and easy to find.
- Authors or contributors to references on the site are clearly identified.
- References and sources for information are listed.
- Experts have reviewed the site's content for accuracy and completeness.

Box 1-1 summarizes some important criteria for evaluation of Internet resources.

Safety Concerns and Supplies

A comprehensive laboratory safety program is essential for ensuring the safety of employees in the clinical laboratory area. The Occupational Safety & Health Administration (OSHA) mandates specific laboratory practices that must be incorporated into the laboratory safety policy. The safety policy should include procedures and precautions for use and maintenance of equipment. Safety equipment

---

BOX 1-1
Evaluation Criteria for Internet Sources

Authority: Who is the author? Does the author list his or her occupation and credentials?
Affiliation: What company or organization sponsors the site?
Currency: When was the information created or updated?
Purpose: What is the purpose of the site (inform, persuade, explain)?
Audience: Who is the intended audience?
Comparison: How does the information compare with other similar works?
Conclusion: Is this site appropriate for research?

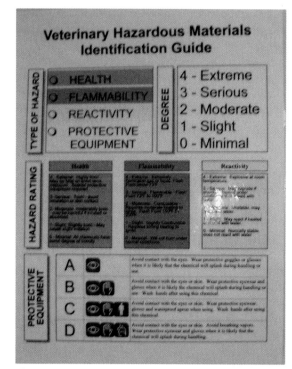

Figure 1-2. Sign explaining how to read hazardous material symbols.

and supplies, such as eyewash stations, fire extinguishers, spill clean-up kits, hazardous and biohazard waste disposal containers, and protective gloves, must be available. All employees working in the clinical laboratory must be aware of the location of these items and thoroughly trained in their use (Fig. 1-2). Laboratory safety policies must be in writing and placed in an accessible location within the clinical laboratory area. Signs should be posted to notify employees that eating, drinking, applying cosmetics, and adjusting contact lenses in the laboratory are prohibited.

LABORATORY MEASUREMENT AND MATHEMATICS

Veterinary technicians require knowledge and skill at performing a variety of calculations in the clinical laboratory. Reagent solutions might need to be prepared or diluted, samples must be measured and sometimes diluted, and results must be calculated.

All these mathematical operations require that the veterinary technician have a thorough understanding of the metric system as well as a strong background in basic algebra.

The Metric System

Although several systems of measurement are used in veterinary medicine, most of the calculations performed in veterinary practice involve units in the metric system. The metric system uses powers of 10 as a base for different units in the system. The metric system is a decimal system of notation with only three basic units for weight, volume, and length. Various values can be expressed in the metric system by adding prefixes to the basic units that designate multiples or fractions of the basic units. To work in the metric system, some of the more commonly used prefixes and their abbreviations must be memorized.

The three basic units of measure are summarized below:

Measurement	Unit	Symbol
Length	Meter	m
Mass	Gram	g
Volume	Liter	l or L

The **metric system** uses multiples or powers of 10 to describe magnitudes greater than or less than the basic units of meter, gram, and liter. The prefixes for the multiples and submultiples of basic units are provided in Table 1-1. For example, the **kilo**gram is 1000 grams, and the **milli**gram is 1/1000 gram.

Consistency is important in all use of numbers, but especially in the metric system. Although the unit gram may be abbreviated gm or Gm, the correct use is g. In addition, for example, 100 **centi**meters is 1 **meter,** and 1000 **meters** is 1 **kilo**meter. Volume examples include 10 **deci**liters in 1 **liter,** 10 **liters** in 1 **deca**liter, and 10 **deca**liters in 1 **hecto**liter.

To minimize errors and misinterpretations of numbers, a few general rules for use of the metric system must be learned. The one rule most often encountered is the unit equivalence of the cubic centimeter and the milliliter. In the metric system, these two units are both used for volume and

TABLE 1-1

Prefixes for the Multiples and Submultiples of Basic Units

Power of 10	Prefix	Symbol
10^{12}	tera	T
10^{9}	giga	G
10^{6}	mega	M
10^{3}	kilo	K
10^{2}	hecto	h
10^{1}	deca or deka	da
10^{-1}	deci	d
10^{-2}	centi	c
10^{-3}	milli	m
10^{-6}	micro	mc or μ
10^{-9}	nano	n
10^{-12}	pico	p
10^{-15}	femto	f
10^{-18}	atto	a

designate the same volume. This is because the metric measure of a liter is defined as a volume of 1000 cubic centimeters (cc) or a volume of 10 cm × 10 cm × 10 cm. Although the terms milliliter and cubic centimeter are often used interchangeably, milliliter is the correct designation for use in medicine.

As with all decimal units, any decimal number that has no whole number to the left of the decimal point should have a zero inserted as a placeholder. Zeroes should not be added after decimal numbers to avoid confusion in medication orders. Fractions are not written in the metric system. Always use decimal numbers to express numbers that are less than one.

Dilutions

The veterinary technician may be asked to prepare dilutions of reagents or patient samples in the clinical laboratory. Concentrations of dilutions are usually expressed as ratios of the original volume to the new volume. A ratio is the amount of one thing relative to another or the number of parts relative to a whole. Ratios may be written in a number of ways; for example, 1/2 = 1:2 = 0.5. These terms express the ratio that is one in two, or one to two, or one half. All three ratios are equal. The terms of a ratio are either abstract numbers (no units) or are of the same units. The only ratio usually expressed as a decimal in veterinary technology is specific gravity. Specific gravity is a ratio expressed in decimal form that represents the weight of a substance relative to the weight of the same volume of water.

To prepare a 1:10 dilution of a patient sample, combine 10 microliters (μL) of sample with 90 μL of distilled water. This represents a dilution that is 10:100, which reduces mathematically to 1:10. Results from any tests on this 1:10 dilution must then be multiplied by 10 to yield the correct result for the undiluted sample.

Serial dilutions are sometimes needed when performing certain immunologic tests or when preparing manual calibration curves for some equipment. The dilutions are prepared as described above, and the concentration of substance in each dilution is calculated. For example, if a standard solution of bilirubin contains 20 mg/dl and is diluted 1:5, 1:10, and 1:20, the concentration of each dilution would then be 4 mg/dl, 2 mg/dl, and 1 mg/dl, respectively.

EQUIPMENT AND INSTRUMENTATION

The size of the veterinary practice and the tests routinely performed in the laboratory determine the equipment and instrumentation needed. Minimal equipment includes a microscope, refractometer, microhematocrit centrifuge, and clinical centrifuge. Additional instrumentation needed, including blood chemistry analyzers, cell counters, and incubators, depends on the type and size of the practice, geographic locale of the practice, and the special interests of practice personnel.

Microscope

A high-quality binocular, compound light microscope is essential, even in the smallest laboratory (Fig. 1-3). It may be used to evaluate blood, urine, semen, exudates, and transudates; other body fluids; feces; and other miscellaneous specimens. It also

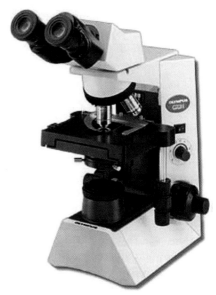

Figure 1-3. A binocular microscope for use in the veterinary clinical laboratory. (Courtesy of B. Mitzner, DVM.)

may be used to detect internal and external parasites and initially characterize bacteria. Ideally, the practice should maintain two microscopes. One should be used for performing routine parasite studies and procedures that use corrosive or damaging materials. The second microscope should be reserved for use with cytology and hematology evaluations.

A compound light microscope is so named because it generates an image by using a combination of lenses. Compound light microscopes have many components and a light path. The optical tube length is the distance between the objective lens and the eyepiece. In most microscopes this distance is 160 mm. The mechanical stage holds a glass slide to be evaluated. The microscope should have a smoothly operating mechanical stage to allow easier manipulation of the sample. Left- or right-handed stages are generally available. Coarse and fine focus knobs are used to focus the image of the object being viewed.

The compound light microscope consists of two separate lens systems: the ocular system and the objective system. The ocular lenses are located in the eyepieces and most often have a magnification of 10×. This means that the ocular lens magnifies an object 10 times. A monocular microscope has one eyepiece, whereas a binocular microscope, the most commonly used type, has two eyepieces.

Most compound light microscopes have three or four objective lenses, each with a different magnification power. The most common objective lenses are 4× (scanning), 10× (low power), 40× (high dry), and 100× (oil immersion). The scanning lens is not found on all microscopes. An optional fifth lens, a 50× (low oil immersion), is found on some microscopes.

Total magnification of the object being viewed is calculated by multiplying the ocular magnification power and the objective magnification power. For example, an object viewed under the 40× objective through a 10× ocular lens is 400 times larger in diameter than the unmagnified object:

$$10\times \text{ (ocular lens)} \times 40\times \text{ (objective lens)} =$$
$$400\times \text{ (total magnification)}$$

The microscope head supports the ocular lenses and may be straight or inclined. A microscope with an inclined head has ocular lenses that point back toward the user. This minimizes the need to bend over the microscope to look through the lenses. A binocular head is needed for nearly all routine laboratory evaluations. Trinocular heads are also available and can be used for training purposes or client education. The nosepiece holds the objective lenses and should always rotate easily and provide ready access to the objective lenses for cleaning. The ocular lenses must be compatible with the objectives in use, so be cautious about buying objectives and oculars from different sources. Wide-field objectives provide a larger visual field area than the standard type and are recommended when the user spends long periods looking through the microscope because they tend to reduce fatigue. High-eyepoint oculars are for individuals who need or prefer to keep their eyeglasses on while using the microscope; however, those who do not wear eyeglasses may find these advantageous as well.

The most important components of the microscope are the objective lenses. Objective lenses are characterized as one of three types: achromatic, semiapochromatic, and apochromatic. The latter two are primarily used in research settings and for photomicrography. One type of achromatic lens, known as planachromatic is also available. This lens type, also referred to as flat field, provides a more uniform field of focus from the center to the periphery of the microscopic image. However, high-quality achromatic lenses are also acceptable for most routine veterinary uses.

The resolving power of the microscope is an indicator of image quality and is described by the term *numerical aperture* (NA). The most common type of condenser is the two-lens Abbe type. The NA of the condenser should be equal to or greater than the NA of the highest power objective. The NA or resolving power of the lens system will be no greater than the NA of the highest power objective. This is especially important for objectives with NA greater than 1.0. To obtain the highest resolution from these objectives, a condenser of 1.0 or greater must be used and the condenser must be raised so that it makes contact with the bottom of the slide. Otherwise, air, which has an NA of 1.0, will be part of the systems, relegating it to a maximal resolution of 1.0.

When viewed through a compound light microscope, an object appears upside down and reversed. The actual right side of an image is seen as its left side, and the actual left side is seen as its right side. Movement of the slide by the mechanical stage also is reversed. Travel knobs are used to move the glass slide and thus the object (or portion of the object) to be moved. When the stage is moved to the left, the object appears to move to the right.

The substage condenser consists of two lenses that focus light from the light source on the object being viewed. Light is focused by raising or lowering the condenser. Without a substage condenser, haloes and fuzzy rings appear around the object. The aperture diaphragm is usually an iris type, consisting of a number of leaves that are opened or closed to control the amount of light illuminating the object.

In modern microscopes, the light source is contained within the microscope. The most common light sources found on compound light microscopes are low-voltage tungsten lamps or higher quality quartz-halogen lamps. The light source can be in the base or separate and should have a rheostat to adjust intensity.

Microscope prices vary depending on quality and accessories included. The best microscope for a typical practice is most often neither the most expensive nor the least expensive one. Accessories such as dual-viewing, phase-contrast or darkfield capabilities, digital cameras, and lighted pointers add to the price but also increase the versatility of the microscope (and the diagnostic laboratory). Reconditioned microscopes are sometimes available through medical or optical equipment suppliers and are an economical alternative to purchasing a new microscope.

Care and Maintenance

Regardless of the features of the individual microscope, care must be taken to follow manufacturer's recommendations for use and routine maintenance (Procedure 1-1). Only high-quality lens tissue should be used to clean the lenses. If cleaning solvent is needed, methanol can be used, or a specially formulated lens cleaning solution can be purchased. Excess oil may require the use of xylene for cleaning. However, xylene may also dissolve some of the adhesives used to secure the objective lenses and must therefore be used sparingly. Note that methanol and xylene are flammable and toxic. The microscope should be wiped clean after each use and kept covered when not in use. A dirty field of study may be caused by debris on the eyepiece. The eyepieces should be rotated one at a time while the technician looks through them. If the debris also rotates, it is located on the eyepiece. The eyepiece is cleaned with lens paper. Cleaning and adjustment by a microscope professional should be performed at least annually.

Extra light bulbs should be available. Changing a light bulb requires turning off the power and unplugging the microscope. When the defective bulb has cooled, it should be removed and replaced with a new bulb according to the manufacturer's instructions. Replacement bulbs should be identical to those they are replacing. Avoid touching the replacement bulb directly because oils from the skin can shorten the life of the bulbs.

PROCEDURE 1-1

Operating the Microscope

1. Lower the stage to its lowest point.
2. Turn on the light.
3. Inspect the eyepieces, objectives, and condenser lens and clean as necessary. (Consult the manufacturer's operating manual for any special cleaning instructions.)
4. Place the slide or counting chamber on the stage, appropriate side up.
5. Move the 10× objective into position by turning the turret, not the objective lens.
6. While looking through the eyepieces, adjust the distance between them so that each field appears nearly identical and the two fields can be viewed as one.
7. Use the coarse and fine focus knobs to bring the image into focus.
8. Adjust the condenser and diaphragms according to the manufacturer's instructions. This allows full advantage of the microscope's resolving power.
9. When using the 40× (high-dry) objective:
   - Look for a suitable examination area using the 10× (low-power) objective.
   - Swing the high-dry objective into place.
   - Do not use oil on the slide when using the high-dry objective.
10. When using the 100× (oil-immersion) objective:
    - Locate a suitable examination area using the 10× (low-power) objective.
    - Place a drop of oil on the slide.
    - Swing the oil-immersion objective into place.
11. When finished:
    - Turn the light off.
    - Lower the stage completely.
    - Swing the 43× or 103× objective into place.
    - Remove the slide or counting chamber.
    - Clean the oil-immersion lens if necessary.

Locate the microscope in an area where it is protected from excessive heat and humidity. With proper care, a high-quality microscope can last a lifetime. The microscope should be placed in an area where it cannot be moved frequently, jarred by vibrations from centrifuges or slamming doors, or splashed with liquids. It must be kept away from sunlight and drafts. The microscope is carried with both hands, one hand securely under the base and the other holding the supporting arm.

Calibration of the Microscope

The size of various stages of parasites is often important for correct identification. Some examples are eggs of *Trichuris vulpis* versus eggs of *Capillaria* species and microfilariae of *Dirofilaria immitis* versus microfilariae of *Dipetalonema reconditum*. Calibration of the lenses should be performed on every microscope that is used in the laboratory. Each objective lens must be individually calibrated (Procedure 1-2).

The stage micrometer is a microscope slide etched with a 2-mm line marked in 0.01-mm (10-m) divisions (Fig. 1-4); 1 micrometer (μm) equals 0.001 mm. The stage micrometer is used only once to calibrate the objectives of the microscope. Once the ocular micrometer within the compound microscope has been calibrated at 4×, 10×, and 40×, it is calibrated for the service life of the microscope; the stage micrometer is never used again. The stage micrometer should therefore be borrowed from a university or other diagnostic laboratory rather than purchased.

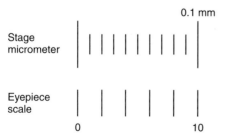

Figure 1-4. Stage micrometer *(upper scale)* and eyepiece scale *(lower scale)* used to calibrate the microscope.

PROCEDURE 1-2

Calibrating the Microscope

1. Start at low power (10×) and focus on the 2-mm line if using the stage micrometer. The 2-mm mark equals 2000 μm.
2. Rotate the ocular micrometer within the eyepiece so that its hatch-mark scale is horizontal and parallel to the stage micrometer (see Fig. 1-4).
3. Align the 0 points on both scales.
4. Determine the point on the stage micrometer aligned with the 10 hatch mark on the ocular micrometer. (In Fig. 1-4, this point is at 0.100 mm on the stage micrometer.)
5. Multiply this number by 100. In this example, 0.100 × 100 = 10 μm. This means that at this power (10×), the distance between each hatch mark on the ocular micrometer is 10 μm. Any object may be measured with the ocular micrometer scale, and that distance is measured by multiplying the number of ocular units by a factor of 10. For example, if an object is 10 ocular units long, then its true length is 100 μm (10 ocular units × 10 μm = 100 μm).
6. Repeat this procedure at each magnification.
7. For each magnification, record this information and label it on the base of the microscope for future reference. The ocular micrometer within the microscope is now calibrated for the duration.
   Objective distance between hatch marks (micrometers):
   4×: 25 μm
   10×: 10 μm
   40×: 2.5 μm

The ocular micrometer is a glass disk that fits into one of the microscope eyepieces. It is sometimes referred to as a reticle. The disks impose an image of a net, scale, or crosshairs over the viewing area. The reticle should be mounted in a separate ocular that can be removed and replaced with a nonreticle assembly for times when the scale is not needed. The disk is etched with 30 hatch marks spaced at equal intervals. The number of hatch marks on the disk may vary, but the calibration procedure does not change. The stage micrometer is used to determine the distance in micrometers between the hatch marks on the ocular microm- eter for each objective lens of the microscope being calibrated. This information is recorded and labeled on the base of the microscope for future reference.

Centrifuge

Another vital instrument in the veterinary practice laboratory is the centrifuge. The centrifuge is used to separate substances of different densities that are in a solution. When solid and liquid components are present in the sample, the liquid portion is referred to as the supernatant and the solid component is referred to as the sediment. The supernatant, such as plasma or serum from a blood sample, can be removed from the sediment and stored, shipped, or analyzed. Veterinary practice laboratories often have more than one type of centrifuge. The micro- hematocrit centrifuge is designed to hold capillary tubes, whereas a clinical centrifuge accommodates test tubes of varying sizes.

Clinical centrifuges used in veterinary labora- tories are one of two types depending on the style of the centrifuge head. A horizontal centrifuge head, also known as the swinging-arm type, has specimen cups that hang vertically when the cen- trifuge is at rest. During centrifugation, the cups swing out to the horizontal position. As the speci- men is centrifuged, centrifugal force drives the particles through the liquid to the bottom of the tube. When the centrifuge stops, the specimen cups fall back to the vertical position.

The horizontal head centrifuge has two disad- vantages. At excessive speeds (greater than 300 revolutions/min), air friction causes heat buildup and can damage delicate specimens. Also, some remixing of the sediment with the supernatant (fluid) may occur when the specimen cups fall back to the vertical position.

The second type of centrifuge head available is the angled centrifuge head (Fig. 1-5). The specimen tubes are inserted through drilled holes that hold the tubes at a fixed angle, usually approximately 52 degrees. This type of centrifuge rotates at higher speeds than the horizontal-head centrifuge, without excessive heat buildup. The angled centrifuge head is usually configured to accommodate just one tube size. Smaller size tubes require the use of an adaptor unless a small-capacity centrifuge is available (Fig. 1-6). Microhematocrit centrifuges are a type of angled centrifuge. The microhematocrit centrifuge is configured to accommodate capillary tubes.

In addition to a standard on/off switch, most centrifuges have a timer that automatically turns the centrifuge off after a preset time. A tachometer or dial to set the speed of the centrifuge is also usually present. Some centrifuges do not have a tachometer and always run at maximal speed. Most centrifuges have speed dials calibrated in revolu- tions per minute (rpm) times 1000. Thus a dial setting of 5 represents 5000 rpm. Some laboratory procedures require that a specific relative centrifu- gal force (RCF) or G-force be used. The calculation for RCF requires measurement of the radius of

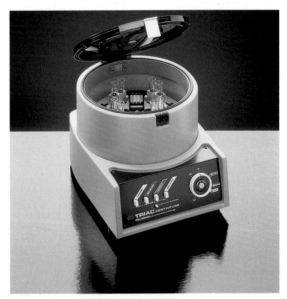

Figure 1-5. This centrifuge is capable of accommo- dating both centrifuge tubes and hematocrit tubes.

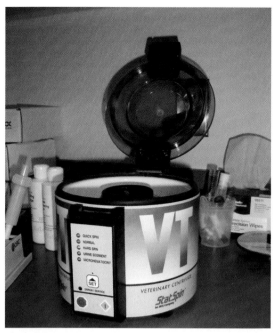

Figure 1-6. The StatSpin centrifuge. This angled-head centrifuge is specifically designed for small sample volumes. (Clover Labs, Sylvania, OH.)

the centrifuge head (r), measured from the center to the axis of rotation. The RCF is then calculated as follows:

$$RCF = 1.18 \times 10^{-5} \times r \times rpm^2$$

A centrifuge also may have a braking device to rapidly stop it. The brake should only be used in cases of equipment malfunction when the centrifuge must be stopped quickly. The centrifuge should never be operated with the lid unlatched. Always load the centrifuge with the open ends of tubes toward the center of the centrifuge head. Tubes must be counterbalanced with tubes of equal size and weight. Water-filled tubes may be used to balance the centrifuge. This ensures that the centrifuge will operate correctly without wobbling and that no liquid is forced from the tubes during operation. Incorrect loading of the centrifuge can cause damage to the instrument and injury to the operator. The centrifuge should be cleaned immediately if anything is spilled inside it. Tubes sometimes crack or break during centrifugation. Pieces

of broken tubes must be removed when the centrifuge stops. If these are not removed, they could permanently damage the centrifuge. The operator's manual should list maintenance schedules of the different components of the centrifuge. Some centrifuges require periodic lubrication of the bearings. Most need the brushes checked or replaced regularly. A regular maintenance schedule prevents costly breakdowns and keeps the centrifuge running at maximal efficiency.

Specimens must be centrifuged for a specific time at a specific speed for maximal accuracy. A centrifuge that is run too fast or for too long may rupture cells and destroy the morphologic features of cells in the sediment. A centrifuge that is run too slowly or for less than the proper time may not completely separate the specimen or concentrate the sediment. Information regarding speed and time of centrifugation should be developed for all laboratory procedures and followed for maximal accuracy.

Refractometer

A refractometer, or total solids meter, is used to measure the refractive index of a solution. Refraction is the bending of light rays as they pass from one medium (e.g., air) into another medium (e.g., urine) with a different optical density. The degree of refraction is a function of the concentration of solid material in the medium. Refractometers are calibrated to a zero reading (zero refractive index) with distilled water at a temperature between 60° F and 100° F. The most common uses of the refractometer are determination of the specific gravity of urine or other fluids and the protein concentration of plasma or other fluids.

The refractometer has a built-in prism and calibration scale (Fig. 1-7). Although refractometers can measure the refractive index of any solution, the scale readings in the instrument have been calibrated in terms of specific gravity and protein concentrations (g/dl). The specific gravity or protein concentration of a solution is directly proportional to its concentration of dissolved substances. Because no solution can be more dilute or have a lower concentration of dissolved substances

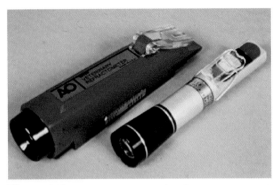

Figure 1-7. Refractometer scale. This instrument is used for measurements of urine specific gravity and total solids in plasma. (From McCurnin DM, Bassert JM: *Clinical Textbook for Veterinary Technicians,* ed 6, St. Louis, 2006, Saunders.)

than distilled water, the scale calibration and readings (either specific gravity or protein concentration) are always greater than zero. The refractometer is read on the scale at the distinct light-dark interface (see Fig. 2-9).

Various refractometer models are available. Most are temperature compensated between 60° F and 100° F. As long as the temperature remains between these two extremes, even as the refractometer is held in the hands, the temperature fluctuation will not affect the accuracy of the reading.

Care and Maintenance

Procedures for use of the refractometer are given in Procedure 1-3. The refractometer should be cleaned after each use. The prism cover glass and cover plate are wiped dry. Lens tissue should be used to protect the optical surfaces from scratches. Some manufacturers suggest cleaning the cover glass and plate with alcohol. The manufacturer's cleaning instructions should be consulted.

The refractometer should be calibrated regularly (weekly or daily depending on use). Distilled water at room temperature placed on the refractometer should have a zero refractive index and therefore read zero on all scales. If the light-dark boundary deviates from the zero mark by more than one-half division, the refractometer should be adjusted by turning the adjusting screw as directed by the manufacturer. The refractometer should not be

PROCEDURE 1-3

Using the Refractometer

1. Inspect and clean the prism cover glass and cover plate.
2. Place a drop of sample fluid on the prism cover glass.
3. Point the refractometer toward bright artificial light or sunlight.
4. Bring the light-dark boundary line into focus by turning the eyepiece.
5. Read and record the result with the appropriate scale (specific gravity, protein).
6. Clean the refractometer according to the manufacturer's recommendations.

used if not calibrated to zero with distilled water. Newer refractometers are digital and contain a microprocessor that provides automatic calibration and temperature monitoring (Fig. 1-8).

Chemistry Analyzers

A variety of different chemistry analyzers are available for use in the veterinary practice laboratory.

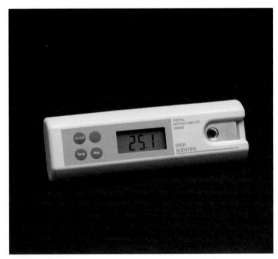

Figure 1-8. Digital refractometer. (Courtesy of B. Mitzner, DVM.)

Veterinarians are better able to diagnose disease and monitor patient therapy when results are available immediately. Most chemistry analyzers used in the veterinary practice utilize the principles of photometry to quantify constituents found in the blood. Analyzers using electrochemical methods are also available for in-house use.

Photometry

Several types of photometers are used in in-house diagnostic equipment (Fig. 1-9). Spectrophotometers are designed to measure the amount of light transmitted through a solution. The basic components of spectrophotometers are the same regardless of the specific manufacturer of the equipment. All spectrophotometers contain a light source, a prism, a wavelength selector, a photodetector, and a readout device (Fig. 1-10). The light source is typically tungsten or halogen lamp. The prism functions to fragment the light into its component wavelength segments. The majority of spectrophotometric tests use wavelengths in the visible portion of the electromagnetic spectrum. A few tests are also available that use wavelengths in the near-infrared and ultraviolet portions of the spectrum. The wavelength selector is usually a cam that only allows one specific wavelength of light to pass into the sample. The photodetector receives whatever light is not absorbed by the sample. The photodetector signal is then transmitted to the readout device. Depending on the model of the instrument, the readout units may be in percent transmittance, percent absorbance, optical density, or concentra-

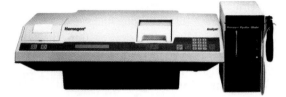

Figure 1-9. The Analyst Blood Chemistry Analyzer. Hemagen Diagnostics Columbia, MD. (Courtesy of B. Mitzner, DVM.)

tion units. Some automated analyzers use variations of the basic photometric procedure. A type of photometer that uses a filter to select the wavelength is referred to as a colorimeter. Another type detects light reflected off a test substance rather than transmitted light. This type is referred to as a reflectometer.

The wavelength used for measurement of a specific blood constituent is chosen on the basis of absorbance properties of the constituent being measured. The wavelength of light chosen for a given measurement is the one that results in the greatest light absorbance (least amount of light transmission) through the sample. For example, if a solution appears blue-green, it will transmit the greatest amount of blue-green light, whereas light in the red portion of the spectrum will be absorbed. Therefore a wavelength in the red portion of the spectrum provides maximal absorbance and would be used for measurement of the component. For a solution to be measured with spectrophotometry, the solution must adhere to

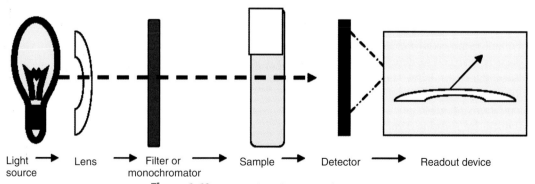

Light source → Lens → Filter or monochromator → Sample → Detector → Readout device

Figure 1-10. Principles of spectrophotometry.

the principle of Beer's law, also known as Beer-Lambert's law. This principle states that a direct linear relationship exists between the concentration of an analyte and light absorption when monochromatic light (light of a single wavelength) is passed through the sample. The law also states that the transmission of monochromatic light through a sample and the concentration of an analyte in the sample have an inverse exponential relationship. The degree of color change is proportional to the solution's concentration.

End Point versus Kinetic Assays

Most photometric analysis procedures use end point readings. That is, the reaction that occurs between the sample and reagent reaches a stable end. The analyzer then uses either a one-point calibration or an internal standard curve to calculate the patient results. Either method requires the use of a standard. A standard is a nonbiologic solution of the analyte, usually in distilled water, with a known concentration. For a one-point calibration, the standard is analyzed in the same manner as a patient sample, and the reaction characteristics are mathematically compared with the patient sample. The specific type of calculation varies depending on the analyzer. In general, however, the ratio of the optical density (O.D.) of the reacted standard is compared with the optical density of the patient sample. An example of this type of calculation is as follows:

$$\text{Patient sample concentration} = \frac{\text{Patient sample O.D.} \times \text{concentration of standard}}{\text{O.D. of standard}}$$

The internal standard curve is created when the analyzer is calibrated. To perform a standard curve, serial dilutions are created of the standard solution, and each is analyzed to determine its absorbance or transmittance of light. The results from each dilution are plotted on a graph as a straight line. The concentrations of subsequent patient samples are determined by locating the intersection of the absorbance of the reacted patient sample with the line on the graph. Analyzers that use standard curve methods must be recalibrated each time new reagent is purchased.

Some analyzers use kinetic methods rather than end point. These are primarily used for enzyme assays or when the reagent is enzyme based. Enzymes induce chemical changes in other substances (called substrates) but are not inherently changed. An enzyme may increase the rate of a biochemical reaction by acting as a catalyst to the reaction. Most enzymes are formed and function intracellularly, so they are found in highest concentrations within cells. For this reason, the blood level of most enzymes is low in a healthy animal. The blood level of an enzyme may be elevated if the enzyme has leaked out of damaged cells or if the cells have increased production of the enzyme and the excess amount has leaked out of the cells into the blood. Each specific enzyme catalyzes the reaction of one specific substrate. Each enzymatic reaction produces a specific product from the interaction of substrate and enzyme. The reaction forms a product but no change in the enzyme.

Because blood levels of enzymes are so low, directly measuring enzyme concentrations is difficult. The tests performed to determine enzyme concentrations in blood indirectly measure the enzyme concentration present by directly measuring the rate of formation of the product of the enzymatic reaction. Kinetic assays do not reach a stable end point. The reaction results are recorded at a specific time after initiation of the reaction even though the reaction continues beyond that time. Measurements not made at the correct time are usually not accurate. One-point calibrations are not generally performed for kinetic measurements. However, several points can be evaluated, and the change in absorbance for both the standard and the patient sample can be used to calculate patient results. When standard curves are created for kinetic methods, the graph is created by choosing the reaction time during which the absorbance would be as close as possible to a straight line. The specific time after initiation of the reaction when the reaction is closest to linear is different for each analyte.

Enzymes are most active when the substrate concentration is high and the product concentration is zero. If the enzyme concentration in the patient sample exceeds the substrate available in the test reagents, the enzyme activity is no longer proportional to the product formed, and the assay is invalid. (The substrate concentration has become a limiting factor to the enzymatic reaction.)

Substrate concentrations must be kept high enough so that they do not invalidate the measurement. Enzymatic/kinetic test kits are manufactured so that a large amount of substrate is initially present to avoid this problem. If the amount of enzyme present in the patient sample is doubled, the rate of the reaction is doubled and the amount of product formed is doubled, as long as time is constant. If the amount of enzyme present in the patient sample is the same but the time is doubled, the amount of product doubles. Therefore if time and enzyme concentration are kept constant, the rate of the reaction may be determined.

Enzyme activity may be inhibited by low temperatures and accelerated by high temperatures. Ultraviolet light and the salts of heavy metals, such as copper and mercury, retard enzymes. Enzymes are proteins and may be denatured by temperature and pH extremes or by organic solvents. Even a small change in an enzyme's polypeptide chain structure may cause it to lose activity, so samples for enzyme assay must be handled with care.

Each enzyme has an optimal temperature at which it works most efficiently. This temperature is typically listed in the instructions that accompany the test kit or analyzer. Most assays are performed at temperatures between 30° C and 37° C (86° F to 98.6° F). For every 10° C (18° F) above the optimal temperature, the enzyme activity doubles. Close monitoring of the incubator or water bath temperature used in enzyme assays is important.

Units of Measurement

Enzyme concentrations are measured as units of activity. These units of measurement may be confusing. For example, enzyme activity is proportional to the enzyme concentration only under certain conditions.

Each investigator who developed an enzymatic analytic method assigned his own unit of measurement to the results, which often reflected the developer's name: Bodansky, Somogyi, and Sigma-Frankel. Because each of the assays was performed

under different conditions (pH, temperature), correlation of the results reported in one unit to those of another became difficult. To avoid this confusion, the International Union of Biochemistry established a unit of enzyme activity known as the *International Unit* (U or IU). According to this system, enzyme concentration is expressed as milliunits per milliliter (mU/ml), units per liter (U/L), or units per milliliter (U/ml). An International Unit is defined as the amount of enzyme that, under given assay conditions, will catalyze the conversion of 1 micromole of substrate per minute. Box 1-2 shows how to convert various units to International Units. Some laboratories have replaced the International Unit system with one better related to the Systeme Internationale (SI) set of basic units, which is based on the metric system. In this system the katal is the basic unit of enzyme activity, the amount of activity that converts 1 mole of substrate per second.

Enzymes usually are named for the substrate on which they act or the biochemical reaction in

---

BOX 1-2
Factors for Converting Various Enzyme Units to International Units

Alkaline Phosphatase
Bodansky units × 5.37 = IU/L
Shinowara-Jones-Reinhart units × 5.37 = IU/L
King-Armstrong units × 7.1 = IU/L
Bessey-Lowry-Brock units × 16.67 = IU/L
Babson units × 1.0 = IU/L
Bowers-McComb units × 1.0 = IU/L

Amylase
Somogyi (saccharogenic) units × 1.85 = IU/L
Somogyi (37° C; 5 mg starch/15 min/100 ml) × 20.6 = IU/L

Lipase
Roe-Byler units × 16.7 = IU/L

Transaminases
Reitman-Frankel units × 0.482 = IU/L
Karmen units × 0.482 = IU/L
Sigma-Frankel units × 0.482 = IU/L
Wroblewsky-La Due units × 0.482 = IU/L

which they participate. Most enzyme names end with the -ase suffix. For example, lipase is an enzyme that catalyzes biochemical reactions that result in the hydrolysis of lipids, or fats, to fatty acids, and lactate dehydrogenase participates in a reaction that involves oxidation, or dehydrogenation, of lactate to pyruvate.

Some enzymes found in different tissues occur as isoenzymes. An isoenzyme is one of a group of enzymes with similar catalytic activities but different physical properties. The serum concentration of an enzyme that occurs as isoenzymes is the total of the concentrations of all the isoenzymes present from various tissues. Identification of which isoenzyme is present in the sample also allows identification of the source of that particular isoenzyme. For example, serum alkaline phosphatase is found in many tissues, particularly osteoblasts, and hepatocytes. If the total serum alkaline phosphatase level is elevated, ascertaining whether the increase is from damaged bone cells or damaged liver cells is impossible. However, if the respective levels of the various isoenzymes of alkaline phosphatase are assayed, levels of the isoenzyme from the damaged tissue are elevated, thus identifying the damaged tissue. The alkaline phosphatase assay performed in the practice laboratory is for total serum alkaline phosphatase because individual isoenzyme assay methods have not yet been developed for the practice laboratory.

Electrochemical Methods

Some analyzers use principles of electrochemistry to determine analyte concentrations. A few analyzers combine electrochemical and photometric methods within self-contained cartridges. Electrochemical methods are used for evaluation of electrolytes and other ionic components. These types of tests vary considerably in configuration but function in a similar manner (Fig. 1-11). Analyzers are designed with specific electrodes that are configured to allow interaction with just one ion. The most common of these systems are known as potentiometers. These systems are designed so that ions diffuse across an area separated by a membrane and the difference in voltage, or electric potential, between the two sides of the membrane

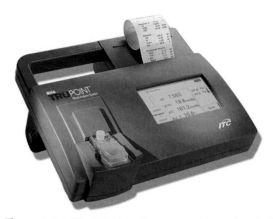

Figure 1-11. The IRMA analyzer uses electrochemical methods to measure blood gases and electrolytes. (International Technidyne. Edison, NJ) (Courtesy of B. Mitzner DVM.)

can be measured. This electrical variation corresponds to the number of active ions present in the sample.

Features and Benefits of Common Chemistry Analyzer Types

Most automated analyzers use liquid reagents, dry reagents, or slides that contain dry reagents. Liquid reagents may be purchased in bulk or in unitized disposable cuvettes. Dry reagents are available in unitized form. Bulk liquid reagents are the least expensive but require additional handling and storage space. Some reagents are flammable and toxic. The purchase of unitized reagents eliminates the hazards associated with handling these reagents. Dry slide reagents pose little or no handling or storage concerns but tend to be more expensive.

Analyzers that use dry systems include those with reagent-impregnated slides, pads, or cartridges. Most of these use reflectance assays. Dry systems tend to have comparatively higher costs associated with them than other analyzer types. Most are not configured for veterinary species and have fairly high incidences of sample rejection, particularly with samples that are lipemic or hemolyzed or are from large animals. However, they do have the benefit of not requiring reagent handling, and performance of single tests is relatively simple. Running profiles on these types of systems tends to be a bit more time-consuming than most other analyzer types. Some dry systems use reagent strips similar to those used for urine chemical testing.

Liquid systems include those that use a lyophilized reagent or an already prepared liquid reagent. The most common type of lyophilized reagent system for veterinary clinical practice uses rotor technology. The rotors consist of individual cuvettes to which diluted samples are added (Fig. 1-12). Cuvettes are optical-quality reservoirs used in the photometer and may be plastic or glass. Rotor-based systems tend to be quite accurate, although some are not configured for veterinary species. They are usually cost-effective for profiles but are not capable of running single tests. Other liquid systems in common use include those with unitized reagent cuvettes or bulk reagent. The unitized systems have the advantage of not requiring reagent handling but tend to be the most expensive of all the liquid reagent systems. In addition, running profiles with these systems is somewhat time-consuming, but single testing is simple. Bulk reagent systems may supply reagent in either concentrated form that must be diluted or working strength. Working strength reagent systems do not usually require any special reagent handling. These analyzers are the most versatile in that they can perform either profiling or single testing with relative ease. Most require little preparation time. However, some have extensive maintenance time, particularly with calibration of test parameters. Some systems that use bulk reagent may have a flow cell instead of a cuvette. Sample and reagent can be aspirated directly through the analyzer without the need for transfer of the reactants into cuvettes.

Dedicated-use analyzers are available for certain tests. These analyzers sample for only one substance, such as blood glucose (Fig. 1-13). Dedicated analyzers can be used if only a single test is requested or in emergency situations. Handheld analyzers for field use are also available (Fig 1-14).

Instrument Care and Maintenance

Chemistry analyzers are sensitive instruments that must be carefully maintained. Veterinary technicians should follow the manufacturer's operating instructions. Instruments generally have a warm-up period to allow the light source, photodetector, and incubator, if present, to reach equilibrium before they are used. Ideally, laboratory personnel should turn on the instrument in the morning and leave it on all day. The instrument is therefore ready to use

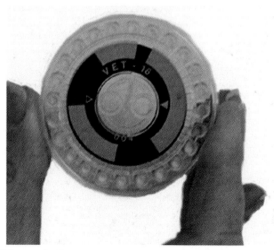

Figure 1-12. Reagent rotor for use in the Analyst Blood Chemistry Analyzer. (Courtesy of B. Mitzner, DVM.)

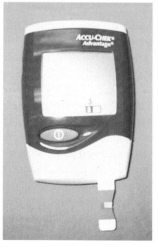

Figure 1-13. This dedicated glucose measuring instrument is available over the counter in many pharmacies. (From Busch SJ: *Small Animal Surgical Nursing: Skills and Concepts,* St. Louis, 2006, Mosby.)

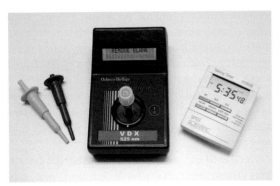

Figure 1-14. This handheld analyzer is used in equine practice to measure sperm count, serum immunoglobulin G, and colostrum immunoglobulin G in the field. (VDx, Inc., Belgium, WI) (Courtesy of B. Mitzner, DVM.)

at any time during the day, especially in emergency situations.

Following the manufacturer's maintenance schedule prolongs the life of the chemistry analyzer. A schedule sheet should be established for each instrument in the laboratory to allow quick and easy review of the maintenance history of any instrument. Most manufacturers have a toll-free number to call if problems arise.

Hematology Analyzers

Instrumentation designed for veterinary hospital use is available to facilitate generation of hematologic data for the complete blood count (CBC). Options are cost-effective and convenient in situations in which at least several CBCs are performed per day. Benefits of instrumentation include reduced labor investment, more complete information, and improvement of data reliability. The brief discussion in this text is not intended to provide an in-depth understanding of instrument system options. Individual users are responsible for becoming familiar with detailed documentation that accompanies specific instruments. Instrumentation for the veterinary hospital falls into three general categories: impedance analyzers, laser-based analyzers, and the quantitative buffy coat analysis system. Some manufacturers now provide analyzers that combine several methods for performing a CBC. One com-

monly available system uses impedance methods for enumeration of cells, as well as laser-based methods for performing the differential white blood cell count (Fig. 1-15). Some hematology analyzers also contain photometric capabilities for evaluation of hemoglobin.

Impedance Analyzers

A number of electronic cell counters used in human medical laboratories have been adapted for veterinary use (Fig. 1-16). This adaptation was necessary because of the variation in blood cell size among different animal species. Some companies have developed dedicated veterinary multispecies hematology systems that count cells and determine the hematocrit, hemoglobin concentration, and mean corpuscular hemoglobin concentration (MCHC). Some also provide a partial white blood cell (WBC) differential count.

Electronic cell counters that use the impedance method are based on passage of electric current across two electrodes separated by a glass tube with a small opening or aperture (Fig. 1-17). Electrolyte fluid on either side of the aperture conducts the current. Counting occurs by moving cells

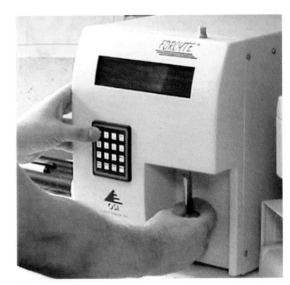

Figure 1-15. The Forcyte hematology analyzer combines impedance and laser-based methods. (Courtesy of Oxford Science, Inc., Oxford, CT.)

allowing the system to catalog cell sizes. Size information may be displayed in a distribution histogram of the cell population. Leukocytes, erythrocytes, and platelets may be enumerated with these systems.

These instruments are calibrated to count cells in specified size ranges, defined by threshold settings, which prevents erroneous interpretation of small debris and electronic noise as cells, and to properly separate cell populations in the same dilution, such as platelets and erythrocytes. Because cell populations vary in size among species, some of the threshold settings are species specific. These settings should be established by the manufacturer and are usually set automatically by system software when the user selects the species for analysis in a software menu. Comprehensive hematology systems designed specifically for veterinary applications are now commonly used in veterinary facilities. These systems incorporate the advantages of individual cell analysis that provides sophisticated information about blood cell populations.

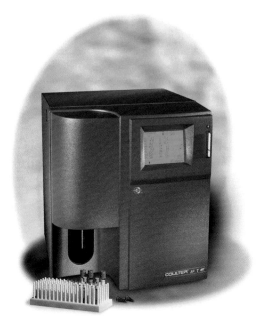

Figure 1-16. The Coulter AcTVet Hematology Analyzer, designed specifically for animal species, uses impedance technology. (Courtesy of Beckman Coulter, Fullerton, CA.)

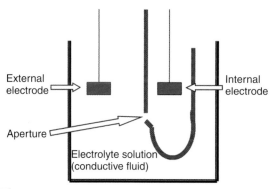

Figure 1-17. Principle of impedance analysis for cell counts.

The blood sample must be diluted to count cells. For WBCs, also known as leukocytes, a dilution is treated with a lytic agent that destroys cell membranes, leaving only nuclei for counting. Erythrocytes, also known as red blood cells (RBCs), may be analyzed on systems that count the RBCs and provide cell size information by using a much greater blood dilution to which no lytic agent is added. Erythrocyte analysis on automated systems provides diagnostic information about cell volume and an alternative method for determining the hematocrit (Hct). The mean corpuscular volume (MCV) may be directly measured from analysis of the erythrocyte volume distribution. The hematocrit is then calculated by multiplying the MCV by the erythrocyte concentration. On more sophisticated systems, the volume distribution curve of the erythrocyte population is displayed. In some analyzers, the red cell distribution width (RDW) may also be provided. This value is determined by mathematic analysis of the distribution and functions as an index of erythrocyte volume heterogeneity. Abnormally high values indicate increased volume heterogeneity and an underlying disturbance of the erythron. When used in

through the aperture by use of vacuum or positive pressure. Because cells are relatively poor conductors of electricity compared with the electrolyte fluid, they impede flow of current while passing through the aperture. These transient changes in current may be counted to determine the blood cell concentration. In addition, the volume or size of the cell is proportional to the change in current, conjunction with the MCV value, the RDW may alert the veterinarian to diseases of erythrocytes that alter RBC size. The same counting and sizing functions exist for counting platelets on more advanced systems.

Many automated hematology systems provide complete analysis of platelet, erythrocyte, and WBC populations, including WBC differential count information. Most provide graphic displays of cell population size analysis. Differential information is calculated from the WBC population size distribution. Normally these systems provide an estimate of the relative percentage of granulated and nongranulated WBCs. This value has limited application in the evaluation of patients with a pathologic condition. Variations in the size of the cells introduce error into this measurement. In addition, numerous morphologic abnormalities can be present and may not be identified with this partial differential count. A thorough examination of the differential blood film must also be included when evaluating patients.

Impedance analyzers are composed of numerous pumps, tubing, and valves that must be maintained. Diluting fluid and dusty glassware may be contaminated with particles large enough to be erroneously counted as cells. The aperture may become partially or totally obstructed. The threshold setting may be improperly set on a counter with a variable threshold control. Cold agglutinins may cause a decreased RBC count because of RBC clumping. Before processing, refrigerated blood samples must be warmed to room temperature. Fragile lymphocytes, as seen with some forms of lymphocytic leukemia, may rupture in the lysing solution used to lyse RBCs. This rupturing can result in a decreased WBC count. The presence of spherocytes (abnormally small, round RBCs) may alter the mean corpuscular volume, thus reducing the calculated hematocrit. Elevated serum viscosity may interfere with cell counts. Platelet counts obtained from impedance counters are affected by platelet clumping and are often inaccurate.

Quantitative Buffy Coat System

The quantitative buffy coat system (QBC, Becton Dickinson, Franklin Lakes, NJ) uses differential centrifugation and estimation of cellular elements by measurements on an expanded buffy coat layer in a specialized microhematocrit tube. It provides a hematocrit value and estimates of leukocyte concentration and platelet concentration. It extrapolates tube volumes to an estimate of concentration based on fixed cell volumes. Partial differential count information is provided in the form of total granulocytes and lymphocyte/monocytes categories. One limitation of these leukocyte groupings is that abnormalities such as left shift and lymphopenia may be undetected unless the blood film is examined as defined for the minimum CBC. These systems are best used as screening tools because they provide an estimation of cell numbers rather than an actual cell count.

Laser-Based Analyzers

These types of analyzers use laser beams to determine the size and density of solid components. Cells scatter light differently depending on the presence or absence of granules and nuclei. The degree and direction of light scatter allows enumeration of monocytes, lymphocytes, granulocytes, and erythrocytes. When certain dyes are added to the sample, variation in laser light scatter can also allow enumeration of mature and immature erythrocytes (Fig. 1-18).

Instrument Care and Maintenance

Electronic cell counters, similar to chemistry analyzers, are sophisticated instruments that require careful maintenance. The manufacturer's recommendations for routine maintenance should be followed. Daily maintenance for many electronic cell counters requires flushing the entire system with bleach and fresh diluting solution to keep the aperture open. Background counts are periodically performed to make sure the diluting solution is not contaminated or the glassware and tubing are not dirty. The vacuum pump must be checked at regular intervals to ensure that the proper amount of blood and diluting fluid is being drawn into the counter.

Incubators

A variety of microbiology tests require the use of an incubator. Incubators for the in-house veterinary practice laboratory are available in a variety of sizes

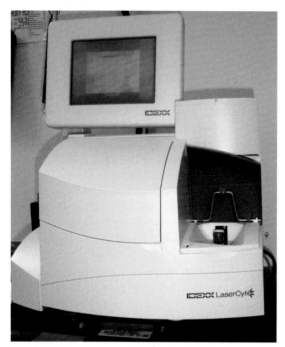

Figure 1-18. A laser-based analyzer for use in the veterinary practice laboratory.

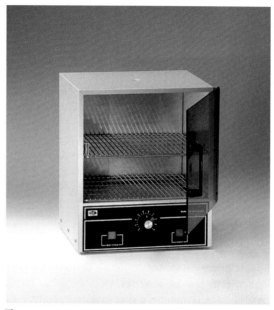

Figure 1-19. Small incubator for use in the veterinary practice laboratory. (Courtesy of B. Mitzner, DVM.)

and configurations. The incubator must be capable of sustaining a constant 37° C. The incubator should be either fitted with a thermometer or should have one placed inside the chamber to monitor temperature (Fig. 1-19). Heat should be provided by a thermostatically controlled element. A small dish of water should also be placed inside to maintain proper humidity. Some incubators have built-in humidity controls, but this type of equipment tends to be expensive. Larger laboratories may have incubators that automatically monitor temperature and humidity, as well as carbon dioxide and oxygen levels.

Pipettes

Although most test kits and analyzers contain their own specific pipettes and pipetting devices, some additional pipettes and pipetting devices may be needed in the veterinary practice laboratory. The primary types of pipettes used in the practice laboratory are transfer pipettes and graduated pipettes. Transfer pipettes are used when critical volume measurements are not needed. These pipettes may be plastic or glass, and some can deliver volumes by drops. Graduated pipettes may contain a single volume designation or have multiple gradations. Pipettes with single gradations are referred to as volumetric pipettes and are the most accurate of the measuring pipettes. Larger volumetric pipettes are usually designated as TD pipettes, which means that the pipette is designed "to deliver" the specific volume. A small amount of liquid should remain in the tip of the pipette after the volume has been delivered. Volumetric pipettes designed to deliver microliter volumes are designated TC, meaning that the pipette is designed "to contain" the specified volume. These pipettes must only be used to add specified volumes to other liquids. The pipette then must be rinsed with the other liquid to deliver the specified volume accurately. The small volume of fluid left in the tip of the pipette is then blown out of the pipette. Pipettes that contain multiple gradations are marked as either TD or "TD with blow out" depending on whether the fluid remaining in the tip of the pipette should remain or be blown out. TD with blow-out pipettes usually contain a double-etched or frosted band at the top.

The pipette chosen for a specific application should always be the one that is the most accurate and that measures volumes closest to the volume needed. For example, a 1-ml pipette, rather than a 5-ml pipette, should be chosen if the volume needed is 0.8 ml. Pipettes are also designed for measuring liquids at specified temperatures, normally room temperature. Liquids that are significantly colder or warmer will not measure accurately. Pipetting devices must also be used correctly, and fluid must not be allowed to enter the pipetting device. Never pipette any fluid by placing your mouth directly on the pipette.

Miscellaneous Equipment and Supplies

Some clinical chemistry and coagulation tests may require the use of a water bath or heat block capable of maintaining a constant temperature of 37° C. Slide dryers can be a useful addition to the busy veterinary practice laboratory. Aliquot mixers can also be helpful by keeping items well mixed and ready for use.

Quality Assurance

Quality assurance refers to the procedures established to ensure that clinical testing is performed in compliance with accepted standards and that the process and results are properly documented. Unlike human medical laboratories, veterinary facilities are not subject to regulations that require quality assurance programs. However, without a comprehensive quality assurance program, accuracy and precision of laboratory test results cannot be verified. A comprehensive quality assurance program addresses all aspects of the operation of the clinical laboratory. This includes qualifications of laboratory personnel, standard operating procedures for care and use of all supplies and equipment, sample collection and handling procedures, methods and frequency of performance of quality control assays, and record-keeping procedures.

Accuracy, Precision, Reliability

Accuracy, precision, and reliability are terms frequently used to describe quality control and are the standards for any quality control program. Accuracy is how closely results agree with the true quantitative value of the constituent. Precision is the magnitude of random errors and the reproducibility of measurements. Reliability is the ability of a method to be accurate and precise. Factors that affect accuracy and precision are test selection, test conditions, sample quality, technician skill, electrical surges, and equipment maintenance.

Test selection refers to the principle of the test method. Many of the tests used in veterinary laboratories were adapted from human medical laboratory tests. Additionally, the clinical significance of test results may vary among different species. Regardless of the test method used, care must be taken to follow the analytical procedure exactly. Any deviation can seriously affect the accuracy of results. Sample quality also greatly affects quality of test results. Samples that are lipemic, icteric, or hemolyzed may require special handling before use with most clinical analyzers. Collection of blood samples from properly fasted animals using appropriate techniques and equipment will minimize this significant source of error. Although not an obvious source of error, electrical power surges and dropouts can significantly alter equipment function. Repeated surges shorten the life of light sources in diagnostic equipment. All electrical equipment should be connected to a device designed to protect it from surges and electrical dropout. Human error is perhaps the most difficult testing parameter to control. Personnel responsible for performance of clinical testing must be appropriately trained in test principles and procedures. Mechanisms should be in place to provide for the continual education of all clinical laboratory personnel. Maintenance of equipment must also be included in quality control programs. A regular, written schedule of equipment maintenance allows changes in equipment function to be detected before obvious errors occur. Always follow manufacturer's recommendations for routine maintenance of instruments and equipment.

Analysis of Control Materials

Control serum is used for technician and instrument assessment. Producing valid results with control materials provides assurance that the procedure was performed correctly and that all components (reagents, equipment, etc.) are functioning correctly. Controls are handled exactly as are patient test samples and should be regularly assayed (with each test batch, daily, or weekly) at the same time patient serum samples are assayed (Fig. 1-20). The frequency of control testing depends on the laboratory's goals. To ensure reliability, control samples must be tested when a new assay is set up, a new technician runs the test, a new lot number of reagents is used, or an instrument is known to perform erratically. Ideally, a control sample is tested with each batch of patient samples. A problem with a particular assay may require an increase in the frequency of control testing.

After the assay is completed, the control value should fall within the manufacturer's reported range. If it does not, the assays of the patient and control samples must be repeated. The results of the analysis of control serum are recorded on a

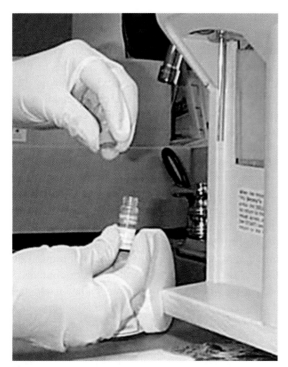

Figure 1-20. Control materials provided by the instrument manufacturer are assayed in the same manner as a patient sample.

chart or log for each assay (Fig. 1-21). The values for tests performed on control serum should not vary significantly each time the tests are performed. Data may be analyzed in two ways: the detection of shifts or trends and the determination of whether results for control samples are within the range established by the manufacturer. If a control serum result does not fall within the range, it should be retested. If it still fails to fall in the range, the reagents, instrument, and technique must be checked. When control values are successively distributed on one or the other side of the mean, the mean has shifted and a systematic error is involved.

Depending on the chemistry analyzer or electronic cell counter in the laboratory, an individual quality control program uses a number of solutions. Control serum consists of pooled, freeze-dried serum from many patients (usually human) that must be accurately rehydrated before use. Assayed control serum has been analyzed repeatedly for each of the many constituents present in serum (e.g., glucose, urea nitrogen, calcium). Data are statistically analyzed, and a range of acceptable values for each constituent is established. The accepted ranges are specific for each test method and equipment manufacturer. The manufacturer of the control serum provides a chart listing the range, or lowest acceptable value to highest acceptable value obtained during the many assays, and the mean, or average value, for each constituent.

Controls with both normal and abnormal concentrations of constituents should be evaluated because an assay method may not perform the same at all concentrations tested by a particular method. Normal control serum has constituent concentrations that approximate levels normal for that constituent. Abnormal control serum has constituent concentrations that are either higher or lower than normal. These abnormal concentrations represent concentrations seen clinically in disease conditions. If an abnormal concentration of a constituent is found in a patient sample, the results may be trusted if the abnormal control serum concentration was assayed as "in range."

Individual laboratories may produce their own control serum. Serum samples obtained from at least 20 clinically healthy animals of one species are pooled and analyzed numerous times in the

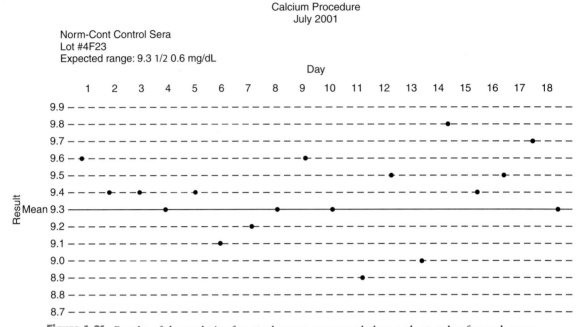

Figure 1-21. Results of the analysis of control serum are recorded on a chart or log for each assay.

laboratory. Data collected from these tests can be statistically analyzed to establish appropriate ranges and mean values. This procedure is time-consuming, especially for smaller laboratories. For this reason, purchasing commercial control sera is much more convenient.

Some manufacturers provide a quality control service in which test samples are sent to many laboratories for assay each month. The results from all the laboratories are collected and compared. From these results the manufacturer can identify laboratories with accuracy problems.

Errors

Many factors other than disease influence the results of laboratory tests. These factors may be preanalytical, analytical, or postanalytical. Postanalytical factors are primarily related to data entry and record keeping.

Preanalytical Variables

Preanalytical factors may be biologic or non-biologic. Biologic variables are factors that are inherent to the patient, such as breed, age, and gender. Because these cannot be controlled, they must be considered by the veterinarian when evaluating test results. Other biologic variables involve factors that can be controlled when drawing the blood sample, such as ensuring the animal is properly fasted. Nonbiologic variables are those related to clerical errors and sample collection and handling. The latter are usually postanalytical errors. Clerical errors are avoidable and include incorrect labeling, delays in transporting samples, incorrect calculations, transcription errors, and sampling the wrong patient. A well-trained and conscientious staff produces few clerical errors. Some of the most common problems related to sample handling are mislabeling and incomplete or incorrect requisition forms. All tubes, slides, and sample containers should be labeled with the owner's last name and the patient's name, species, identification number if available, and date.

Analytical Variables

Analytical variables affect the procedure by which the analyte is measured by the instrument. The specific impact on a test result will differ between laboratories depending on the type of instrumentation. Improperly maintained instruments can cause errors that are evident as shifts or trends in results obtained with a specific assay method. They often result in gradual changes, causing the mean value of results to shift in one direction (elevated or decreased). Some factors causing systematic errors include inaccurate standard sera, reagent instability, and method nonspecificity (using a test method unsuitable for the constituent being assayed).

Random errors are caused by variation found in glassware and pipettes, electronic and optic variations of instruments, and variation in temperature controls and timing. These errors occur in all parts of a system and increase the variability of results.

Applied Quality Control

Instrument maintenance is required to prolong the life of the instrument and prevent expensive downtime. All instruments are accompanied by an owner's manual. If the manual has been misplaced, the manufacturer should be contacted for a replacement. The manual lists the instrument components that must be inspected and attended to regularly. A notebook listing a schedule with the types of maintenance required for each instrument facilitates instrument maintenance. A page is dedicated to each instrument and includes the following:

- Instrument name
- Serial number
- Model number
- Purchase date
- Points to be checked
- Frequency of checks
- Record of test readings
- Changes made to restore accuracy and precision of readings
- Cost and time associated with necessary repairs and restoration
- Name or initials of the person performing the maintenance

Results obtained with control serum are recorded and kept in a permanent record. The veterinary technician should graph results so that changes or trends can be visually detected (see Fig. 1-21).

If attention is paid to detail and as many sources of all three types of error as possible can be eliminated, the laboratory can provide reliable results. Sloppy, inattentive work habits can lead to diagnostic and therapeutic disasters that may result in the death of an animal. Careful attention to detail ensures the veterinarian has all the correct information needed to make a proper diagnosis, prescribe appropriate treatment, and offer an educated prognosis.

LABORATORY RECORDS

Laboratory records are divided into internal and external record systems. Complete, up-to-date records are necessary for both systems. Numerous computer systems are now available for almost all the records generated in the veterinary clinic or hospital. Patient information, inventory, ordering information, sales records, and laboratory data can be stored on a computer. Clinics using a computer system should be sure to keep backup records in case of computer failure or damage from computer viruses.

Internal Records

By using internal records, the laboratory tracks assay results and obtains methods. The records consist of standard operating procedures (SOP) and quality control data and graphs. The SOP contains the instructions for all analyses run in the laboratory. Each procedure is described on a separate page. The easiest way to maintain the book is to insert the instruction sheets accompanying each commercial test kit in a three-ring binder, along with pages for any other procedures performed in the laboratory. Each procedure not performed with commercial kits is described on a separate page, including the name of the test, synonyms (if any) for the test, the rationale, reagent list, and step-by-step instructions for a single analysis. Individual pages can be inserted into plastic overlays for protection. The SOP book is reviewed periodically and updated as needed. Those who keep an SOP book on a computer should make sure an up-to-date hard copy backup is available.

External Records

Laboratory personnel communicate with people throughout the veterinary clinic or hospital and in other laboratories through the use of external records. These consist of request forms that accompany the sample to the laboratory, report forms for assay results, laboratory log books with individual test results, and a book containing pertinent information on samples sent to reference laboratories. In a clinic or hospital with an internal computer network, all personnel can access much of this information as needed.

Information provided on a request form includes the patient's full identification (including identification number, if available) and presenting signs, date and method used to obtain the sample, pertinent history, tests desired, any special notes regarding sample handling, and to whom and by what method results are to be reported (telephone, fax, e-mail, or written report).

The report form should include complete patient identification and presenting signs, test results (including appropriate units), and notation of any extraordinary observations or explanatory comments, if applicable. For additional backup, the laboratory staff should keep a log book to record test results. If the original laboratory report form is lost in transit, the results are retrievable.

Recommended Reading

Bellamy JE, Olexson DW: *Quality assurance handbook for veterinary laboratories,* Ames, IA, 2000, Iowa State Press.

Glick M, Ryder K: *Interferographs: user's guide to interferences in clinical chemistry instruments,* ed 2, Indianapolis, 1991, Science Enterprises.

Kerr MG: *Veterinary laboratory medicine: clinical biochemistry and haematology,* ed 2, 2002, Blackwell.

Lake T: *Dosage calculations for veterinary nurses and technicians,* St Louis, 2004, Elsevier.

CHAPTER 2

Hematology and Hemostasis

Elaine Anthony, Margi Sirois

KEY POINTS

- Hematopoiesis refers to the production of blood cells and platelets and includes erythropoiesis (production of erythrocytes), leukopoiesis (production of leukocytes), and thrombopoiesis (production of platelets).
- Sites for blood collection vary in different species, but the jugular vein is the vessel of choice for blood collection in most mammals.
- The preferred method of blood collection is the Vacutainer system.
- The preferred anticoagulant for hematology testing is ethylenediamine tetraacetic acid (EDTA); the preferred anticoagulant for coagulation testing is citrate.
- The complete blood count includes total red blood cell and white blood cell counts, packed cell volume, hemoglobin concentration, erythrocyte indices, and the differential blood cell count.
- Other tests that may be added to the complete blood count include the plasma protein concentration and reticulocyte count.
- Histograms provide a graphic presentation of the numbers of cells and platelets and can be used to aid in quality assurance.
- A differential white blood cell count, evaluation of the morphologic characteristics of red and white blood cells, and platelet estimate are vital parts of the complete blood count.

- Changes in leukocyte morphologic features may affect the nucleus and/or cytoplasm or involve inclusions within the cell.
- Changes in erythrocyte morphologic features affect the cell size, shape, color, and/or arrangement.
- Reticulocytes are immature red blood cells that require staining with a supravital stain for identification.
- Bone marrow samples may be collected by core sampling or aspiration techniques.
- A variety of techniques can be used to prepare bone marrow samples, with the compression smear the most common method.
- When examining bone marrow samples, evaluate cellular morphologic characteristics and determine the relative percentages of nucleated cells and adipocytes, the relative percentages of erythroid and myeloid cells, and the ratio of myeloid cells to erythroid cells.
- Blood coagulation proceeds through mechanical and chemical phases.
- Commonly performed tests for blood coagulation include the platelet count, activated clotting time, and buccal mucosa bleeding time. Additional tests are used in specific circumstances.

Hematology testing represents an important role of the veterinary technician: to provide accurate and reliable clinical laboratory test results to the veterinarian. An understanding of the principles of the various hematology tests and methods to ensure accuracy of results is vital. The recent focus on economic health of the veterinary clinic has also provided an opportunity for veterinary technicians to perform additional diagnostic testing, improve overall animal care, and provide an additional source of revenue for the clinic.

A complete hematology profile is indicated for diagnostic evaluation of disease states, well-animal screening (e.g., geriatric), and as a screening tool before surgery. The complete blood count (CBC) includes red and white blood cell counts, hemoglobin concentration, packed cell volume, differential white blood film examination, and calculation of absolute values and erythrocyte indices. Additional tests that may be needed include reticulocyte counts, measurement of total solids, and thrombocyte (platelet) estimates. Bone marrow evaluation is sometimes needed for definitive diagnosis and prognosis in some patients. In some patients, additional information on the hematopoietic and hemostatic systems are needed and bone marrow evaluation must be performed. Specific indications include unexplained nonregenerative anemia, leukopenia, thrombocytopenia, and pancytopenia (decreased numbers of all cell lines). Bone marrow evaluation is also used to confirm certain infections (e.g., ehrlichiosis) and diagnose hematopoietic neoplasms (e.g., lymphoproliferative disorders). Tests of the hemostatic systems (blood coagulation) include the thrombocyte count, bleeding time test, prothrombin time, and activated clotting time tests.

HEMATOPOIESIS

Hematopoiesis refers to the production of blood cells and platelets. Whole blood is composed of fluid and cells. The fluid component is plasma; the cellular component is made up of red blood cells (RBCs), also called erythrocytes; white blood cells (WBCs), also called leukocytes; and platelets, also called thrombocytes. An understanding of the overall process in the production of these components will aid in their evaluation. The process begins in early embryonic life and involves a number of complex chemical pathways and various organs. Some variations in the processes exist between juvenile and adult animals. Hematopoietic activity in the prenatal animal occurs in a variety of organs, including the liver, spleen, thymus, and red bone marrow. In the adult animal, the red bone marrow is the primary site for production and maturation of all the blood cells and platelets. However, during periods of hematopoietic stress, the liver and spleen may revert to their fetal role and produce blood cells in the adult.

Erythropoiesis (the production of erythrocytes), leukopoiesis (the production of leukocytes), and thrombopoiesis (the production of platelets) involve different pathways and chemical messengers. However, all the blood cells arise from the same pluripotent hematopoietic stem cell. In response to interaction with various chemical messengers, referred to as cytokines, the stem cells begin to differentiate into one of two types: myeloid or lymphoid. Further differentiation in response to additional cytokines results in commitment to forming specific cell types. Nearly two dozen different cytokines have been identified. The primary cytokine responsible for the production of RBCs is erythropoietin (EPO). EPO is primarily produced by certain cells in the kidney in response to decreased oxygen tension. The cells produce EPO, which then circulates in the blood to the bone marrow, where it binds to receptors on the surface of erythroid precursor cells, causing them to divide and mature. Lesser amounts of EPO are also produced in hepatocytes. The stimulus for production of leukocytes and thrombocytes is less understood. The hormones leukopoietin and thrombopoietin are involved, as are numerous additional cytokines. Figure 2-1 summarizes the stages in early hematopoiesis. Some references refer to the early progenitor lines (myeloid, lymphoid) as colony-forming units and the later stages as blast-forming units.

The myeloid line differentiates into erythroblasts, which give rise to the erythrocytes; megakaryoblasts, which give rise to platelets; and the myeloblast, which gives rise to the granulocytic

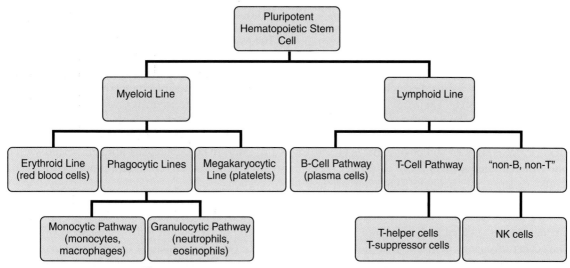

Figure 2-1. Summary of the stages of early hematopoiesis.

leukocytes and the monocytes. The lymphoid line differentiates into the lymphoblast, which gives rise to the various populations of lymphocytes.

COLLECTION AND HANDLING OF BLOOD SAMPLES

When preparing to collect blood, the technician should first determine what specific test procedures will be needed. This will determine, in part, the equipment and supplies needed and the choice of a particular blood vessel from which to collect the sample. The sample must be drawn before the initiation of any medical treatment. If treatments have been given, these must be noted on the blood sample collection record. Some test methods cannot be accurately performed once the patient has received certain pharmaceutical therapies.

The preferred blood source is almost always venous blood. Jugular blood collection is most appropriate in common veterinary species. In some species there are no readily accessible veins, or the collection of venous blood would be excessively traumatic to the animal. It may be necessary to collect peripheral or capillary blood samples in those cases. Commonly used blood collection sites

TABLE 2-1

Commonly Used Blood Collection Sites

Canine	Cephalic vein
	Jugular vein
	Saphenous vein
Feline	Cephalic vein
	Jugular vein
Equine	Jugular vein
Bovine	Caudal vein
	Mammary vein
	Jugular vein
Avian	Wing vein
	Toenail clip
Rabbit	Ear vein
	Toenail clip
Rodents	Tail vein
	Cardiac puncture

Reprinted from Sirois M: *Veterinary clinical laboratory procedures,* St Louis, 1995, Mosby.

are summarized in Table 2-1. The blood collection site must be cleaned and swabbed with alcohol before collection. The alcohol should be allowed to dry before proceeding with the sample collection. The animal must be restrained, preferably with minimal manual restraint. Every effort should be made to minimize stress in the patient because it often compromises the sample.

Collection Equipment

Traditionally samples have been collected by using a needle and syringe. When this method is used, the needle chosen should always be the largest one that the animal can comfortably accommodate. The syringe chosen should be one that is closest to the required sample volume. Use of a larger syringe could collapse the patient's vein. The preferred method of blood collection is the use of a vacuum system (Fig. 2-2). This system is composed of a needle, needle holder, and collection tubes. The collection tubes may be plain sterile tubes or may contain anticoagulants. The tubes are available in sizes ranging from a few microliters to 15 ml. The correct size tube must be used to minimize damage to the sample or the possibility of collapsing the vein. The tubes should be allowed to fill to the correct volume, based on the strength of the vacuum pressure in the tube, to ensure the appropriate ratio of anticoagulant and blood. An advantage of this system is that multiple samples can be collected directly into the collection tubes without multiple venipuncture procedures. Sample quality is best when samples are collected with vacuum tubes using proper techniques.

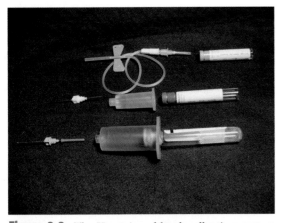

Figure 2-2. The Vacutainer blood collection system consists of a needle, holder, and collection tube. Several types of systems are available.

Whole Blood

The veterinary technician obtains a whole blood sample by withdrawing the blood into a suitable container with the proper anticoagulant to prevent clotting. As soon as the blood is collected, the blood and anticoagulant are mixed with a gentle rocking motion. Shaking the sample vigorously causes hemolysis, which in turn can affect the results of the assays when chemicals normally found within the erythrocytes are released into the plasma.

Plasma and Serum

Plasma is the fluid portion of whole blood in which the cells are suspended. It is composed of approximately 90% water and 10% dissolved constituents such as proteins, carbohydrates, vitamins, hormones, enzymes, lipids, salts, waste materials, antibodies, and other ions and molecules. Serum is plasma from which fibrinogen, a plasma protein, has been removed. During the clotting process, the soluble fibrinogen in plasma is converted to an insoluble fibrin clot matrix. When blood clots, the fluid that is squeezed out around the cellular clot is serum. Specific protocols for obtaining serum and plasma samples are located in Chapter 3.

Anticoagulants

Hematology testing primarily uses whole blood samples. Hemostatic testing uses both whole blood and blood plasma. Anticoagulants are required when whole blood or plasma samples are needed. An anticoagulant is a chemical that, when added to a whole blood sample, prevents or delays clotting (coagulation) of the sample. The choice of a particular anticoagulant should be made on the basis of the tests needed. Some anticoagulants may affect assays, so the test procedure should be consulted for the proper anticoagulant. Some anticoagulants can interfere with certain coagulation tests. Regardless of the anticoagulant chosen, the sample and anticoagulant must be well mixed (by gentle inversion) before use. Samples that are not tested within 1 hour of collection should be refrigerated. Refrigerated samples must be brought back to room temperature and remixed by gentle inversion before analysis. Whole blood should not be frozen because blood cells lyse during the freezing and thawing processes. Table 2-2 summarizes commonly used anticoagulants.

Heparin

Heparin is a suitable anticoagulant for most tests that require plasma samples, particularly blood chemistry analyses. Heparin anticoagulant should never be used for differential blood film analysis because the anticoagulant interferes with the staining of WBCs. Heparin is available as a sodium, potassium, lithium, or ammonium salt. Heparin acts by preventing conversion of prothrombin to thrombin during the clotting processes. Because heparin can cause clumping of WBCs and interferes with the normal staining pattern of the WBCs, it should not be used for analyses of WBCs.

Heparin should be used at a ratio of 20 U/ml of blood to be collected. For small sample volumes, a convenient method for using heparin is to coat the inside walls of a syringe with liquid heparin before the sample is drawn from the patient. Vacuum collection tubes containing the proper amount of heparin are commercially available. These tubes are most convenient when many heparinized samples are needed.

Ethylenediamine Tetraacetic Acid

Ethylenediamine tetraacetic acid (EDTA) is the preferred anticoagulant for hematologic studies because it does not alter cell morphology. It should not be used if plasma samples are to be used for chemical assays. EDTA is available as sodium or potassium salt and prevents clotting by forming an insoluble complex with calcium, which is necessary for clot formation. EDTA tubes are available in either liquid or powder forms. The liquid form creates some dilution of the sample. To prevent clotting, EDTA is added at 1 to 2 mg/ml of blood to be collected. Vacuum collection tubes containing the proper amount of EDTA are commercially available. Excess EDTA causes cells to shrink and invalidates most cell counts performed with automated analyzers.

Oxalates and Citrates

Oxalates are available as sodium, potassium, ammonium, or lithium salts. Citrates are available as sodium or lithium salts. They prevent clotting by forming insoluble complexes with calcium, which is necessary for clot formation. Potassium oxalate is the most commonly used oxalate salt. To prevent clotting, it is used at 1 to 2 mg/ml of blood to be collected. Sodium citrates are also commonly used, especially in transfusion medicine. Vacuum collection

TABLE 2-2

Commonly Used Anticoagulants

Name	Mode of Action	Advantages	Disadvantages	Uses
Heparin	Antithrombin	Reversible, nontoxic	Clumps WBCs, expensive	Critical RBC measurements
EDTA (potassium, sodium)	Chelates calcium	Best preservation	Irreversible, shrinks cells	Hematology
Oxalates (potassium, sodium, lithium)	Chelates calcium	Temporary	Variable effects	Coagulation
Citrates (sodium, lithium)	Chelates calcium	Nontoxic, reversible	Interferes with blood chemistry	Coagulation Transfusions
Fluorides (sodium)	Chelates calcium	Inhibits cell metabolism	Interferes with enzymatic tests	Preserves blood glucose

Reprinted from Sirois M: *Veterinary clinical laboratory procedures,* St Louis, 1995, Mosby.

tubes containing the proper amount of oxalate and citrate anticoagulants are commercially available. Unfortunately oxalates also may bind metallic ions necessary for enzyme activity. Potassium oxalate may inhibit lactate dehydrogenase and alkaline phosphatase activity. Also, because it is a potassium salt, it cannot be used with blood samples to be assayed for potassium. Sodium citrates similarly interfere with sodium assays, as well as many of the commonly performed blood chemistry tests.

Sodium Fluoride

Sodium fluoride, best known as a glucose preservative, also has anticoagulant properties. As an anticoagulant it is used at 6 to 10 mg/ml of blood to be collected. Vacuum collection tubes containing the proper amount of sodium fluoride for anticoagulation are commercially available. Sodium fluoride also may be added to other samples as a glucose preservative even if a different anticoagulant is present. For glucose preservation, sodium fluoride is used at 2.5 mg/ml of blood. Sodium fluoride interferes with many of the enzymatic tests performed on blood serum.

SAMPLE VOLUME

The amount of blood collected from an animal depends on the quantity of serum or plasma required for the assay and the hydration status of the patient. For example, a well-hydrated animal with a packed cell volume (PCV) of 50% should yield a blood sample that is 50% cells and 50% fluid. A 10-ml blood sample should yield 5 ml of fluid. In dehydrated animals, hemoconcentration results in a smaller ratio of fluid to cells. A dehydrated animal with a PCV of 70% yields a blood sample that is 70% cells and 30% fluid. This means that only 3 ml of fluid is obtained from a 10-ml blood sample.

As a rule of thumb, enough blood should be collected to yield enough serum, plasma, or whole blood to run all the planned assays three times. This allows for technician error, instrument failure, or the need to dilute a sample without having to collect another sample from the animal.

Blood samples must be adequately mixed before the performance of any tests; inadequate mixing results in erroneous data. For example, RBCs in horses start to settle within seconds, and a PCV performed on an unmixed sample may be erroneous. Tubes of blood may be mixed by gentle inversion for several seconds by hand or by placement of the tube on a commercially available tilting rack or rotator.

THE COMPLETE BLOOD COUNT

A CBC provides a minimum set of values that may be determined reliably and cost-effectively in the hospital setting. The CBC can be performed manually or by automated analyzers. A variety of procedures are available for both methods.

The CBC should consist of the following basic information:

- Total RBC count
- PCV
- Plasma protein concentration
- Total WBC count
- Blood film examination: differential WBC count, erythrocyte and leukocyte morphology, platelet estimation
- Reticulocyte count when the patient is anemic
- Hemoglobin concentration
- Erythrocyte indices

Quality Control

Automated analyzers can provide accurate and cost-effective results. However, care should be taken in choosing the most appropriate instrument for a clinic. Hematology analyzers for use in veterinary facilities employ impedance methods, buffy coat analysis, or laser methods when evaluating a sample. Each method has specific advantages and disadvantages. Regardless of which analyzer is used, an understanding of the test principles for the specific analyzer is essential. Knowing the limitations of the analytical system enhances the validity of the test results. Regular quality control is also essential for ensuring the accuracy of test results.

In addition to the routine care and maintenance of equipment used in hematology testing, the test results themselves can be used as a type of quality control. Hematology tests often overlap somewhat in the information they provide. The test results can then be used to confirm that other results are accurate. For example, if the PCV is low, the total RBC count should also be low and evidence of decreased total RBCs should be present on the differential blood film. Similarly, if the mean corpuscular volume (MCV) calculation indicates that cells are microcytic, this should also be evident on the blood film. Recall from Chapter 1 that cell counters often use the size of the particles passing through the apparatus as a method of counting cells. If significant macrocytosis is present in a sample, this could lead to a decreased RBC count because some cells may be counted as other cell types rather than as RBCs. All these tests serve as a type of internal quality control in hematology testing.

Cell Counts

Counting of erythrocytes and leukocytes is a routine part of the CBC. Cell counts can be performed by manual or automated methods. The total WBC (leukocyte) count is one of the most useful values determined in a CBC. Total RBC (erythrocyte) and platelet (thrombocyte) counts, although more difficult and less accurate, may also be performed manually with a hemacytometer or by automated methods. Manual cell count methods usually use the Unopette system (Becton, Dickinson and Co., Franklin Lakes, NJ) (Fig. 2-3). This system includes a pipette that holds a predetermined amount of blood and a reservoir that contains a diluting and lysing agent.

The most commonly used WBC counting Unopette system uses a 20-μl (microliter) pipette and 3% acetic acid as a diluent. The RBC counting system uses a 10-μl sample pipette and 0.85% saline as a diluent (the RBCs are not lysed in this count). Unopette systems contain a premeasured volume of diluent and provide a specific dilution ratio. The appropriate amount of blood is added to the diluent, or lysing solution. After approximately 10 minutes, the reservoir is inverted several times to mix the cells evenly and is converted to a dropper assembly. Once filled with the appropriate

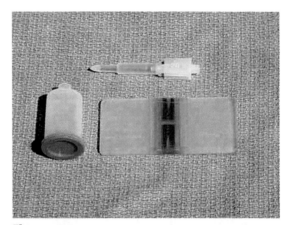

Figure 2-3. The hemocytometer and Unopette reservoir and pipette used for counting of WBCs and platelets.

volume of blood and mixed, a small amount of the blood-diluent mixture is placed on a hemocytometer. This is commonly called "charging" the hemacytometer. Proper filling is important for accurate cell counts. The area under the cover glass should be filled completely without the sample overflowing into the moat around the grid area. If the sample overflows, the hemacytometer should be cleaned and refilled with the sample.

Hemacytometers are counting chambers used to determine the number of cells per microliter (μl, sometimes referred to as cubic centimeters) of blood. Several models are available, but the most common type used has two identical sets of fine grids of parallel and perpendicular etched lines called *Neubauer rulings* (Fig. 2-4). Each grid is divided into nine large squares. The four-corner squares are divided into 16 smaller squares, and the center square, referred to as the "super square," is divided into 400 tiny squares (25 groups of 16 each). The area of each grid (Neubauer ruling) is designed to hold a precise amount of sample (0.9 μl). Each of the nine squares on the Neubauer grid holds 0.1 μl. Knowing the number of cells in set parts of the grid and the amount of sample in that area is the basis for calculating the number of cells per microliter of blood. Mechanical counters are available to track of the number of each cell observed.

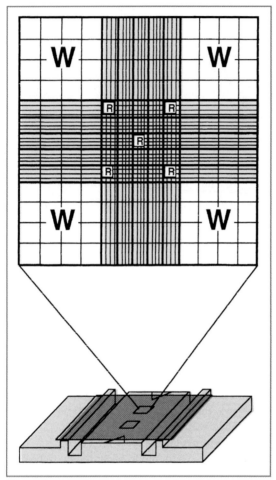

Figure 2-4. Neubauer hemacytometer. The large *W*s indicate the squares that are counted for a total white blood cell (WBC) count with the 1:20 dilution WBC Unopette system. The small *R*s indicate the squares that are counted for a red blood cell (RBC) count with the RBC Unopette system. (From McCurnin DM and Bassert JM: *Clinical textbook for veterinary technicians,* ed 6, St Louis, 2006, Saunders.)

The iris diaphragm of the microscope must be closed to a point at which the cells are most visible. The hemacytometer and cover slip are composed of optical-quality glass and must be free of dust and grease. The hemacytometer, with cover slip applied, is loaded with the diluted solution and placed on the microscope, and the counting grid is found by using the 40× or 43× objective lens. For WBC counts, cells are counted in the nine primary squares with the 10× objective. The count should proceed in an orderly fashion, starting at one end of the square, going across to the other side, then down one microscopic field and back across until all cells within the square are counted. Cells that are touching the line between two squares are counted with that square if they are touching either the top or left line. Do not count cells touching the bottom or right lines.

The number of cells counted from both sides of the hemacytometer are added and divided by two. The average number obtained is then divided by dilution and volume factors; counts are expressed as cells per microliter of blood. Cell counts should not vary more than 10% among the individual grid squares. Variations of more than 10% usually indicate improper filling of the hemacytometer.

For WBC counts using the standard 1/100 dilution, the cells in all nine squares on both sides of the hemacytometer are counted and averaged. For example, if a WBC count is performed and 80 and 76 cells are counted on all nine squares on each side of the hemacytometer, respectively, the average number is 78 cells. This is divided by the dilution ratio (1/100) and the volume factor that represents the volume of nine squares. For this example, the final cell count would be reported as 8.6×10^3/µl (78 divided by $1/100 \times 0.9$). A mathematic approximation of this calculation involves simply multiplying the average number of cells by 110. An alternate method involves counting the four corner squares and center square on each side of the hemacytometer and multiplying the total number of cells by 100. This method is less accurate when the usual 1/100 dilution is used but can be accomplished more quickly.

For RBC counts, the center and four corner squares within the super square are counted. The number counted is divided by the dilution and volume factors. The standard dilution for RBC counts is 1/200; the volume factor is 0.02. This can be mathematically manipulated to a multiplication factor of 10,000. For example, if an average of 450 cells is counted, the RBC count would be recorded as 4,500,000, or 4.5×10^6/µl.

RBC counts may also be estimated by dividing the PCV by six. For example, if the PCV is 36, the estimated RBC count is 36/6 = 6 million RBCs/μl. The Unopette system also provides a method for manually counting platelets, as described later.

Packed Cell Volume (PCV)

The PCV (also called microhematocrit) is the percentage of whole blood composed of erythrocytes or RBCs. Whole blood is collected in an anti-coagulant, such as EDTA or heparin, and placed in a capillary tube (75 mm). Microhematocrit tubes should be filled approximately three fourths full, with one end plugged with clay sealant (Fig. 2-5), placed in a centrifuge with the plugged end facing outward, and then centrifuged in a microhemato-crit centrifuge for 2 to 5 minutes (Fig. 2-6). Of the blood cells, RBCs have the highest specific gravity and gravitate to the bottom of the tube, appearing as a dark red layer. Any measuring device, such as

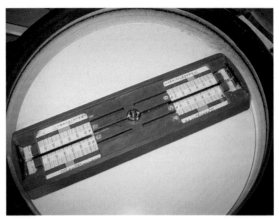

Figure 2-6. Microhematocrit tubes are placed with the clay plug toward the outside of the centrifuge. Two tubes placed opposite each other are required to balance the centrifuge. (From Busch SJ: *Small Animal Surgical Nursing: Skills and Concepts,* St. Louis, 2006, Mosby.)

a ruler, can be used to determine the PCV. Special hematocrit tube reader cards are available, many of which have a linear scale, so the amount of blood in the tube need not be exact. The bottom of the RBC layer should be at the zero line and the top of the plasma on the top line. The percentage can then be read as the line level with the top of the RBC layer (Fig. 2-7).

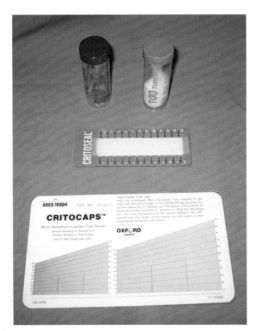

Figure 2-5. Heparinized *(red)* and plain *(blue)* microhematocrit tubes, PCV card reader, and clay used to seal the microhematocrit tube. (From Busch SJ: *Small Animal Surgical Nursing: Skills and Concepts,* St. Louis, 2006, Mosby.)

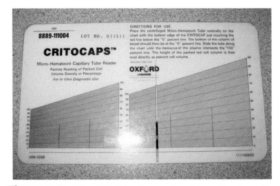

Figure 2-7. The PCV is determined by aligning the top of the clay plug on the zero line and locating the intersecting line where the packed red cells and buffy coat meet. (From Busch SJ: *Small Animal Surgical Nursing: Skills and Concepts,* St. Louis, 2006, Mosby.)

A whitish-gray layer just above the RBC layer is termed the buffy coat and consists of WBCs and platelets. The height of the buffy coat layer can provide a rough estimate of the total WBC count. The presence of increased numbers of nucleated RBCs imparts a reddish tinge to the buffy coat. The plasma is the clear-to-yellow fluid at the top. Plasma obtained by this method can be used to determine the plasma protein concentration by refractometry. Plasma color and transparency may be helpful in the determination of a diagnosis and should be recorded. Normal plasma is clear and a pale straw-yellow color (Fig. 2-8). Serum that appears cloudy is described as lipemic. This may be the result of a pathologic condition or may be seen as an artifact if the patient was not properly fasted before blood collection. A reddish-tinged plasma layer is described as hemolyzed. This may also be an artifact if the blood sample was not properly collected and handled or can be evidence of a pathologic condition, such as hemolytic anemia. Plasma that appears deep yellow is described as icteric and can be seen in animals with liver disease or hemolytic anemia. Abnormal plasma colors must be noted because the color can interfere with the chemical analyses if photometric methods are used for evaluation of plasma constituents.

The macrohematocrit method for determining PCV is not commonly performed because it requires a large amount of blood, generally a minimum of 10 ml. The blood is placed in a Wintrobe tube and centrifuged for 10 minutes at 18,000 rpm. The scale on the Wintrobe tube is read at the level of the packed RBCs, and that number is multiplied by 10 to determine the PCV.

Plasma Protein Concentration

Although not specifically considered a hematologic test, the materials needed for plasma protein concentration are already available as the result of performing the PCV. Plasma protein concentration estimation by refractometry is an important component of the CBC in all species. The plasma used to determine the PCV is collected by breaking the hematocrit tube just above the buffy coat–plasma interface. The plasma is allowed to flow onto the refractometer prism (Fig. 2-9). The refractometer is then held to a bright light and the reading is made at the dividing line between the bright and dark field. The protein value (in grams per deciliter) is read directly from a scale inside the refractometer. Lipemic plasma contains chylomicrons that cause the light to diffract in many different directions and usually results in a false increase in the total protein reading.

Hemoglobin Testing

The protein molecule hemoglobin is the functional unit of the erythrocyte. The molecule consists of two main components: the heme portion, which contains iron, and the globin portion, which is composed of paired chains of amino acids. The synthesis of hemoglobin occurs during maturation of the

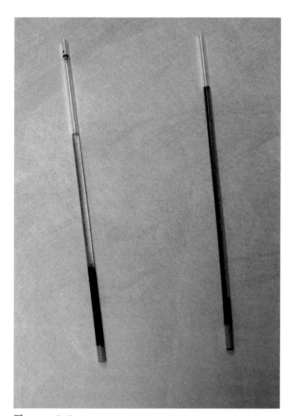

Figure 2-8. Icteric *(left)* and hemolyzed *(right)* plasma in a PCV tube.

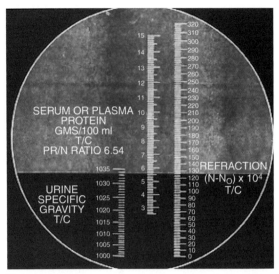

Figure 2-9. The reading scale within the refractometer. (From McCurnin DM, Bassert JM: *Clinical Textbook for Veterinary Technicians,* ed 6, St. Louis, 2006, Saunders.)

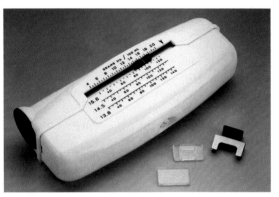

Figure 2-10. The hemoglobinometer uses a color-matching method for determining hemoglobin concentration in a sample of lysed RBCs.

RBCs in the bone marrow. Once in circulation, different forms of hemoglobin can exist. Hemoglobin bound to oxygen is referred to as oxyhemoglobin. When the oxygen is delivered to the tissues by the RBCs, carbon dioxide binds in place of the oxygen. The carbon dioxide is then replaced again by oxygen during respiration. Other forms of hemoglobin that may also be present include methemoglobin and sulfhemoglobin. Both of these forms are inefficient at oxygen transport. Sulfhemoglobin results from normal RBC aging processes. Methemoglobin occurs naturally both in plasma and within RBCs but can be converted to hemoglobin and used for oxygen delivery. Carboxyhemoglobin results from exposure to carbon monoxide. Hemoglobin and methemoglobin have a much higher affinity for carbon monoxide than for oxygen or carbon dioxide. Therefore the reaction that creates carboxyhemoglobin is irreversible.

A variety of methods are available for determination of hemoglobin. The oldest methods use color matching of lysed RBCs (Fig. 2-10). Some automated analyzer types provide only an estimate of the hemoglobin concentration based on the RBC count.

Most automated analyzers determine hemoglobin concentration by mixing a small amount of blood with a solution to lyse the blood cells and then comparing the color of the sample with a standard. Exposure to cyanide converts all forms of hemoglobin to cyanmethemoglobin. Lysing solutions that contain small amounts of cyanide function to convert all forms of hemoglobin to cyanmethemoglobin and therefore provide a measure of all forms of hemoglobin in the sample. A number of automated and semiautomated analyzers are dedicated to hemoglobin measurement. Most of these use a modification of the cyanmethemoglobin photometric procedure and are quite accurate if properly maintained. Small dedicated analyzers are also available. Some of these provide results only for oxyhemoglobin and use simple color-matching technology. Other types use photometric procedures calibrated to approximate the cyanmethemoglobin procedure.

Erythrocyte Indices

Determination of erythrocyte indices is helpful in the classification of certain types of anemia. The erythrocyte indices include the mean corpuscular volume (MCV), mean corpuscular hemoglobin (MCH), and MCH concentration mean corpuscular hemoglobin concentration (MCHC). The indices can provide an objective measure of the size of the RBCs and their average hemoglobin concentration. The accuracy of the calculation depends on the accuracy of the individual measurements of total RBC count, PCV, and hemoglobin concentration. Values for erythrocyte indices should always be compared with the morphologic features of the cells on the blood smear. For example, a low value for MCH should be evident as erythrocytes that appear more pale than normal (hypochromic) on the blood smear.

Mean Corpuscular Volume

MCV is the measure of the average size of the erythrocytes. MCV is calculated by dividing the PCV by the RBC concentration and multiplying by 10. The unit of volume is the femtoliter (fl).

For example, if a dog has a PCV of 42% and an RBC count of 6.0 million/μl, the MCV is 70 fl.

Many of the automated hematology analyzers determine the MCV electronically and use that measurement to calculate the PCV.

Mean Corpuscular Hemoglobin

MCH is the mean weight of hemoglobin (Hb) contained in the average RBC. It is calculated by dividing the hemoglobin concentration by the RBC concentration and multiplying by 10:

$$MCH = \frac{Hb(g/dl)}{RBC\ (\times 10^9/\mu l)} \times 10$$

Mean Corpuscular Hemoglobin Concentration

MCHC is the concentration of hemoglobin in the average erythrocyte (or the ratio of weight of hemoglobin to the volume in which it is contained). The MCHC (in grams per deciliter) is calculated by dividing the hemoglobin concentration (in grams per deciliter) by the PCV (percentage) and multiplying by 100.

$$MCHC = \frac{Hb(g/dl)}{PCV\%} \times 100$$

For example, if a dog has a hemoglobin concentration of 14 g/dl and a PCV of 42%, the MCHC is 33.3 g/dl. The normal range for MCHC is 30 to 36 g/dl for all mammals, with the exception of some sheep and all members of the family Camellidae (camels), which have MCHC values of 40 to 45 g/dl.

Histograms

Many automated analyzers offer histograms of the cell counts and platelet counts. A histogram is a graph that provides a visual report of the sizes (on the x-axis) and numbers (on the y-axis) of the various cellular components. The histogram can be used to verify results of the differential blood cell film and provide an indication of any problem with test results. For example, when megathrombocytes or platelet aggregates are present, the WBC count performed on most automated analyzers will be falsely elevated because those large platelets are usually counted as leukocytes. The histogram can provide evidence of this anomaly because the WBC curve on the histogram will be altered (Fig. 2-11).

Preparation of Blood Films

The blood film is used to perform the differential WBC count; estimate platelet numbers; and evaluate the morphologic features of WBCs, RBCs, and platelets.

Peripheral blood films can be prepared by using either a wedge smear technique or a cover slip technique.

Wedge smears are prepared by placing a small drop of blood on a clean glass microscope slide. The end of a second slide is placed against the surface of the first slide at a 30-degree angle and drawn back into the drop of blood. The angle of the second slide can be modified to account for changes in consistency of blood from an anemic patient (Fig. 2-12 and Procedure 2-1). When the blood has spread along most of the width of the spreader slide, it is then pushed forward with a steady, even, rapid motion. The slide should be gently waved in the air to allow it to air dry quickly. A properly prepared blood film is thin, with even distribution of cells.

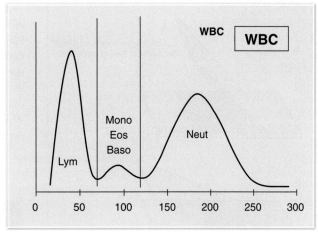

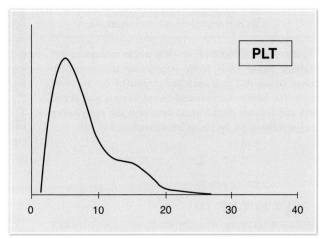

Figure 2-11. Histograms. **A,** Normal WBC histogram. **B,** Platelet histogram. **C,** Platelet histogram with evidence of platelet aggregates. (Courtesy of B. Mitzner, DVM.)

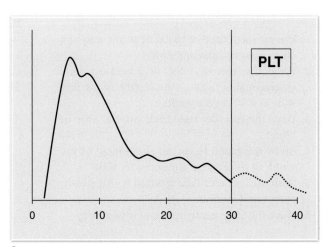

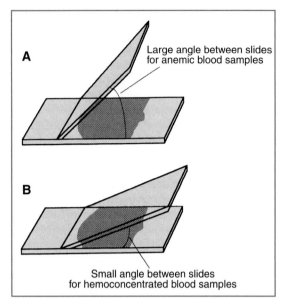

Coverslip smears are made by putting one drop of blood in the center of a clean square cover slip. Place a second cover slip diagonally on top of the first, causing the blood to spread evenly between the two surfaces. Then pull the cover slips apart in a single smooth motion before the blood has completely spread (Fig. 2-13 and Procedure 2-2). Wave the smears gently in the air to promote drying.

Figure 2-12. Difference in slide angle necessary for making blood films from anemic or hemoconcentrated blood. **A,** Large angle for anemic blood. **B,** Small angle for hemoconcentrated blood. (From McCurnin DM and Bassert JM: *Clinical textbook for veterinary technicians,* ed 6, St Louis, 2006, Saunders.)

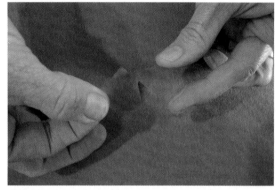

Figure 2-13. Preparing a blood film by the coverslip method.

PROCEDURE 2-1

Preparation of Wedge Film Blood Smear

1. Place a small drop of blood near one end of a clean glass microscope slide.
2. Place the narrow edge of a second slide (spreader slide) against the surface of the first slide at a 30-degree angle
3. Draw the spreader slide back into the drop of blood.
4. Allow the blood to spread along most of the width of the edge of the spreader slide
5. Push the spreader slide forward with a steady, even, rapid motion.
6. Wave the slide gently to allow it to air dry

PROCEDURE 2-2

Preparation of Coverslip Blood Smear

1. Place a small drop of blood in the center of a clean, square coverslip.
2. Place a second coverslip diagonally on top of the first
3. Allow the blood to spread evenly between the two surfaces until the blood almost fills the area between the coverslips
4. Pull the coverslips apart in a single smooth motion
5. Wave the coverslips gently to allow them to air dry

Staining Blood Films

After they air dry, the films must be stained to clearly distinguish the individual cells and identify any abnormal cellular characteristics. Blood films can be stained with any of the Romanowsky-type stains. The commonly available Romanowsky stains include Wright's stain and Wright-Giemsa stain. Romanowsky stains are available either in one-step or three-step formulations. The components of the stain may vary somewhat but usually include a fixative and buffered solutions of eosin and methylene blue. The fixative used is usually 95% methanol. The eosin component is buffered at an acidic pH and stains the basic components of the cells, such as hemoglobin and eosinophilic granules. The methylene blue component is buffered to an alkaline pH and stains the acidic components of the cell, such as leukocyte nuclei. A one-step stain that gives acceptable results is Diff-Quik (Dade Behring, Deerfield, IL). When a three-step stain is used, the slide is rinsed with distilled water between each of the three components. Care must be taken to avoid dripping water into any of the stain components or the stain will become degraded. A final rinse with distilled water should be done on all slides and then the slides allowed to dry before microscopic examination of the smear.

Table 2-3 lists problems related to staining. Cells appear dark if overstained, whereas extensive rinsing may cause them to look faded. Changing stains regularly is necessary for consistent results and the prevention of stain precipitation on the film. Stains can also be filtered to remove excess debris. Refractile artifacts on RBCs are another common problem. These are usually caused by moisture in the fixative solution. Take care not to confuse these artifacts with cellular abnormalities.

Performing the Differential Cell Count

Although most veterinary hematology analyzers provide at least a partial differential WBC count, a blood film must still be prepared and evaluated. A large number of abnormalities will not be routinely reported by automated analyzers, including the following:

Nucleated RBCs	Toxic granulation
Megaplatelets	Platelet clumps
Heinz bodies	Polychromasia
Target cells	Hemoparasites
Lupus erythematosus cells	Bacteria
Left shift	Hypersegmentation
Lymphoblasts	Basophils

Examining the slides the same way each time is important to avoid making mistakes in counting cells or missing important observations. Always begin the examination by scanning the slide under low power magnification (100×). A general assessment of overall cell numbers can be obtained. The entire slide should then be scanned for the presence of platelet clumps, large abnormal cells, and microfilariae. Locating the feathered edge and monolayer is performed next at high power magnification (Fig. 2-14). The feathered edge area of the blood film contains cells that are usually greatly distorted and erratically distributed. The monolayer is the area of the blood film where the cells are evenly and randomly distributed and not distorted. Once these two areas are identified, the technician focuses on one microscopic field in the monolayer just adjacent to the feathered edge. The differential count is performed in the smear monolayer by using oil-immersion (1000×) magnification. A minimum of 100 WBCs are counted, identified, and recorded during this count. Because 100 WBCs are counted, the number of each WBC type observed is recorded as a percentage. This is called the *relative WBC count*. Various counting devices are available to help perform the differential WBC count (Fig. 2-15).

Quantifying Morphologic Changes

In addition to enumerating each type of WBC, the differential blood count requires that the morphologic features of the cells be evaluated and the platelet count be estimated. The presence of any abnormal cells or toxic changes should be semiquantified. Two methods are commonly used for assessing the degree of morphologic changes. One method uses a scale of 1+, 2+, 3+, and 4+ to indicate the relative percentage of cells with the morphologic change. The designation 1+ generally

TABLE 2-3

Troubleshooting Staining Problems

Problem	Solution
Excessive Blue Staining (RBCs May Be Blue-Green)	
Prolonged stain contact	Decrease staining time
Inadequate wash	Wash longer
Specimen too thick	Make thinner smears if possible
Stain, diluent, buffer or wash water too alkaline	Check with pH paper and correct pH
Exposure to formalin vapors	Store and ship cytologic preparations separate from formalin containers
Wet fixation in ethanol or formalin	Air dry smears before fixation
Delayed fixation	Fix smears sooner if possible
Surface of the slide was alkaline	Use new slides
Excessive Pink Staining	
Insufficient staining time	Increase staining time
Prolonged washing	Decrease duration of wash
Stain or diluent too acidic	Check with pH paper and correct pH; fresh methanol may be needed
Excessive time in red stain solution	Decrease time in red solution
Inadequate time in blue stain solution	Increase time in blue stain solution
Mounting cover slip before preparation is dry	Allow preparation to dry completely before mounting cover slip
Weak Staining	
Insufficient contact with one or more of the stain solutions	Increase staining time
Fatigued (old) stains	Change stains
Another slide covered specimen during staining	Keep slides separate
Uneven Staining	
Variation of pH in different areas of slide surface (may be caused by slide surface being touched or slide being poorly cleaned)	Use new slides and avoid touching their surface before and after preparation
Water allowed to stand on some areas of the slide after staining and washing	Tilt slides close to vertical to drain water from the surface or dry with a fan
Inadequate mixing of stain and buffer	Mix stain and buffer thoroughly
Precipitate on Preparation	
Inadequate stain filtration	Filter or change the stain(s)
Inadequate washing of slide after staining	Rinse slides well after staining
Dirty slides used	Use clean new slides
Stain solution dries during staining	Use sufficient stain and do not leave it on slide too long
Miscellaneous	
Overstained preparations	Destain with 95% methanol and restain; Diff-Quik–stained smears may have to be destained in the red Diff-Quik stain solution to remove the blue color; however, this damages the red stain solution
Refractile artifact on RBC with Diff-Quik stain (usually caused by moisture in fixative)	Change the fixative

From Cowell RL, Tyler RD, Meinkoth JH: *Diagnostic cytology and hematology of the dog and cat,* ed 2, St Louis, 1999, Mosby.

Push blood film

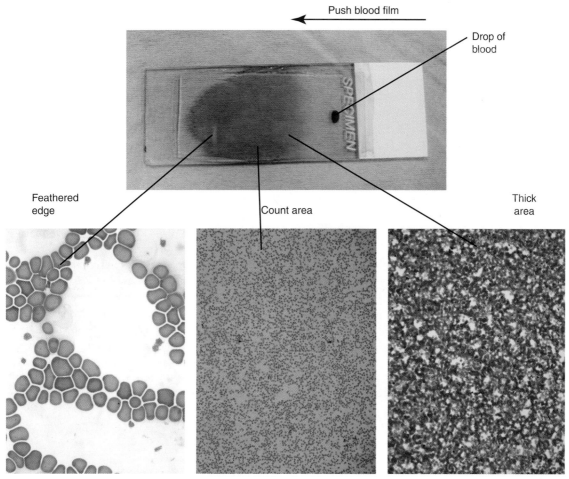

Drop of blood

Feathered edge

Count area

Thick area

Figure 2-14. Gross and microscopic views of different areas on a blood film. The blood film on the glass slide at the top was made by pushing the blood from the drop (indicated *drop of blood*) at the right to the left *(large arrow)*. The three major areas of the blood film *(feathered edge, count area, thick area)* are indicated by the lines connected to the respective microscopic views.

equates to 5% to 10% of the cells being affected, 2+ indicates 10% to 25%, 3+ indicates approximately 50%, and 4+ indicates more than 75% of the cells are affected. These are subjective assessments. Another method uses the designations "slight," "moderate," or "marked" to indicate approximately 10%, 25%, and more than 50% of cells as affected, respectively.

Absolute Values

Once the relative percentages of each cell type have been determined, the absolute value of each cell type must be calculated. This is accomplished by multiplying the total WBC count by the percentage of each cell type. For example, if 80% neutrophils are counted on the differential blood film and the total WBC count was 6000/μl, the

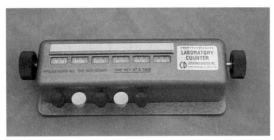

A

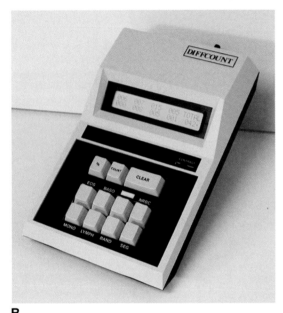

B

Figure 2-15. A standard **(A)** and electronic **(B)** tabulator used for the differential blood cell count. (Courtesy of B. Mitzner, DVM.)

absolute value for neutrophils is 4800 neutrophils/ μl of blood.

White Blood Cells

Mature and immature neutrophils, lymphocytes, monocytes, eosinophils, and basophils make up the leukocytes (WBCs) found in the blood of most mammals. Each type of cell plays an important role in the body's defense system, and the total concentration of each type is extremely valuable in the diagnosis of various diseases.

Definitions

The following are some definitions of hematologic terms used in this section:

-penia: Decreased number of cells in the blood. For example, neutropenia refers to decreased numbers of neutrophils in the blood. Lymphopenia describes decreased numbers of lymphocytes in the blood.

-philia or -cytosis: Increased number of cells in the blood. For example, neutrophilia refers to increased numbers of neutrophils in the blood. Leukocytosis refers to increased numbers of leukocytes in the blood.

Left shift: Increased numbers of immature neutrophils in the blood.

Leukemia: Neoplastic cells in the blood or bone marrow. Leukemias are often described as leukemic, subleukemic, or aleukemic, indicating the variation in the tendency for neoplastic cells to be released in the blood.

Leukemoid response: Condition that can be mistaken for leukemia. It is characterized by marked leukocytosis (more than 50,000/μl) and is usually the result of inflammatory disease.

Morphologic Features of Mammalian Leukocytes in Peripheral Blood

Neutrophil. The nucleus of neutrophils is irregular and elongated; true filaments between nuclear lobes are rare (Fig. 2-16). The presence of three to five nuclear lobes is characteristic of mammalian neutrophils. The nucleus of equine neutrophils has heavily clumped, coarse chromatin. The cytoplasm stains pale pink with fine, diffuse granules. Bovine neutrophils have darker-pink cytoplasm.

In avian, reptile, some fish, and some small mammal species (e.g., rats, rabbits, guinea pigs), the cell that is functionally equivalent to the neutrophil is referred to as a heterophil. Heterophils have distinct eosinophilic granules in their cytoplasm (Fig. 2-17). They are sometimes referred to as pseudoeosinophils.

Band Neutrophil. The nucleus of band neutrophils is horseshoe shaped, with large round ends

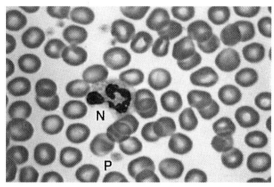

Figure 2-16. A canine neutrophil *(N)* and platelet *(P)* in a blood smear from a normal patient.

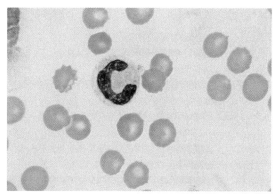

Figure 2-18. A canine band neutrophil. (From Cowell RL, Tyler RD, and Meinkoth JH: *Diagnostic Cytology and Hematology of the Dog and Cat,* ed 2, St. Louis, 1999, Mosby.)

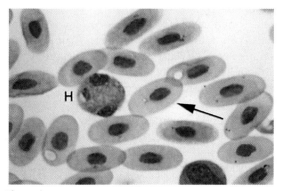

Figure 2-17. Nucleated erythrocytes in a blood film from a reptile. A heterophil *(H)* is also present.

coarsely clumped, and the cytoplasm is light blue and quite scanty. Chromocenters, or areas of condensed chromatin, should not be confused with nucleoli; chromocenters appear as dark clumps within the nucleus. Medium-size to large lymphocytes are 9 to 11 µm in diameter, with more abundant cytoplasm. The cytoplasm may contain pink-purple granules. Normal bovine lymphocytes may contain nucleolar rings and may be large and difficult to distinguish from neoplastic lymphoid cells (Fig. 2-21).

(Fig. 2-18). Although slight indentations may be present in the nucleus, if the constriction is greater than one third the width of the nucleus, the cell is usually classified as a segmented neutrophil. The designation of a neutrophil as a band or a mature segmented cell is somewhat subjective. Each facility should clearly state the criteria for which a neutrophil will be designated a band and apply that criteria consistently to all samples. If in doubt over whether a particular cell is a band or a mature segmented cell, the cell is best classified as a mature cell. More immature neutrophils (myelocytes, metamyelocytes) are rare in peripheral blood (Fig. 2-19).

   Lymphocyte. Small lymphocytes are approximately 7 to 9 µm in diameter and have a slightly indented nucleus (Fig. 2-20). The chromatin is

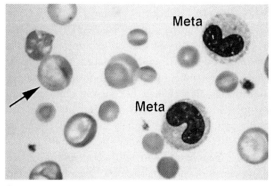

Figure 2-19. Metamyelocytes on a blood film from a dog with regenerative anemia. Polychromatophilic RBCs *(arrow)* are also present, along with several spherocytes.

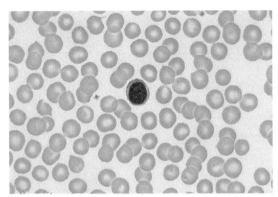

Figure 2-20. A small, mature lymphocyte in blood from a normal canine. (From Cowell RL, Tyler RD, and Meinkoth JH: *Diagnostic Cytology and Hematology of the Dog and Cat,* ed 2, St. Louis, 1999, Mosby.)

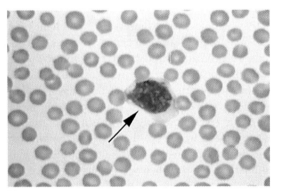

Figure 2-21. Normal bovine blood film with a large lymphocyte.

Monocyte. Monocytes are large cells that contain variably shaped nuclei (Fig. 2-22). The nucleus is occasionally the shape of a kidney bean but is often elongated and lobulated. The nuclear chromatin is more diffuse in monocytes than in neutrophils, in which it is coarsely clumped. The cytoplasm of monocytes is blue-gray and may contain vacuoles and/or small, fine, pink granules (Fig. 2-23). Monocytes may be difficult to distinguish from band neutrophils, large lymphocytes, or metamyelocytes that are toxic. If a left shift is not present, the cells in question are probably monocytes.

Eosinophil. Eosinophils contain a nucleus similar to that of neutrophils, but the chromatin is

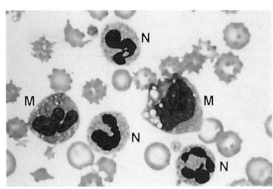

Figure 2-22. Normal canine monocytes *(M)* and neutrophils *(N)*.

usually not as coarsely clumped. The shape of the eosinophilic granules varies considerably among species (Fig. 2-24). The granules in canine eosinophils often vary in size with small and large granules within the same cell, and stain less intensely than those of other species; they usually are hemoglobin colored. Feline eosinophils contain granules that are small, rod shaped, and numerous. Equine eosinophil granules are large and round to oval, staining an intense orange-red. Eosinophil granules in cattle, sheep, and pigs are round and much smaller than those in horses. They are large, round, uniform in size, and stain an intense pink.

Basophil. The nucleus of basophils is similar to that of monocytes. Basophil granules in dogs

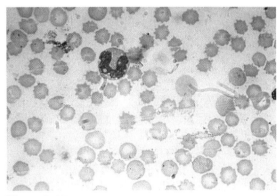

Figure 2-23. A normal canine monocyte showing the characteristic kidney bean–shaped nucleus and vacuoles.

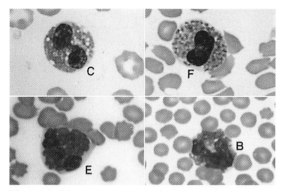

Figure 2-24. Canine *(C),* feline *(F),* equine *(E),* and bovine *(B)* eosinophils demonstrating the variable size, shape, and color of granules in different species.

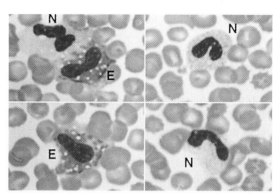

Figure 2-26. Nuclear hyposegmentation in neutrophils *(N)* and eosinophils *(E)* from a dog with Pelger-Huët anomaly (Wright's stain).

are few in number and stain purple to blue-black. Equine and bovine basophil granules are usually more numerous and may completely pack the cytoplasm. Feline basophil granules are round, stain light lavender (Fig. 2-25), and rarely contain dark granules.

Morphologic Abnormalities Seen in WBCs.

Nuclear Hyposegmentation. Pelger-Huët anomaly is a congenital defect characterized by hyposegmentation of all granulocyte nuclei. Nuclear chromatin appears condensed but unsegmented. Cytoplasm of affected cells appears normal (Fig. 2-26).

Hyposegmentation may simply reflect early release of band neutrophils. Pseudo–Pelger-Huët

anomaly has been reported and is either a variant of a normal inflammatory response or may be caused by an idiosyncratic drug reaction. In general, in pseudo–Pelger-Huët anomaly, fewer neutrophils are hyposegmented than in the congenital anomaly.

Nuclear Hypersegmentation. Canine and feline neutrophils with five or more lobes are considered hypersegmented (Fig. 2-27). This is usually attributable to aging of neutrophils, either in vivo—as would be seen with endogenous or exogenous glucocorticoids, which prolong the half-life of circulating neutrophils—or in vitro, as a result of prolonged storage of blood before making blood films. Hypersegmented neutrophils also are seen

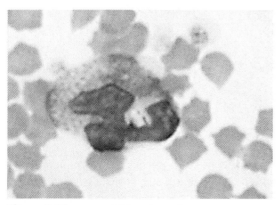

Figure 2-25. Normal feline basophil.

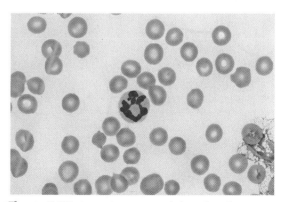

Figure 2-27. A canine neutrophil with a hypersegmented nucleus. (From Cowell RL, Tyler RD, and Meinkoth JH: *Diagnostic Cytology and Hematology of the Dog and Cat,* ed 2, St. Louis, 1999, Mosby.)

in blood films from poodles with poodle macrocytosis.

Toxic Change. The most common disease-induced cytoplasmic changes in neutrophils are referred to as toxic changes and are associated with conditions such as inflammation, infection, and drug toxicity. These changes are more significant when they occur in dogs; if severe they often suggest bacterial infection. However, toxic changes are seen quite commonly in cats that are not severely ill. Types of toxic change include cytoplasmic basophilia; Döhle's bodies; vacuoles, or "foaminess" (Fig. 2-28) and, rarely, intensely stained primary granules, referred to as toxic granulation (Fig. 2-29). Affected cells may also appear much larger than normal segmented neutrophils (Fig. 2-30). These "toxic" changes are thought to be caused by decreased time of neutrophil maturation within the marrow.

Intracytoplasmic Neutrophil Inclusions in Infectious Diseases. Canine distemper inclusions may appear in RBCs or neutrophils and are pale blue to magenta. Rickettsial inclusions (*Ehrlichia* species) may be seen within the cytoplasm of neutrophils (Fig. 2-31), as are the gametocytes of *Hepatozoon canis*.

"Atypical" and "Reactive" Lymphocytes. Azurophilic granules in the cytoplasm of lymphocytes (Fig. 2-32) are often associated with chronic antigenic stimula-

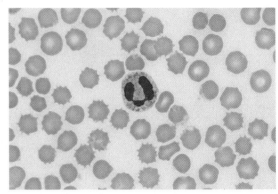

Figure 2-29. A neutrophil with toxic granulation. (From Cowell RL, Tyler RD, and Meinkoth JH: *Diagnostic Cytology and Hematology of the Dog and Cat,* ed 2, St. Louis, 1999, Mosby.)

tion, especially in canine ehrlichiosis. Azurophilic granules may be present in normal bovine lymphocytes. Atypical lymphocytes may also have cleaved nuclei and/or show evidence of asynchronous maturation of the nucleus and cytoplasm. "Reactive" lymphocytes (Fig. 2-33) have increased basophilia in the cytoplasm; may have more abundant cytoplasm; and sometimes contain a larger, more convoluted nucleus. These changes are usually caused by antigenic stimulation secondary to vaccination or infection.

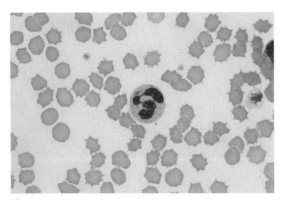

Figure 2-28. A toxic neutrophil showing cytoplasmic basophilia and a large Döhle's body. The RBCs are crenated. (From Cowell RL, Tyler RD, and Meinkoth JH: *Diagnostic Cytology and Hematology of the Dog and Cat,* ed 2, St. Louis, 1999, Mosby.)

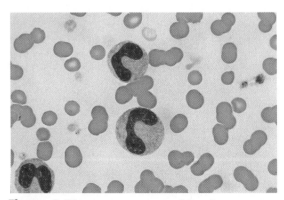

Figure 2-30. A giant neutrophil adjacent to a normally proportioned feline neutrophil. (From Cowell RL, Tyler RD, and Meinkoth JH: *Diagnostic Cytology and Hematology of the Dog and Cat,* ed 2, St. Louis, 1999, Mosby.)

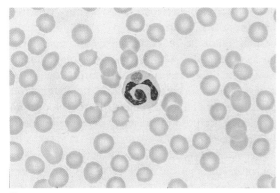

Figure 2-31. A canine neutrophil containing an *Ehrlichia* morula. (From Cowell RL, Tyler RD, and Meinkoth JH: *Diagnostic Cytology and Hematology of the Dog and Cat,* ed 2, St. Louis, 1999, Mosby.)

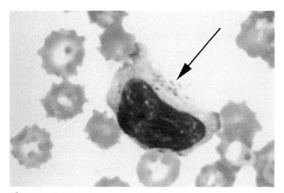

Figure 2-32. An atypical lymphocyte containing azurophilic granules in a canine blood film.

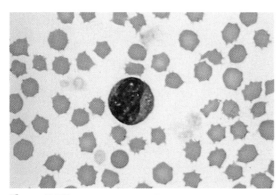

Figure 2-33. A reactive lymphocyte in a canine blood film. Numerous acanthocytes are also present.

Lysosomal Storage Disorders. In this group of rare inherited diseases a substance is abnormally stored within cells, usually because of an intracellular enzyme deficiency. Numerous types have been reported in animals. Clinical signs vary depending on the specific enzyme deficiency. Most types have either skeletal abnormalities or progressive neurologic disease. Because most cells of the body are affected, the stored substance often may be seen in leukocytes, usually monocytes, lymphocytes, or neutrophils. The appearance of the leukocytes varies depending on the type of lysosomal storage disease. Lymphocytes may be vacuolated or contain granules; neutrophils may also contain granules (Fig. 2-34).

Birman Cat Neutrophil Granulation Anomaly. Neutrophils from affected cats contain fine eosinophilic to magenta granules. This anomaly is inherited as an autosomal-recessive trait. Neutrophil function is normal and affected cats are healthy. This granulation must be distinguished from toxic granulation and the granulation seen in neutrophils of cats with mucopolysaccharidosis and GM_2 gangliosidosis, two of the lysosomal storage disorders.

Chédiak-Higashi Syndrome. Neutrophils in cats with Chédiak-Higashi syndrome have large, fused 0.5- to 2-μm lysosomes within the cytoplasm and stain lightly pink or eosinophilic (Fig. 2-35). Approximately one in three or four neutrophils contains fused lysosomes. Granules of eosinophils appear slightly plump and large. These cats have a slight

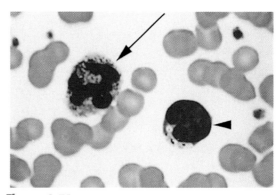

Figure 2-34. A feline lymphocyte containing vacuoles and granules *(arrowhead)* and a neutrophil with toxic granulation *(arrow).*

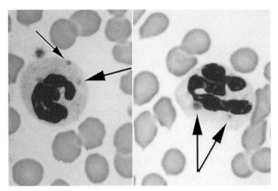

Figure 2-35. Blood film from a cat with Chédiak-Higashi syndrome. Note the large pink granules *(arrow)*.

tendency to bleed because platelet function is abnormal. Although neutrophil function is also abnormal, affected cats are generally healthy.

Smudge Cells. Smudge cells, sometimes referred to as basket cells, are degenerative leukocytes that have ruptured (Fig. 2-36). Their presence is not considered significant unless large numbers are present. Small numbers of smudge cells can be produced as an artifact when blood is held too long before making the smear or excess pressure is used when making the smear. Large numbers of smudge cells are associated with leukemia.

Morphology of Mammalian Erythrocyte in Peripheral Blood. Normal erythrocyte morphologic features vary among different species of domestic animals. Normal canine erythrocytes are a biconcave disk shape and have a distinct area of central pallor. Feline erythrocytes are round with no central pallor. Unlike the RBCs of mammals, avian RBCs are nucleated. The morphologic characteristics of erythrocytes can be categorized according to cell arrangement on the blood film, size, color, shape, and presence of structures in or on erythrocytes.

Cell Arrangement. Rouleaux formation is a grouping of erythrocytes in stacks (Fig. 2-37). Increased rouleaux formation is seen with increased fibrinogen or globulin concentrations. Rouleaux is accompanied by an increase in the erythrocyte sedimentation rate. Marked rouleaux formation is seen in healthy horses. Rouleaux may be seen as an artifact in blood that is held too long before preparing the blood film and in blood that has been refrigerated.

Agglutination of erythrocytes must be distinguished from rouleaux formation (Fig. 2-38). Agglutination occurs in immune-mediated disorders in which antibody coats the erythrocyte, resulting in bridging and clumping of RBCs. It is sometimes observed macroscopically and microscopically. To differentiate rouleaux from agglutination, add a drop of saline to a drop of blood and examine the sample microscopically for agglutination. Rouleaux will disperse in saline.

Size. Anisocytosis is a variation in the size of RBCs (Fig. 2-39) and may indicate the presence of

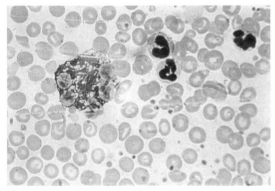

Figure 2-36. A smudge cell and several neutrophils in a canine blood film.

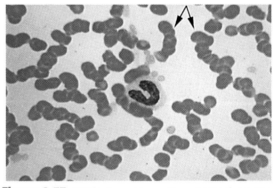

Figure 2-37. Marked rouleaux in a normal equine blood film. A neutrophilic band cell is also present.

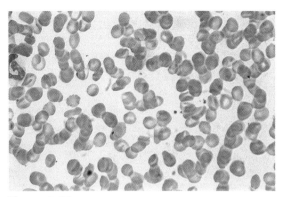

Figure 2-38. Autoagglutination on a canine blood film.

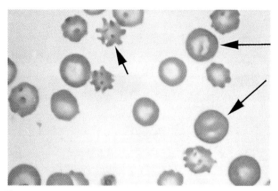

Figure 2-40. Macrocytic polychromatophilic RBCs *(long arrows)* and acanthocytes *(small arrow)* are present in this canine blood film.

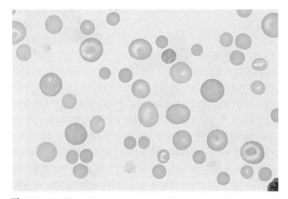

Figure 2-39. Mixed anisocytosis in a canine blood film. Several target cells are also present. (From Cowell RL, Tyler RD, and Meinkoth JH: *Diagnostic Cytology and Hematology of the Dog and Cat,* ed 2, St. Louis, 1999, Mosby.)

organelles remaining within the cytoplasm; therefore these are young cells. This is the same cell that, when stained with new methylene blue or brilliant cresyl blue, may appear as a reticulocyte.

Hypochromasia is a decreased staining intensity caused by insufficient hemoglobin within the cell (Fig. 2-41). The cell will normally appear more darkly stained along the periphery gradually tapering to a much paler central region. Iron deficiency is the most common cause, although macrocytic erythrocytes often appear hypochromic because of their large diameter. Hypochromic cells should be distinguished from bowl-shaped or "punched-out" cells, which are produced as an

macrocytes (large cells) or microcytes (small cells) or both. Anisocytosis is a common finding in normal bovine blood. Macrocytes are RBCs that are larger than normal, with an increased MCV. Macrocytes are usually young, polychromatophilic erythrocytes (reticulocytes). Microcytes are RBCs with a diameter less than that of normal erythrocytes, with a decreased MCV. Microcytic cells may be seen with iron deficiency.

Color. Polychromasia or polychromatophilic erythrocytes are RBCs exhibiting a bluish tint when stained with Romanowsky (Wright's type) stain (Fig. 2-40). The blue tint is due to the presence of

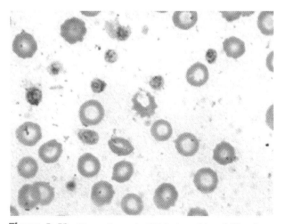

Figure 2-41. Hypochromic RBCs in a blood film from a dog with iron-deficiency anemia.

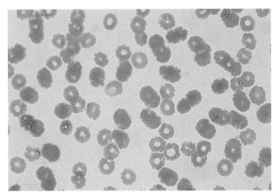

Figure 2-42. The punched-out appearance to many of these RBCs is an artifact caused by inadequate drying of the blood film.

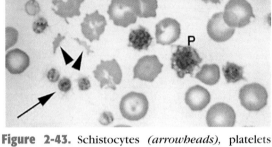

Figure 2-43. Schistocytes *(arrowheads)*, platelets *(arrow)*, and giant platelets *(P)* are seen on this blood film from a dog with iron-deficiency anemia.

artifact with improper smear technique (Fig. 2-42). Animals with true hypochromasia almost always have microcytosis, as determined by a decreased MCV. Normochromia is a normal staining intensity.

Hyperchromatophilic refers to cells that appear more darkly stained than normal cells. This gives the appearance that the cells are oversaturated with hemoglobin. Because the RBC has a fixed maximum capacity for hemoglobin, oversaturation cannot occur. These cells are usually microcytes or spherocytes.

Shape. Abnormally shaped erythrocytes are called poikilocytes. This terminology is not helpful because it does not suggest a specific diagnosis. The origin of the abnormal shape depends in part on the species being examined. Shape and color changes are considered important when they are associated with specific disorders. The term poikilocytosis should be used only when the morphologic abnormality cannot be described using more specific terms.

Schistocytes (Fig. 2-43), which are RBC fragments, are usually formed as a result of shearing of the red cell by intravascular trauma. Schistocytes may be observed with disseminated intravascular coagulopathy (DIC) when erythrocytes are broken by fibrin strands, with vascular neoplasms (e.g., hemangiosarcoma), and with iron deficiency. Animals with DIC usually have concurrent thrombocytopenia.

Acanthocytes, or spur cells, are irregular, spiculated red cells with a few unevenly distributed surface projections of variable length and diameter (Fig. 2-40) and are seen in patients with altered lipid metabolism, such as may occur in cats with hepatic lipidosis and, occasionally, in dogs with liver disease. They are seen quite consistently in dogs with hemangiosarcoma of the liver. The presence of acanthocytes in middle-age to old large-breed dogs with concurrent regenerative anemia is suggestive of hemangiosarcoma.

Echinocytes (burr cells) are spiculated cells with numerous short, evenly spaced, blunt to sharp surface projections of uniform size and shape. Echinocyte formation can be an artifactual, in vitro process associated with slow drying of blood films; it is then termed crenation. Echinocytes can also be produced as an artifact if the EDTA tube is underfilled. Echinocytes have also been associated with renal disease and lymphosarcoma in dogs, after exercise in horses, and with rattlesnake envenomation in dogs (Fig. 2-44).

Drepanocytes, or sickle cells, are observed in the blood of normal deer and angora goats. This is thought to be an in vitro phenomenon resulting from low oxygen tension (Fig. 2-45).

Keratocytes are commonly referred to as "helmet cells," "blister cells," or "bite cells." The presence of keratocytes has been associated with hemangiosarcoma, neoplasia, glomerulonephritis, and various

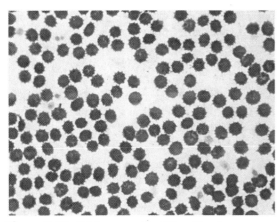

Figure 2-44. Echinocytes in a feline blood smear.

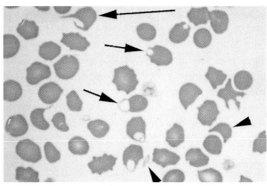

Figure 2-46. Numerous keratocytes *(arrows)* and a schistocyte *(arrowhead)* are present in this blood film from a cat with iron-deficiency anemia.

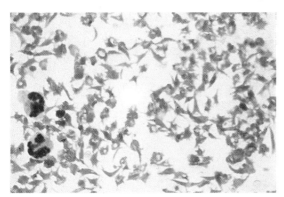

Figure 2-45. Drepanocytes (sickle cells) in a blood film from a normal deer.

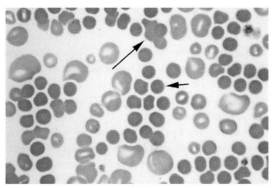

Figure 2-47. Anisocytosis and spherocytes *(short arrow)* are present in this canine blood film. A cluster of agglutinated cells *(long arrow)* is also present.

hepatic diseases. The cell may appear to contain a vacuole. Keratocytes are believed to form from intravascular trauma involving bisection of the cell by fibrin strands. The opposing sides of the cell may then adhere to each other and form a pseudovacuole (Fig. 2-46).

Spherocytes are darkly staining red cells with reduced or no central pallor (Fig. 2-47). Spherocytes are not easily detected in species other than dogs. They have a reduced amount of membrane surface area as a result of partial phagocytosis by macrophages, which occurs because of antibody and/or complement on the surface of the RBC. Spherocytes are significant in that they suggest immune-mediated destruction of RBCs, resulting in hemo-

lytic anemia. They also may be seen after transfusion with mismatched blood. Immune-mediated hemolytic anemia is usually a regenerative anemia, with marked polychromasia and high reticulocyte count. However, in some instances the anemia is nonregenerative as a result of antibodies against RBC precursors within the bone marrow. In these cases, spherocytes are often difficult to detect because the presence of large polychromatophilic cells facilitates recognition of the small spherocytes. Although spherocytes have a decreased diameter and appear small, their volume is normal, and dogs with immune-mediated hemolytic anemia do not have decreased MCV.

Codocytes are also referred to as leptocytes. This group of cells is characterized by an increased membrane surface area relative to the cell volume. They may take a variety of shapes. Target cells are leptocytes with a central area of pigment surrounded by a clear area and then a dense ring of peripheral cytoplasm (see Fig. 2-39). A few may be seen in normal blood smears and may also be associated with anemias, liver diseases, and some inherited disorders. Leptocytes may also appear as folded cells and stomatocytes. Folded cells have a transverse, raised fold extending across the center of the cell and a clear, slitlike pale region in the center of the cell (Fig. 2-48). Folded cells and stomatocytes are considered an artifact if the areas of pallor are all perpendicular to the feathered edge. Barr cells are also referred to as knizocytes. This type of leptocyte appears to have a bar of hemoglobin across the center of the cell.

Anulocytes are bowl-shaped erythrocytes that form as a result of loss of membrane flexibility that does not allow the cell to return to a normal shape after passing through a capillary. These cells may be seen in any acute disease.

Dacryocytes are teardrop-shaped cells seen in myelofibrosis and certain other myeloproliferative diseases. These may be produced as an artifact but can be identified by the direction of the elongated tail. Dacryocytes produced as artifact have their tails pointing in the same direction.

Oval, elliptical, or elongated erythrocytes may be seen in various types of anemia. These are some-times referred to as *pencil cells*. In the llama and other members of the camel family, these are the predominant cell type and do not indicate a pathologic condition. Normal goat and sheep blood may also contain oval-shaped erythrocytes. Hemoglobin pigment may appear evenly disbursed throughout the cell or concentrated at each end of the oval, with a central area of pallor (Fig. 2-49).

Inclusions.

Nucleated erythrocytes. In mammals, nucleated erythrocytes represent early release of immature cells during anemia but also may be occasionally observed in nonanemic animals (Fig. 2-50). All RBCs of nonmammalian species, such as birds and reptiles, contain nuclei (see Fig. 2-17). Nucleated

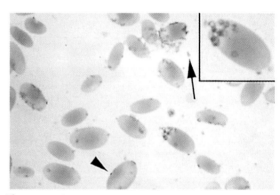

Figure 2-49. *Eperythrozoa* organisms in a blood film from a camel. Note the oval RBCs, which are normal in this species.

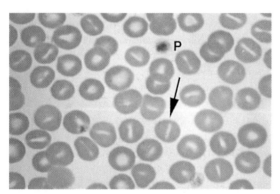

Figure 2-48. Folded cells and stomatocytes *(arrow)* and a platelet *(P)* on a canine blood film.

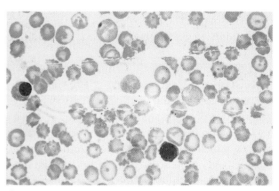

Figure 2-50. Nucleated RBCs in a canine blood film.

RBCs (NRBCs) are included in the total WBC count performed by hemacytometers and electronic cell counters. When performing a differential cell count, NRBCs may be counted separately and reported as NRBCs/100 WBCs. The number of NRBCs encountered while counting 100 WBCs is incorporated into the following equation to calculate a corrected leukocyte count:

$$\text{Corrected WBC count} = \frac{\#\ \text{RBCs}}{\text{Observed WBC count} - \frac{\#\ \text{RBCs}}{100\ \text{WBCs}}}$$

Basophilic stippling, or the presence of small, dark-blue bodies within the erythrocyte, is observed in Wright's-stained cells and represents residual RNA. It is common in immature RBCs of ruminants and occasionally in cats during a response to anemia and is usually characteristic of lead poisoning when seen in dogs (Fig. 2-51).

Howell-Jolly bodies are basophilic nuclear remnants seen in young erythrocytes during the response to anemia (Fig. 2-52). As cells containing nuclear remnants pass through the spleen, phagocytic cells remove the remnants. Consequently, increased numbers may be seen after removal of the spleen or with splenic disorders.

Heinz bodies are round structures representing denatured hemoglobin caused by certain oxidant drugs or chemicals. The denatured hemoglobin becomes attached to the cell membrane and appears as a pale area with Wright's stain (Fig. 2-53). When stained with new methylene blue (same technique used for reticulocytes), the Heinz bodies

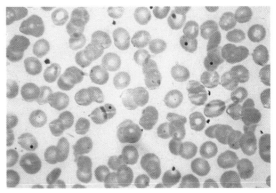

Figure 2-52. Howell-Jolly bodies on a canine blood film.

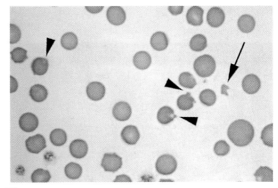

Figure 2-53. Heinz bodies *(arrowheads)* on a feline blood film stained with Wright's stain.

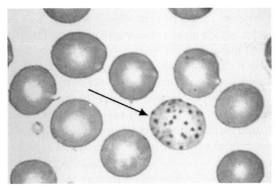

Figure 2-51. Basophilic stippling of an RBC *(arrow)* from a dog with lead poisoning.

appear blue (Fig. 2-54). In dogs, they are 1 to 2 μm in diameter. Unlike other domestic animals, normal cats have Heinz bodies in as many as 5% of their RBCs, and Heinz bodies are often increased in concentration with diseases such as lymphosarcoma, hyperthyroidism, and diabetes mellitus in cats.

Reticulocytes are immature erythrocytes that contain organelles (ribosomes) that are lost as the cell matures (Fig. 2-55). These organelles account for the diffuse blue-gray or polychromatophilic staining of immature cells with Wright's stain. Romanowsky stain does not stain these cellular components. A supravital stain, such as new methylene blue or brilliant cresyl blue, must be used. Supravital stains contain no fixatives. When reticulocytes are stained with supravital stain, the

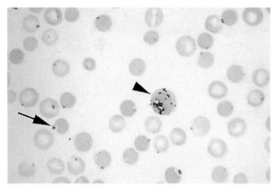

Figure 2-54. Heinz bodies *(arrow)* on a feline blood film stained with new methylene blue. A reticulocyte *(arrowhead)* is also present.

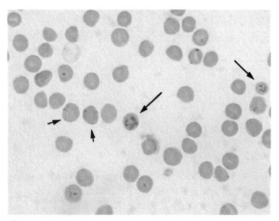

Figure 2-55. Feline blood smear with both punctuate *(short arrows)* and aggregate reticulocytes *(long arrows)*. (From McCurnin DM, Bassert JM: *Clinical Textbook for Veterinary Technicians,* ed 6, St. Louis, 2006, Saunders.)

organelles clump into visible granules referred to as reticulum. This reticulum is present as aggregates or chains of blue granules. The stain must be fresh and should be filtered before use. This will help minimize artifacts such as stain precipitate and bacteria that are present in these supravital stains.

Several methods can be used to prepare reticulocyte smears. Special reticulocyte kits are available, or blood can be stained by placement of a few drops of blood and an equal number of drops of new methylene blue or brilliant cresyl blue stain in a small test tube. The mixture is allowed to stand for approximately 15 minutes. Alternatively, the stain can also be added to a drop of blood directly on a glass slide. The stain and blood should be well mixed and allowed to stand for several minutes before creating the blood film. A drop of the mixture is then used to prepare a conventional air-dried blood film, which can then be examined or counterstained with Wright's stain. Staining intensity of reticulocytes may be enhanced by placing the prepared reticulocyte slide in 95% methanol for a few seconds followed by 5 seconds in the methylene blue component of Diff-Quick Stain.

Cats, unlike other species, have two morphologic forms of reticulocytes. The aggregate form contains large clumps of reticulum, is similar to reticulocytes in other species, and is the same cell that stains polychromatophilic with Wright's stain. The punctate form, unique to cats, contains two to eight small, singular, basophilic granules. These cells do not stain polychromatophilic with Wright's stain. In normal, nonanemic cats, approximately 0.4% of the RBCs are aggregate reticulocytes, whereas 1.5% to 10% of the RBCs are punctate reticulocytes. For a meaningful reticulocyte count in cats, only the aggregate form of reticulocyte should be counted.

A reticulocyte count is an expression of the percentage of RBCs that are reticulocytes. The percentage of reticulocytes per 1000 erythrocytes is determined using the oil-immersion lens. A reticulocyte count should be performed on the blood of all anemic domestic animals except horses, which do not release reticulocytes from the bone marrow even in the face of regenerative anemia. Reticulocyte concentration is useful in assessing the bone marrow's response to anemia.

Reticulocyte counts should be interpreted according to the degree of anemia because fewer mature erythrocytes are present in anemic animals, and reticulocytes are released earlier and persist longer than in normal animals. Higher percentages may be seen in hemolytic than in hemorrhagic types of anemia. Although reticulocytes are often reported as a percentage, a more useful method is to calculate a corrected reticulocyte count and a reticulocyte production index.

A corrected reticulocyte count is calculated by multiplying the observed reticulocyte percentage by the observed hematocrit/normal hematocrit. For dogs, 45% is used as the normal hematocrit; 35% is used for cats. For example, if a dog has a PCV of 15% and an observed reticulocyte count of 15%, the corrected reticulocyte count is as follows:

$$15\% \times 15\%/45\% = 5\%$$

A reticulocyte production index is calculated by dividing the corrected reticulocyte percentage by the maturation time of the reticulocyte for the observed patient's hematocrit. Maturation time values are based on the patient hematocrit (Table 2-4). For the previous example, if the dog corrected reticulocyte count is 5%, the reticulocyte production index is 5/2.5 = 2.5, indicating that the patient is producing reticulocytes at a rate 2.5 times more quickly than normal.

Parasites. Parasites may be present in or on erythrocytes. Stain precipitate and drying artifacts are sometimes confused with red cell parasites. Drying artifact usually appears refractile (Fig. 2-56). The most commonly seen blood parasites in small animals are *Ehrlichia* and *Haemobartonella*. Occasionally a microfilaria of *Dirofilaria immitis* may be seen on a peripheral blood film (Fig. 2-57).

Haemobartonella felis is a fairly common parasite of feline erythrocytes. The disease is referred to as hemobartonellosis, or feline infectious anemia. Recent information derived from DNA sequence analysis has shown that these bacteria are most closely related to the genus Mycoplasma, and many authors now classify the organism as *Mycoplasma*

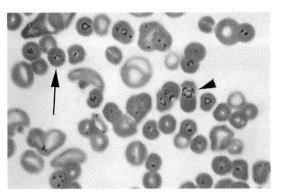

Figure 2-56. Drying artifacts. These will appear refractile under the microscope.

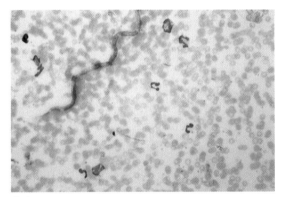

Figure 2-57. Microfilaria of *Dirofilaria immitis* in a canine blood film.

haemofelis. The organisms appear as small (0.2 to 0.5 μm), coccoid, rod-shaped, or ringlike structures that stain dark purple with Wright's stain (Fig. 2-58). They most frequently appear as short rods on the periphery of RBCs. The parasitemia is cyclic; if hemobartonellosis is suspected, the blood should be examined several times at different times of the day before the infection is ruled out. Whole blood that has not been in contact with anticoagulant is preferred for examination of suspected hemobartonellosis. The organisms often detach from the surface of the RBC when in anticoagulant. *Haemobartonella canis* infection is rare in dogs and usually is observed only in splenectomized or immunosuppressed dogs. The organism most commonly appears as a chain of small cocci or rods that

TABLE 2-4

Reticulocyte Maturation Index	
Patient Hematocrit	**Maturation Time**
45%	1
35%	1.4
25%	2
15%	2.5

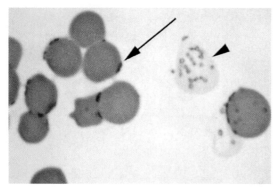

Figure 2-58. *Haemobartonella/Mycoplasma* organisms on the periphery of erythrocytes.

stretch across the surface of the erythrocyte. The chains may appear to branch.

A variety of species of *Ehrlichia* are capable of infecting dogs. *Ehrlichia platys* affects only platelets and causes infectious cyclic thrombocytopenia. Other *Ehrlichia* species may infect any of the leukocytes. *Ehrlichia canis* commonly infects monocytes and neutrophils (Fig. 2-59). *Ehrlichia* parasites belong to a group of rickettsial organisms. Nomenclature of the various species has changed significantly in recent years as additional information on the biochemistry of the organisms is uncovered. Many authors refer to some *Ehrlichia* species as *Anaplasma*. The organism is transmitted by the brown dog tick and appears as small clus-

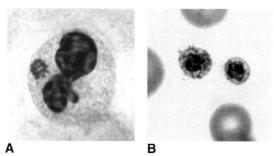

A   **B**

Figure 2-59. A, *Ehrlichia equi* morula in the cytoplasm of a neutrophil. **B,** Two platelets containing *Ehrlichia platys* morulae, (From Harvey JW: *Atlas of Veterinary Hematology: Blood and Bone Marrow of Domestic Animals,* St. Louis, 2001, Saunders.)

ters, called *morulae* (3 to 6 μm), in the cytoplasm. The disease may result in neutropenia, thrombocytopenia, and anemia. Chronically affected animals may be severely anemic, with marked leukopenia and thrombocytopenia, but sometimes the only hematologic abnormality is lymphocytosis. The total plasma protein level usually is increased. The organisms are best demonstrated during the acute phase but usually are present in small numbers. Films made from the buffy coat may aid diagnosis. However, in most cases organisms are not seen and the diagnosis is made by immunologic testing.

Eperythrozoonosis in swine, cattle, and llamas is quite similar to hemobartonellosis; the organisms are closely related. *Eperythrozoa* appear as small (0.8 to 1.0 μm) cocci, rods, or rings on the RBC surface or free in the plasma. The ring form is most common (see Fig. 2-49).

Anaplasma marginale is an intracellular blood parasite that causes anaplasmosis in cattle and wild ruminants. It appears as small, dark-staining cocci at the margin of RBCs and must be differentiated from Howell-Jolly bodies because their sizes are similar. Early in the course of the disease as many as 50% of RBCs may contain parasites. By the time the anemia is severe, usually less than 5% of RBCs are affected.

Cytauxzoon felis is a rare cause of hemolytic anemia in cats. The organism appears as small (1.0 to 2.0 μm), irregular ring forms within erythrocytes, lymphocytes, and macrophages.

Babesiosis of cattle is caused by *Babesia bigemina* and *B. bovis*. The disease is also called Texas fever, redwater fever, and cattle tick fever. *Babesia* spp. appear as large (3 to 4 μm), pleomorphic, teardrop-shaped intracellular organisms, frequently seen in pairs (Fig. 2-60). Babesiosis in horses (piroplasmosis) is caused by *B. equi* and *B. caballi,* which are similar to *B. bigemina.* Babesiosis is rare in horses, and the few cases reported in the United States have been seen in the South, especially Florida. Babesiosis in dogs is caused by *B. canis* and *B. gibsoni.* They are also similar in appearance to *B. bigemina,* but *B. gibsoni* is slightly smaller and appears as rings. Only a small percentage of erythrocytes may be affected. The organisms are more commonly observed in RBCs at the feathered edge.

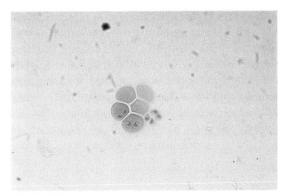

Figure 2-60. *Babesia* organisms in bovine RBCs.

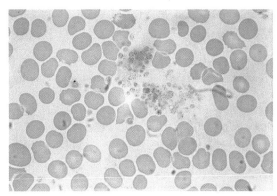

Figure 2-61. A platelet clump in a canine blood film.

Platelet Estimate

Platelets (thrombocytes) are an important component of hemostasis. One procedure for platelet evaluation is examination of the blood film. When platelet numbers appear decreased, determining platelet concentration by a more quantitative procedure is appropriate. Platelet numbers should be evaluated in the counting area of the blood film. The numbers of platelets in a minimum of 10 microscopic fields should be counted. The size of the oil-immersion field depends on the type of microscope used. With the use of older microscopes, an average of three to five or more platelets per oil-immersion field is considered adequate. When using newer models, 8 to 10 platelets per oil-immersion field are more common in normal patients. Platelet estimates can also be reported as the average number seen in 10 microscopic fields or as the range seen in 10 fields. The presence of an average of seven or range of 7 to 21 platelets is reported as adequate. To get an indirect measure of platelet number, count the number of platelets seen per 100 WBCs on the differential blood film. This number is then used to calculate the platelet estimate with the following equation:

$$\frac{\text{thrombocytes}}{100 \text{ leukocytes}} \times \frac{\text{WBC count}}{\mu L} = \text{thrombocytes}/\mu L$$

Platelet clumping is common in cats. If clumps are observed (Fig. 2-61), platelets are probably adequate in number. The presence of unusually large platelets (megathrombocytes) (Fig. 2-62), may sug-

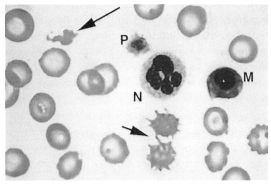

Figure 2-62. A megathrombocyte *(P)*, acanthocyte *(short arrow),* and schistocyte *(long arrow)* on a canine blood film.

gest early release of platelets from the bone marrow and should be noted. Platelets, especially in cats, may be larger than erythrocytes. If decreased platelet numbers are suspected on the basis of the blood film examination, a platelet count is indicated.

Erythrocyte Osmotic Fragility

The osmotic fragility (OF) test provides a measure of the RBC ability to withstand hemolysis in varying concentrations of saline solution. The OF test measures the amount of hemolysis that occurs in varying concentrations of saline solution compared with a normal control. This test may add some useful information in the differentiation among some forms of anemia in the dog and cat. It is not routinely performed in veterinary medicine except at veterinary research and referral centers. OF is commonly measured by the Unopette RBC OF test kit. The kit contains reservoirs with differing concentrations of buffered saline solutions. RBCs that are lysed in the hypertonic solutions release hemoglobin. The amount of hemoglobin released is measure by photometric techniques. The percent hemolysis in each of the saline solutions is calculated. The mean OF is expressed as the concentration of saline in which 50% hemolysis occurs. Although the exact relationship between the OF result and the cell's ability to survive in vivo is not well characterized, a relationship exists between abnormal OF test results and decreased survival time for red cells. Increased resistance to hemolysis is noted in a variety of conditions that cause an increase in the surface-to-volume ratio of the red cell (e.g., some forms of liver disease, iron deficiency). Reticulocytes are also more resistant to hemolysis because of their greater surface area. Decreased resistance to hemolysis is seen in patients with autoimmune hemolytic anemia and parasitic infections such as haemobartonellosis, babesiosis, and infection with hookworms.

BONE MARROW EVALUATION

Collection of Bone Marrow Samples

Bone marrow evaluation is a valuable tool in diagnosis and prognosis in specific cases. The need for bone marrow evaluation is usually determined by the findings of the differential count from a peripheral blood cell sample. When the differential blood cell count demonstrates ambiguous or unexplained abnormal results, bone marrow evaluation is usually needed to provide sufficient detail for the diagnostician. Specific indications for bone marrow evaluation include persistent, unexplained pancytopenia, neutropenia or thrombocytopenia, and/or nonregenerative anemia. Less-common indications for bone marrow evaluation include the presence of cells with abnormal morphologic features or the unexplained presence of immature

cells on the differential blood film (e.g., nucleated RBCs, left shift). Bone marrow evaluation is also used to stage neoplastic disease and diagnose specific parasitic diseases (e.g., leishmaniasis, ehrlichiosis). Bone marrow evaluation may be contraindicated in some cases, particularly when hemostatic defects are present.

Samples may be collected by aspiration or removal of a bone marrow core. Proper restraint is crucial for biopsy of the bone marrow in dogs and cats. Sedation or local anesthesia may be needed when the patient is resistant to manual restraint. General anesthesia may be used but is complicated because patients undergoing bone marrow evaluation are usually compromised and represent a significant anesthetic risk. Aseptic technique is vital throughout the procedure.

All necessary equipment and supplies should be gathered before beginning the procedure. For collection of bone marrow aspirate samples, prepare syringes with EDTA solution by drawing 0.5 ml saline into the syringe and dispensing it into an empty small EDTA blood collection tube. Withdraw the mixture and then repeat the procedure. This creates a diluted EDTA flush to use on the syringe and bone marrow needle. Gather slides and set them on an incline. Usually, about 10 slides should be prepared. Other equipment needed includes a #11 scalpel blade, sterile skin preparation supplies, and suture material (if needed). Special bone marrow needles are preferred, although an 18-gauge hypodermic needle may be used in cats with thin bones. Bone marrow needles have a stylet that serves to prevent occlusion of the needle with bone and surrounding tissue as it is inserted into the marrow cavity. Needle types used for bone marrow collection include the Rosenthal, Illinois sternal, and Jamshidi needles (Fig. 2-63). Bone marrow needles are available as disposable products.

Aspiration Biopsy

Several sites can be used for an aspiration biopsy, including the head of the humerus, iliac crest, or femoral canal. The most common collection site in cats is the femoral head. The easiest site to localize in dogs is the humeral head. Even in obese dogs

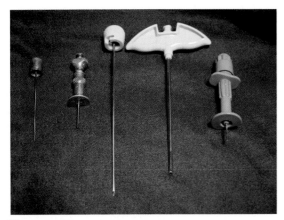

Figure 2-63. Bone marrow needles *(left to right):* Rosenthal stylet, Rosenthal needle, Jamshidi needle and stylet, Illinois needle.

and cats this site is easily identified because little overlying muscle or fat is present. The site of entry is the craniolateral side of the proximal humerus, distal to the greater tubercle. An obvious flat surface lies just subcutaneously at the site of entry. The site must be aseptically prepared and draped. A stab incision is made at the site with a sterile scalpel blade, and the needle inserted with the stylet in place (Fig. 2-64). Slight pressure should be placed on the side of the needle against the stylet to avoid blockage of the needle with bony material. A slight caudoventral angle introduces the

needle into the head of the humerus. The needle and stylet are then advanced until the cortex of the humerus is reached. The needle is then rotated while slight forward pressure is applied. This allows the needle to penetrate the cortical bone and keeps the needle in place. The stylet is then removed and a syringe is attached. A large syringe (10 ml) is usually preferred to allow for a greater negative pressure. The syringe plunger is rapidly and vigorously withdrawn until blood enters the hub of the needle. Firm restraint is essential at this stage because disruption of nerves in the area may cause momentary discomfort to the animal. As soon as material is present in the hub of the needle, pressure should be released to minimize hemodilution of the sample. Ideally the stylet should be replaced and the needle left in place until smears are prepared to ensure that an adequate sample has been obtained. A small suture may be needed to close the site. Bone marrow aspirate samples clot rapidly, so smears must be made immediately or the sample mixed with 0.5 ml of 2% to 3% EDTA in saline. Even when smears are made immediately, placing a small amount of EDTA in the syringe and needle before beginning the collection procedure may be helpful.

Core Biopsy

In most situations, better-quality samples and greater diagnostic information are obtained if a core sample of marrow is collected in addition to an aspiration biopsy. Always use different sites for each collection when collecting both an aspirate and a core sample. This will ensure that the procedures do not introduce artifact into the next sample. Core samples allow the architecture of the cells to remain intact, although morphologic features of individual cells are more difficult to assess than with an aspiration sample. In addition, some parasites may be visible within macrophages of the bone marrow and will be more easily seen with a core biopsy. Overall cellularity of the marrow is most accurately determined with a core sample because it is not diluted with blood. The procedure is generally the same as for aspiration biopsy, with the following exceptions. The core sample is collected with a 16 to 18 gauge Jamshidi

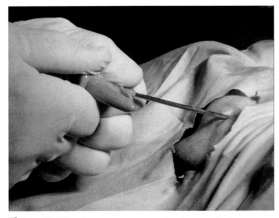

Figure 2-64. Bone marrow aspiration technique.

needle. The most commonly used site for collection is the iliac crest. Once the needle is introduced into the cortical bone, it should be moved forward approximately 1 inch and rotated back and forth to cut the piece of bone from the cortex. The needle is then removed and the stylet used to expel the core sample through the proximal (hub) end of the needle. Forcing the sample back through the narrow distal end of the needle introduces pressure artifact into the sample. An impression smear (see Chapter 9) should be made from the sample before placing it in formalin. Never place smears from aspirate samples in proximity to formalin-preserved specimens. Formalin fumes interfere with staining of cytology specimens.

Preparing Marrow Smears

Bone marrow samples must be made immediately if not mixed with EDTA at the time of collection. If EDTA has been used, smears must be made within 1 hour of collection. Marrow smears of aspirate samples can be prepared in a similar manner to peripheral blood. Two to 12 slides are prepared so that additional samples are available if additional testing (e.g. immunofluorescence assay [IFA]), special staining) is needed. Aspiration samples should be pushed out of the hub of the needle by using pressure from the syringe. Bone marrow samples are thicker than blood and should contain particles or spicules. Excess blood and/or EDTA in the sample can be removed by tilting the slide to allow it to run off. Alternatively, the sample can be expelled into a Petri dish and the bone marrow spicules removed with a small plastic pipette or capillary tube.

Line smears, starfish smears, and squash preps (compression smears) can also be used for bone marrow samples. A modified compression technique may provide the most useful sample. The compression prep method has been widely used for many years for preparation of cytology specimens (see Chapter 9). The technique is similar to that used for cover slip preparation of peripheral blood films. Bone marrow smears must be rapidly air dried and stained, usually with a Romanowsky-type stain. Staining time must be increased depending on the cellularity and thickness of the sample. One slide is usually stained with hemosiderin to identify iron particles in the marrow sample. Hematoxylin-eosin stain is preferred for core biopsy samples, although Giemsa stain may also be used. Recent advances in cytochemistry and immunochemistry have also provided a large number of alternative staining techniques. These techniques use methods that can bind with surface molecules unique to specific cell types and have simplified definitive identification of cells in bone marrow.

Evaluation of Bone Marrow Films

A systematic approach should be used when evaluating a bone marrow film. Bone marrow status should never be evaluated without the results of a differential WBC count from a concurrent peripheral blood film. Stained bone marrow smears must first be examined at low power (100×) magnification. This initial examination is used to evaluate the adequacy of the preparation. If the sample is not stained properly or cells are not easily distinguished, another slide should be obtained. Assuming the preparation is adequate, the low power examination can provide an indication of overall cellularity of the bone marrow. In adult animals, normal bone marrow generally contains approximately 50% nucleated cells and 50% fat. Marrow samples from juvenile mammals are usually 25% fat, whereas geriatric animals usually have marrow consisting of approximately 75% fat. The marrow sample is described as acellular (aplasia), hypercellular (hyperplasia), or hypocellular (hypoplasia) on the basis of the proportion of nucleated cells versus fat present. Although the adipocytes are dissolved during fixation of samples, the marrow contains what appear to be large vacuoles, representing the ruptured adipocytes. Samples are then further characterized by describing the type of cells present (e.g., hypoplasia/myeloid). Neoplasia is a possibility if all the cells look alike. A systematic approach to bone marrow evaluation is summarized in Procedure 2-3.

PROCEDURE 2-3

Evaluating Bone Marrow Aspirate

Low power examination
1. Evaluate adequacy of preparation
2. Determine relative percentages of nucleated cells and adipocytes

High power examination
1. Determine relative percentages of erythroid and myeloid cells using method preferred:
   a. Count 500 cells and classify all cell types and calculate M:E ratio or;
   b. Categorize 500 cells and calculate an erythroid and myeloid maturation index or;
   c. Categorize 200 cells and calculate myeloid and erythroid left shift indexes
2. Evaluate for presence of hemosiderin
3. Describe cellular morphology

Cells in Bone Marrow

Once overall cellularity is determined, the sample is examined at higher magnification ($400\times$ to $450\times$) to determine the relative percentages of erythroid and myeloid cells. One method requires counting and classifying 500 cells. Myeloid cells are relatively large and pale-staining cells, whereas erythroid cells are smaller and have clumped basophilic nuclei. Cells of the erythroid series include the rubriblast, prorubricyte, rubricyte, and metarubricyte. The rubriblast contains a nucleolus and a small amount of basophilic cytoplasm. Prorubricytes are smaller than rubriblasts, with a slightly more condensed nucleus and intensely blue cytoplasm. Cells in the rubricyte stage initially have basophilic cytoplasm and moderate clumping of the nucleus. As the cell matures, the morphologic characteristics of rubricytes are distinguished by marked nuclear clumping and pink cytoplasm because of the incorporation of hemoglobin. Metarubricytes are the smallest cells in the erythroid series and have a condensed nucleus and deep red cytoplasm. Cells in the

myeloid series include the myeloblast, promyelocyte, myelocyte, and metamyelocyte. Myeloblasts are larger than rubriblasts and have a prominent nucleolus and pale blue cytoplasm. A few reddish granules may be evident in the cytoplasm. The promyelocyte is a large, pale-staining cell with prominent reddish cytoplasmic granules. Myelocytes are smaller cells with a round nucleus. Granules characteristic of the mature neutrophil, eosinophil, and basophil begin to appear during the myelocyte stage. The metamyelocyte is similar in appearance to the myelocyte except that the nucleus is indented. Band cells are also present in bone marrow and have a horseshoe-shaped nucleus with parallel sides. Mature, segmented neutrophils, eosinophils, and basophils are also present in small numbers (Fig. 2-65).

Rubricytes and metarubricytes usually comprise 80% to 90% of the erythroid cells. Metamyelocytes, bands, and segmented myeloid cells comprise approximately 80% to 90% of the myeloid cells. The ratio of myeloid cells to erythroid cells (M/E ratio) is determined by counting 500 nucleated cells and classifying them as erythroid or myeloid. Normal M/E ratios should be between 0.75:1.0 and 2.0:1.0. Normal values for differential counting of bone marrow cells vary considerably among different species. Because the complete differential count of a marrow smear is time-consuming, several modifications to the differential cell count are used. Some laboratories use a system that classifies cells into one of eight categories: immature myeloid, mature myeloid, immature erythroid, mature erythroid, eosinophilic, monocytoid, lymphocytic, and plasma cells. In this classification scheme, immature cells include the myeloblasts, promyelocytes, rubriblasts, and prorubricytes. Several alternate systems for evaluation of bone marrow cells are used. One system involves classifying cells into groups and then calculating an erythroid maturation index and myeloid maturation index. An additional system is used that calculates a left shift index for both myeloid and erythroid cell lines. The erythroid left shift index involves counting and classifying 200 cells as either immature (rubriblasts, prorubricytes, and early rubricytes) or mature (late

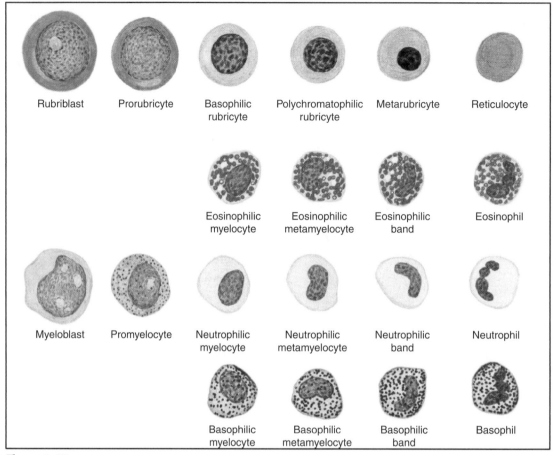

Figure 2-65. Maturation of myeloid and erythroid cells. (Drawing by Dr. Perry Bain. From Meyer DJ, Harvey JW: *Veterinary Laboratory Medicine: Interpretation and Diagnosis,* ed 3, St. Louis, 2004, Saunders.)

rubricytes and metarubricytes) and dividing the percentage of immature by mature erythroid cells. The myeloid left shift index is calculated by dividing the percentage of all immature granulocytes (myeloblast through band cell) by the percentage of mature granulocytes in a 200–cell count differential.

Megakaryocytes are not evenly distributed in a bone marrow aspirate. They are very large cells containing multiple fused nuclei and are often seen in clusters, particularly at the edges of the slide (Fig. 2-66). Megakaryocytes may number 8 to 10 per low power field, although 2 to 3 per low power field is more common. Generally, more than 10 per

low power field would indicate an increase in this cell line.

Other cell types present in bone marrow samples include macrophages, lymphocytes, plasma cells, mast cells, osteoblasts, and osteoclasts. Osteoblasts appear similar to plasma cells except that they are much larger and contain paler-appearing nuclear material. They also tend to be found in clusters when seen in samples collected by aspirate techniques. Plasma cells are slightly larger than lymphocytes with a greater nucleus-to-cytoplasm ratio. Plasma cells often have a perinuclear clear area around the eccentrically located nucleus and distinctly basophilic cytoplasm

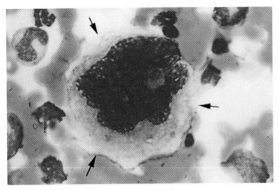

Figure 2-66. A megakaryocyte in a canine bone marrow aspirate sample.

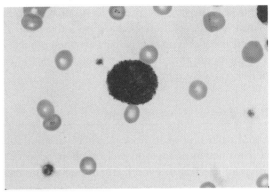

Figure 2-68. A mast cell in a feline blood film. (From Cowell RL, Tyler RD, and Meinkoth JH: *Diagnostic Cytology and Hematology of the Dog and Cat,* ed 2, St. Louis, 1999, Mosby.)

(Fig. 2-67). Inclusions containing immunoglobulin are often present. These inclusions are commonly referred to as Russell bodies and the cell referred to as a Mott cell. Osteoclasts contain multiple nuclei and may appear somewhat fused and similar in appearance to megakaryocytes except that the megakaryocyte nucleus is multilobed. Osteoclasts are seen most often in samples from young, actively growing animals. The cytoplasm is blue and may contain granular material of variable sizes that stains a deep red. Macrophages in bone marrow samples often contain phagocytized material that may aid in diagnosis. In core biopsy samples, macrophages are seen in the center of clusters of erythropoietic areas. These erythropoietic "islands" are usually disrupted during aspiration biopsy.

Lymphocytes are produced in the bone marrow but are usually present in low numbers. Immature stages (lymphoblasts and prolymphocytes) are difficult to distinguish from rubriblasts and prorubricytes. Reactive lymphocytes and normal, mature lymphocytes may also be present and appear as they would if seen in peripheral blood samples. Mast cells are characterized by abundant, small, metachromatic cytoplasmic granules (Fig. 2-68).

Hemosiderin is present in macrophages in bone marrow and is also found free of cells. It is easily identifiable as small gray to black granules when traditional blood film stains are used. Prussian blue stain may also be used to demonstrate the presence of this iron store. Hemosiderin is almost always absent in bone marrow preparations from cats. A decrease or absence of hemosiderin is significant in most other species.

Reporting of Results

Results of bone marrow evaluation include at minimum the overall cellularity and either M/E ratio, maturation index, or left shift index. If a complete differential count of marrow cells is not possible, the sample is usually described in narrative form and any unique patterns or morphologic abnormalities described. When present, stainable iron (hemosiderin), increased presence of mitotic figures, increased presence of osteoblasts,

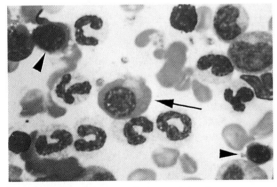

Figure 2-67. A plasma cell *(arrow)* in a bone marrow aspirate from a normal dog.

osteoclasts, mast cells, presence of phagocytized material, and metastatic cells from other organs should also be recorded. The data are then reported along with the concurrent differential count from a peripheral blood film.

Disorders of Bone Marrow

Abnormalities seen in bone marrow samples can be classified as changes in cell numbers or in cell morphologic features and maturation. Samples can be characterized as either increased or decreased cellularity of all cell types, or increased or decreased cellularity of one cell type. In addition, abnormal hematopoiesis when cellularity is normal can also occur. A glossary of terms used to describe these abnormalities is presented in Table 2-5.

Inflammatory conditions may also be evident on examination of a bone marrow aspirate. These conditions are classified according to the primary cell type(s) present as one of four types: fibrinous, chronic, chronic granulomatous, and chronic pyogranulomatous. Fibrinous inflammation typically involves infiltration of the bone marrow with fibrin exudate without the presence of inflammatory cells. Chronic inflammation is a hyperplastic condition characterized by increased numbers of plasma cells, mature lymphocytes, and/or mast cells.

TABLE 2-5

Terminology of Bone Marrow Aspirate

Term	Definition
Aplasia	Less than 25% myeloid cells
Basophilic hyperplasia	Basophilia in bone marrow and peripheral blood
Dyserythropoiesis	Abnormal erythrocyte morphology
Dysgranulopoiesis (Dysmyelopoiesis)	Abnormal granulocyte morphology
Dysmegakaryopoiesis (Dysthrombopoiesis)	Increased megakaryocytes in bone marrow with thrombocytopenia
Emperipolesis	Presence of intact, viable blood cells within the cytoplasm of megakaryocytes
Eosinophilic hyperplasia	Eosinophilia in bone marrow and peripheral blood
Erythroid hyperplasia	Normal or increased cellularity with normal or increased absolute neutrophil count
Erythroid hypoplasia	Normal or decreased cellularity with normal or decreased absolute neutrophil count
Granulocytic hyperplasia	Normal or increased cellularity with normal or increased PCV and high M/E ratio
Hyperostosis	Thickening of cortical bone
Hypocellular	Decrease in overall cellularity
Megakaryocytic hyperplasia	Increase in numbers of megakaryocytes in bone marrow
Monocytic hyperplasia	Increased presence of precursors cells of the monocyte series
Myelodysplasia	Atypical cells with less than 30% blast cells present
Myelofibrosis	Increased presence of fibrous tissue that displaces hematopoietic tissue
Neoplasia	Atypical cells with greater than 30% blast cells present
Neutrophilic hyperplasia, effective	Neutrophilia in bone marrow and peripheral blood
Neutrophilic hyperplasia, ineffective	Neutrophilia in bone marrow concurrent with neutropenia in peripheral blood
Osteosclerosis	Thickening of the trabecular bone
Reactive macrophage hyperplasia	Increased presence of active macrophages, often containing phagocytized material

Chronic granulomatous inflammation is characterized by increased numbers of macrophages. If both macrophages and neutrophils are present, the condition is described as pyogranulomatous.

Neoplasia

Neoplastic disorders of hematopoiesis are classified as either lymphoproliferative or myeloproliferative. The common term used to describe the presence of neoplastic blood cells in bone marrow and peripheral blood is leukemia. When blast cells comprise more than 30% of marrow cells, the condition is often described as acute. Chronic forms of leukemia are characterized by the presence of more mature cells (fewer than 30% blast cells) that have neoplastic characteristics in blood and bone marrow. Chronic myeloid leukemia can develop into a condition called myelofibrosis. In this condition, much of the bone marrow is replaced by scar tissue incapable of producing blood cells.

Myeloproliferative disease is a progressive leukemic disorder that can be of the following types: acute myeloid leukemia, chronic granulocytic leukemia, chronic eosinophilic leukemia, chronic basophilic leukemia, chronic myelomonocytic leukemia, essential thrombocythemia, or primary erythrocytosis (polycythemia vera). Acute myeloid leukemia is further classified according to the types of cells and their relative differentiation as one of nine subtypes (Table 2-6). The classification involves determination of the percentage of nucleated cells and the degree of differentiation, or commitment toward development into a specific cell type. Forms of chronic myeloid leukemia are less common than acute myeloid leukemia. They are classified according to the primary cell type involved and are often accompanied by a left shift. Essential thrombocythemia is extremely rare. This chronic condition is characterized by significant increases in platelet count and marked increases in megakaryoblasts and megakaryocytes in the bone marrow. Primary erythrocytosis is unique in that the maturation patterns and mature cells produced appear normal, although their numbers are greatly increased. This disorder is thought to result from mutation of erythroid stem cells that causes the cells to be hyperresponsive to EPO or capable of proliferation independent of EPO concentration.

Lymphoproliferative disease, or lymphocytic leukemia, comprises nearly 10% of hematopoietic tumors diagnosed in dogs. Lymphoproliferative disorders include acute lymphocytic leukemia, chronic lymphocytic leukemia, and plasma cell myeloma. Increased numbers of plasma cells seen in bone marrow samples are also referred to as multiple myeloma. Acute lymphocytic leukemia is characterized by the presence of lymphoblasts and/or prolymphocytes in blood and/or bone marrow. Chronic lymphocytic leukemia is characterized by

TABLE 2-6

Classification of Acute Myeloid Leukemias

Traditional Terminology	Subtype	Characteristics
Reticuloendotheliosis	AML-AUL	Predominance of undifferentiated blast cells
Granulocytic leukemia	AML-M1	Myeloblastic leukemia with differentiation to the granulocytic series
Granulocytic leukemia	AML-M2	Myeloblastic leukemia with neutrophilic differentiation
Myelomonocytic leukemia	AML-M4	Combination of myeloblasts and monoblasts
Monocytic leukemia	AML-M5a	Monocytic leukemia with >80% monoblasts and promonocytes
Monocytic leukemia	AML-M5b	Monocytic leukemia with 30%-80% monoblasts and promonocytes
Erythroleukemia	AML-M6	Combination of myeloblasts and rubriblasts
Erythremic myelosis	AML-M6Er	Erythroid leukemia
Megakaryoblastic leukemia	AML-M7	Increased megakaryoblasts in peripheral blood and bone marrow

the presence of greater than 30% mature lympho-cytes in the bone marrow. Leukemia can also arise from other cell lines, causing myelogenous or monocytic disease. Primary bone tumors are those that originate in the bone. The most common type of primary bone tumor is osteosarcoma. Osteo-sarcoma arises from osteoblasts and can spread rapidly to other parts of the body. Malignant histio-cytosis is a malignant condition characterized by increased proliferation of neoplastic macrophages. Erythrophagocytosis may be seen with this condi-tion. Mast cell leukemia is seen in dogs and cats, although it is not common.

Classification of Anemia

The function of RBCs, or erythrocytes, is to trans-port and protect hemoglobin, the oxygen-carrying pigment. Daily production of erythrocytes equals the daily loss from destruction of aged cells in a healthy animal. If RBC production is decreased or destruction and/or loss is increased, anemia results. Anemia is a condition of reduced oxygen carrying capacity of erythrocytes. It may result from a reduced number of circulating RBCs, reduced PCV, or a reduced concentration of hemoglobin. Anemia may be classified according to bone marrow response as either regenerative or nonregenerative or according to RBC size and hemoglobin con-centration (MCV, MCHC).

Classification by Bone Marrow Response

This classification is most clinically applicable because it distinguishes between regenerative and nonregenerative anemia. In regenerative anemia, the bone marrow responds to anemia by increasing erythrocyte production and releasing immature erythrocytes. These immature RBCs, that is, poly-chromatophilic RBCs or reticulocytes, can be observed on the blood film and indicate that the marrow is responsive. The ability of bone marrow to respond indicates that the cause of the anemia is probably either blood loss (hemorrhage) or blood destruction (hemolysis). In nonregenerative anemia, the bone marrow is unable to respond to the anemic state and reticulocytes are absent on blood films, suggesting bone marrow dysfunction.

A bone marrow aspiration biopsy is then indicated once common endocrine and metabolic causes of nonregenerative anemia are excluded.

Classification by RBC Size and Hemoglobin Concentration

Anemia can be classified as normocytic (RBCs of normal size), macrocytic (RBCs larger than normal), or microcytic (RBCs smaller than normal). Normo-cytic anemia is characterized by RBCs of normal size and is secondary to a variety of chronic dis-orders. In domestic animals, the most common cause of macrocytic anemia is the transitory increase in RBC size seen with regenerative anemia (reticulocytosis). In human beings, macrocytic anemia is frequently associated with vitamin B_{12} and folic acid deficiencies. These conditions are rarely, if ever, seen in domestic animals.

Microcytic anemia is almost always the result of iron deficiency. Division of immature erythrocytes stops when a critical concentration of hemoglobin is reached. With inadequate iron for hemoglobin synthesis, extra division may occur, resulting in smaller erythrocytes. Although chronic blood loss is the most common cause of iron deficiency in adult animals, inadequate dietary iron results in iron-deficiency anemia in young nursing animals such as kittens and baby pigs.

Anemia may be hypochromic (reduced hemo-globin concentration) or normochromic (normal hemoglobin concentration). A hyperchromic state is not possible. Newly released polychromatophilic erythrocytes (reticulocytes) are hypochromic because the full concentration of hemoglobin is not yet attained. Macrocytic hypochromic anemia suggests regeneration. Iron deficiency also results in hypochromic anemia but is also characterized by microcytosis. Most other types of anemia are normochromic.

EVALUATION OF COAGULATION

Hemostasis is the ability of the body's systems to maintain the integrity of the blood and blood vessels. It involves a number of complex pathways, platelets, and coagulation factors. Any alteration in these parameters can result in a bleeding disorder.

Coagulation of blood proceeds through a mechanical phase and a chemical phase. The mechanical phase is initiated when a blood vessel is ruptured or torn. The exposed blood vessel subendothelium is a charged surface, and platelets are attracted to this surface. As platelets congregate at the site, they undergo morphologic and physiologic changes. These changes cause the platelets to adhere to each other as well as the blood vessel endothelium. This also causes platelets to release the initiating factor for the chemical phase of hemostasis. The chemical phase is referred to as the coagulation cascade and involves a number of coagulation factors (Table 2-7). Each factor participates in a chemical reaction that serves to initiate the next reaction in the pathway. The end result of the coagulation cascade is the formation of a mesh of fibrin strands that forms the clot. The final phase of hemostasis involves degradation of the fibrin clot.

Various coagulation tests have been developed to evaluate specific portions of the hemostatic mechanisms. Some tests measure just the mechanical phase of hemostasis. Others can measure specific parts of the chemical phase. All patients should be evaluated for coagulation defects before undergoing surgery. Most coagulation tests can be completed with minimal time and equipment and are relatively inexpensive. Figure 2-69 summarizes the chemical phase of the blood coagulation process.

Coagulation Tests

Blood samples for coagulation tests should be collected carefully, with minimal tissue damage and minimal venous stasis. Samples should never be collected through indwelling catheters. The preferred anticoagulant for coagulation tests is sodium citrate. Samples for whole blood clotting time and

TABLE 2-7

Blood Coagulation Factors

Designation	Synonym
Factor I	Fibrinogen
Factor II	Prothrombin
Factor III	Tissue thromboplastin
Factor IV	Calcium
Factor V	Proaccelerin
Factor VI	Proconvertin
Factor VII	Antihemophilic factor
Factor VIII	Christmas factor, plasma thromboplastin
Factor IX	Smart-Prower factor
Factor X	Plasma thromboplastin antecedent
Factor XI	Hageman factor
Factor XII	Fibrin-stabilizing factor

Reprinted from Sirois M: *Veterinary clinical laboratory procedures,* St Louis, 1995, Mosby.

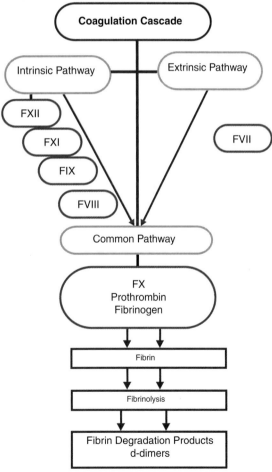

Figure 2-69. A summary of the blood coagulation process.

activated coagulation time do not require an anticoagulant.

Platelet Counting Methods

Platelets counts are best performed by manual methods (e.g., Unopette 5855). Some automated analyzers also perform platelet counts. If a coagulation disorder is suspected, a manual platelet count should be performed because automated counts can be highly inaccurate as a result of platelet clumping and platelet/RBC overlap. Always use a freshly collected blood sample to perform manual platelet counts. Morphologic changes in platelets include aggregation and giant platelets. These abnormalities will not be evident with automated analyzers and must therefore be detected using the differential blood film.

The procedure is similar to counting WBCs. A 20-μl pipette is used with 1% ammonium oxalate as a diluent. The ammonium oxalate hemolyzes the RBCs but preserves the WBCs and platelets. The platelets are counted at 400× magnification in the 25 small squares located in the large center square of the grid. The number of platelets counted is then multiplied by 1000 to calculate the number of platelets per μl of blood. Counting platelets is especially difficult because of their small size and tendency to clump together. Platelets are counted after the WBCs because it takes approximately 10 minutes for the platelets to settle within the hemacytometer counting chamber. The hemacytometer should be placed in a moist chamber while the platelets settle to avoid dehydration of the sample. An inverted petri dish containing damp paper towels may be used for this purpose.

Activated Clotting Time

This test can evaluate every clinically significant clotting factor except factor VII. The test requires a Vacutainer tube that contains diatomaceous earth. The diatomaceous earth causes the activation of the coagulation pathways. The tube must be prewarmed in a 37° C (98.6° F) water bath or heat block. Venipuncture is performed and 2 ml of blood is collected directly into the tube. A timer is started as soon as the blood enters the tube. The tube is mixed once by gentle inversion and

placed in a 37° C incubator or water bath. The tube is observed at 60 seconds and then at 5-second intervals for the presence of a clot. Normal values are approximately 60 to 90 seconds. Severe thrombocytopenia (fewer than 10,000 platelets/μl) and abnormalities associated with the intrinsic coagulation cascade prolong the activated clotting time.

Whole Blood Clotting Time

The whole blood clotting time (Lee-White method) is a test of the intrinsic clotting mechanism. The whole blood clotting time tests are not commonly performed because the activated clotting time is more sensitive. The test is performed by collecting 3 ml of blood in a plastic syringe, noting the time blood first appears in the syringe (by using a stopwatch). Immediately place 1 ml of blood in each of three 10- × 75-mm tubes that have been rinsed with saline. The tubes are then placed in a 37° C (98.6° F) water bath. The first and then the second tubes are tilted at 30-second intervals until coagulation occurs. The third tube is tilted in a similar manner. The time elapsed between the appearance of blood in the syringe and clot formation in the third tube is the clotting time. The normal whole blood clotting time for dogs is 2 to 10 minutes, horses 4 to 15 minutes, and cattle 10 to 15 minutes.

Buccal Mucosa Bleeding Time

This is a primary assay for the detection of abnormalities in platelet function. The test requires a Simplate I or II (Organon Teknika, Durham, NC) spring-loaded lancet, blotting paper or filter paper, stopwatch, and tourniquet. The patient should be anesthetized and placed in lateral recumbency. A strip of gauze is used to tie the upper lip back to expose the mucosal surface and act as a tourniquet. A 1-mm-deep incision is made with the Simplate device. Standard blotting paper or filter paper is used to blot the incision site (Fig. 2-70). This is done by lightly touching the paper to the drop of blood and allowing the blood to be absorbed without touching the incision. Blotting is repeated every 5 seconds until bleeding has stopped. The normal bleeding time for domestic animals is 1 to 5 minutes. A prolonged bleeding time occurs with

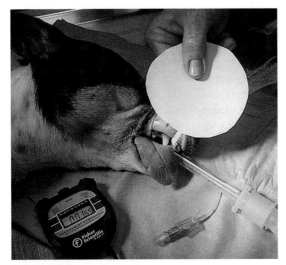

Figure 2-70. The buccal mucosa bleeding time test. (Courtesy B. Miztner, DVM.)

most platelet dysfunction syndromes. It will also be prolonged in thrombocytopenia, so a platelet count must also be performed.

Clot Retraction Test

This procedure allows the evaluation of platelet number and function and intrinsic and extrinsic pathways. Blood is drawn into a plain sterile tube and incubated at 37° C. The tube is examined at 60 minutes and reexamined periodically over a 24-hour period. A clot should be evident in 60 minutes, retracted in approximately 4 hours, and markedly compact at 24 hours.

Fibrinogen Determination

Automated methods for fibrinogen determination involve photometric analysis. These are not commonly performed in veterinary practice. One manual method that may be used for fibrinogen determination involves the use of two hematocrit tubes. The tubes are centrifuged as for a PCV and the total solids on one tube are determined, usually with a refractometer. The second tube is then incubated at 58° C for 3 minutes. The second tube is recentrifuged and the total solids measured. Multiply the total solids in grams per deciliter by

1000 to obtain the concentration in milligrams per deciliter. Fibrinogen is then calculated by the following equation (with all values in milligrams per deciliter):

$$\text{TS mg/dl}_{\text{(non-incubated)}} - \text{TS mg/dl}_{\text{(incubated)}} = \text{Fibrinogen mg/dl}$$

One-Stage Prothrombin Time (OSPT) Test

Prothrombin tests are usually performed by automated analyzers. This test evaluates the extrinsic coagulation pathway. The test uses a citrated plasma sample to which tissue thromboplastin reagent is added. A reagent designed to recalcify the sample is then added. Under normal conditions, a clot should form within 6 to 20 seconds. The normal range for dogs is 7 to 10 seconds. A prolonged OSPT may be associated with severe liver disease, DIC, or hereditary or acquired deficiencies of any factors of the extrinsic coagulation cascade. The test is sensitive to vitamin K deficiency or antagonism, such as warfarin toxicity.

Activated Partial Thromboplastin Time (APTT)

The activated partial thromboplastin time is another test of the intrinsic clotting mechanism. Some methods require multiple reagents. The SCA 2000 (Synbiotics Corporation, San Diego, CA.) is a handheld analyzer that performs both the prothrombin time and activated partial thromboplastin time (Fig. 2-71). Citrated plasma is incubated with an activator of factor XII, platelet substitute (cephaloplastin). After addition of calcium, the

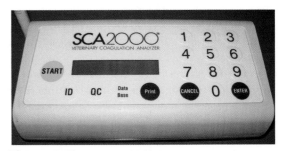

Figure 2-71. The SCA2000 Coagulation Analyzer provides measurements of prothrombin time and activated partial thromboplastin time.

time to form fibrin is determined. A variety of acquired and hereditary disorders, in addition to administration of heparin, can reduce one or more factors necessary for the normal intrinsic coagulation cascade.

PIVKA

The acronym PIVKA refers to *p*roteins *i*nduced (invoked) by *v*itamin *K* *a*bsence. Vitamin K is required to activate coagulation factors II, VII, IX, and X. When vitamin K is deficient, precursor proteins of factors II, VII, IX, and X build up and can be detected by PIVKA or Thrombotest (Axis-Shield PoC Norton, MA). The test can differentiate rodenticide toxicity from primary hemophilia when activated clotting time is prolonged. It is a more sensitive test than prothrombin when time these factors are depleted. PIVKA may become prolonged within 6 hours of ingestion of anticoagulant rodenticides, whereas prothrombin time prolongs within 24 hours and activated partial thromboplastin time within 48 hours.

d-Dimer and Fibrin Degradation Products

Both of these tests are used to evaluate tertiary hemostasis. d-Dimers and fibrin degradation products (or fibrin split products) are formed as a clot is degraded. These tests are therefore useful in identifying the presence of DIC and also provide diagnostic information in cases of liver failure, trauma, and hemangiosarcoma. A canine in-house test is available for d-Dimer analysis.

HEMOSTATIC DEFECTS

Bleeding disorders may be caused by congenital or acquired defects in coagulation proteins, platelets, or the vasculature. Most bleeding disorders found in veterinary species are secondary to some other disease process. Primary coagulation disorders are rare and are usually the result of an inherited defect in production of coagulation factors. Signs of congenital or acquired deficiencies in coagulation proteins usually involve delayed deep tissue hemorrhage and hematoma formation. Clinical signs associated with congenital or acquired defects or deficiencies of platelets include superficial

petechial and ecchymotic hemorrhages, epistaxis, melena, and prolonged bleeding at injection and incision sites. With functional defects or deficiencies in concentration of coagulation proteins, clinical signs usually appear before the animal reaches 6 months of age. The majority of congenital coagulation factor disorders in veterinary species involve a deficiency or abnormality of a single factor.

The most common inherited coagulation disorder of domestic animals is von Willebrand's disease, which is the result of decreased or deficient production of von Willebrand's factor. Von Willebrand's factor circulates with Factor VIII and functions to aid platelet aggregation at the initiation of the coagulation pathways. The disease occurs with relative frequency in Dobermans and has been reported in other canine breeds, as well as rabbits and swine. Several distinct forms of the disease have been identified on the basis of their patterns of inheritance. Other common inherited coagulation factor disorders of veterinary species are listed in Table 2-8.

Secondary coagulation disorders can result from decreased production or increased destruction of platelets, as well as nutritional deficiencies, liver disease, and ingestion of certain medications or toxic substances. Thrombocytopenia refers to a decreased number of platelets and is the most common coagulation disorder seen in small animal veterinary practice. The causes of platelet deficien-

TABLE 2-8

Common Inherited Coagulation Disorders of Dogs

Disorder	Breeds Affected
Prothrombin deficiency	Cocker spaniel, beagle
Factor VII deficiency	Beagle, malamute
Factor VIII deficiency (hemophilia A)	Many breeds
Factor IX deficiency (hemophilia B)	Many breeds
Factor X deficiency	Cocker spaniel
Factor XI deficiency	Great Pyrenees, English Springer spaniel
Factor XII deficiency	Poodle, Shar Pei

cies are often unknown. However, infection with certain bacterial, viral, and parasitic agents can result in thrombocytopenia. Thrombocytopenia can also occur as a result of bone marrow depression that reduces the production of platelets or autoimmune disease that increases the rate of platelet destruction. Because the liver is the site of production of most coagulation factors, any condition that affects liver function can result in a coagulation disorder. Ingestion of toxic substances such as warfarin can also create bleeding disorders. Warfarin inhibits vitamin K function. Because vitamin K is required for synthesis and activation of some coagulation factors, this can create a deficiency in several necessary components of the coagulation cascade. Ingestion of medications such as aspirin can also cause bleeding disorders.

Disseminated Intravascular Coagulation

Although not a disease entity on its own, DIC is associated with many pathologic conditions. DIC is often seen in trauma cases, as well as in a large number of infectious diseases. A large number of events can trigger DIC. The resulting hemostatic disorder may manifest as systemic hemorrhage or microvascular thrombosis. Because the triggering event and the resulting disorder are diverse, the laboratory findings are highly variable. Most patients with DIC have prolonged activated partial thromboplastin time and elevated fibrinogen, as well as significant thrombocytopenia.

Recommended Reading

Cowell R, Tyler R, Meinkoth J: *Diagnostic cytology and hematology of the dog and cat,* ed 2, St Louis, 1999, Mosby.

Meyer DJ, Harvey JW: *Veterinary laboratory medicine: interpretation and diagnosis,* St Louis, 2004, Saunders.

Sirois M: Hematology and hemostasis. In Sirois M: *Principles and practice of veterinary technology*, St Louis, 2004, Mosby.

Thrall MA, Baker DC, Lassen ED: *Veterinary hematology and clinical chemistry,* Philadelphia, 2004, Lippincott Williams & Wilkins.

CHAPTER 3

Clinical Chemistry

Margi Sirois

KEY POINTS

- The availability of affordable in-house analyzers for blood chemistry analysis has improved patient care.
- Clinical chemistry testing usually requires either a serum or plasma sample.
- Protein assays commonly performed in the veterinary practice laboratory are the total protein and albumin tests.
- Tests of the hepatobiliary system commonly performed in the veterinary practice laboratory are alanine aminotransferase, aspartate aminotransferase, bilirubin, and alkaline phosphatase.
- Common tests for kidney function include blood urea nitrogen and creatinine.
- Pancreatic function tests evaluate either the endocrine or the exocrine functions of the pancreas.

- Tests of pancreatic exocrine function include amylase and lipase.
- Pancreatic endocrine function can be evaluated with the glucose, fructosamine, and glycosylated hemoglobin tests.
- Other endocrine function tests (e.g., adrenocorticotropic hormone, thyroid assays) primarily use immunologic methods rather than chemical analyses.
- Electrolyte assays performed in the veterinary practice laboratory include sodium, potassium, and chloride.
- Some electrolyte analyzers can also evaluate calcium, phosphorus, magnesium, and bicarbonate.

n both human and veterinary medical practice, current trends indicate a move toward greater point-of-care capabilities. This translates into better customer service and enhances the practice of veterinary medicine. Determinations of levels of the various chemical constituents in blood can be an important aid in the formulation of an accurate diagnosis, prescription of proper therapy, and documentation of the response to treatment. The chemicals being assayed are generally associated with particular organ functions and may be enzymes associated with particular organ functions or metabolites and metabolic by-products that are processed by certain organs. Analysis of these components usually requires a carefully collected blood serum sample. Plasma may be used in some cases. Chemical measurements should be completed within 1 hour after blood collection. If testing will be delayed, freezing of the sample will preserve the integrity of most of the constituents. Freezing may interfere with some test methods, however. Certain anticoagulants may also interfere with particular chemical analyses. Many factors other than disease influence the results of chemistry tests. These factors may be preanalytical, analytical, or postanalytical (see Chapter 1).

Many veterinary practices own or lease chemistry analyzers to perform routine chemical assays. This focus on in-house laboratory work makes the veterinary technicians' laboratory skills perhaps their biggest asset to the practice.

As the person most likely to be in charge of the laboratory, the veterinary technician must become familiar with the types of analytic instruments available (see Chapter 1), the variety of testing procedures used, and the rationale underlying the analyses. The most important contribution the technician can make to the practice laboratory is accurate and reliable test results. In vitro results must reflect, as closely as possible, the actual in vivo levels of blood constituents.

SAMPLE COLLECTION

Most chemical analyses require collection and preparation of serum samples. Whole blood or blood plasma may be used for some test methods or with specific types of equipment. The instructions accompany the chemistry analyzers and should be consulted for the type of sample required. Collection of a high-quality sample on which to perform an assay has a direct effect on the quality of test results. Most adverse influences on sample quality can be avoided with careful consideration of sample collection and handling.

Specific blood collection protocols vary depending on the patient species, volume of blood needed, method of restraint, and types of samples needed. Chapter 2 contains additional information on blood collection protocols, supplies, and equipment. Blood samples for chemical testing should always be collected before treatment is initiated. Administration of certain medications and treatments may affect results of biochemical testing. Preprandial samples, or samples from an animal that has not eaten for 12 hours, are preferred. Postprandial samples, or samples collected after an animal has eaten, may produce erroneous results. Samples taken after the patient has eaten can produce false values for a number of blood components, including glucose, urea, and lipase. Regardless of the method of blood collection, the sample must be labeled immediately after it has been collected. The tube should be labeled with the date and time of collection, the owner's name, the patient's name, and the patient's clinic identification number. If submitted to a laboratory, include with the sample a request form that includes all necessary sample identification and a clear indication of which tests are requested.

Plasma

Plasma is the fluid portion of whole blood in which the cells are suspended. It is composed of approximately 90% water and 10% dissolved constituents, such as proteins, carbohydrates, vitamins, hormones, enzymes, lipids, salts, waste materials, antibodies, and other ions and molecules. Procedure 3-1 describes obtaining a plasma sample. The sample must not be contaminated with any cells from the bottom of the tube after centrifugation. If the sample cannot be centrifuged within 1 hour, it must be refrigerated. If heparinized plasma has been

PROCEDURE 3-1

Plasma Sample Preparation

1. Collect a blood sample in a container with the appropriate anticoagulant.
2. Mix the blood-filled container with a gentle rocking motion 12 times.
3. Make sure the container is covered to prevent evaporation during centrifugation.
4. Centrifuge (within an hour of collection) at 2000 to 3000 rpm for 10 minutes.
5. With a capillary pipette, carefully remove the fluid plasma layer from the bottom layer of cells.
6. Transfer the plasma to a container labeled with the date, time of collection, patient's name, and case or clinic number.
7. Process immediately or refrigerate or freeze as appropriate.

PROCEDURE 3-2

Serum Sample Preparation

1. Collect a whole blood sample in a container that contains no anticoagulant.
2. Allow the blood to clot in its original container at room temperature for 20 to 30 minutes.
3. Gently separate the clot from the container by running a wooden applicator stick around the wall of the container between the clot and the wall.
4. Cover the sample and centrifuge at 2000 to 3000 rpm for 10 minutes.
5. With a capillary pipette, remove the serum from the clot.
6. Transfer the serum to a container labeled with the date, time of collection, patient's name, and clinic or case number.
7. Refrigerate or freeze the sample as appropriate

stored overnight after separation or has been frozen, the sample should be centrifuged again to remove any fibrin strands that may have formed. Freezing may affect certain test results; the test instructions should be consulted for all the tests that must be run before a plasma sample is frozen.

Serum

Serum is plasma from which fibrinogen, a plasma protein, has been removed. During the clotting process, the soluble fibrinogen in plasma is converted to an insoluble fibrin clot matrix. When blood clots, the fluid that is squeezed out around the cellular clot is serum. Obtaining a serum sample is described in Procedure 3-2. Centrifuging at speeds greater than 2000 to 3000 rpm or for a prolonged time may result in hemolysis. Serum separator tubes (SST) contain a gel that forms a physical barrier between serum or plasma and blood cells during centrifugation. The inside walls of the tube also contain silica particles that assist in clot activation. Blood collected into an SST should be mixed by inverting the tube several times and

then allowing the sample to clot for 30 minutes before centrifugation. SST transport tubes are also available. These contain approximately double the amount of gel in a standard SST. The additional gel barrier helps minimize any interaction between the serum and cells after centrifugation so that test results are not likely to be affected if tests are delayed. Any prolonged delays in testing require that the serum be removed from the SST and placed in a sterile tube. The tube can then be refrigerated or frozen. Freezing may affect some test results; therefore the test instructions should be consulted for all the tests that must be run before a serum sample is frozen.

Factors Influencing Results

Many factors other than disease influence the results of chemistry tests. Hemolysis, lipemia, certain medications, and inappropriate sample handling can all lead to inaccurate results. Effects of sample compromise are summarized in Table 3-1.

TABLE 3-1

Effects of Sample Compromise

Sample Characteristic	Effect	Result
Lipemia	Light scattering	↑
	Volume displacement	↓
	Hemolysis*	↑↓
Hemolysis/blood substitutes	Release of analytes	↑
	Release of ezymes*	↑↓
	Reaction inhibition	↓
	Increased OD (absorbance)	↑
	Release of water	↓
Icterus	Spectral interference	↑
	Chemical interaction	↑
Hyperproteinemia	Hyperviscosity	↓
	Analyte binding*	↑↓
	Volume displacement	
Medications	Reaction interference*	↑↓

*Variable effect depending on analyte and test method.
From Sirois M: *Principles and practice of veterinary technology,* ed 2, St Louis, 2004, Mosby.

Hemolysis

Hemolysis may result when a blood sample is drawn into a moist syringe, mixed too vigorously after sample collection, forced through a needle when being transferred to a tube, or frozen as a whole blood sample. A syringe must be completely dry before it is used because water in the syringe may cause hemolysis. The needle from a syringe should be removed before blood is transferred to a tube. Forcing blood through a small needle opening may rupture cells. When transferring a blood sample to a tube, the veterinary technician should expel the blood slowly from the syringe without causing bubbles to form. Hemolysis can also result when excess alcohol is used to clean the skin and not allowed to dry before beginning the blood collection procedure.

Hemolysis, regardless of cause, can greatly alter the makeup of a serum or plasma sample. For example, fluid from ruptured blood cells can dilute the sample, resulting in falsely lower concentrations of constituents than are actually present in the animal. Certain constituents normally not found in high concentrations in serum or plasma escape from ruptured blood cells, causing falsely elevated concentrations in the sample. Hemolysis may elevate levels of potassium, organic phosphorus, and certain enzymes in the blood. Hemolysis also interferes with lipase activity and bilirubin determinations. Therefore, plasma or serum is frequently the preferred sample over whole blood, and serum is frequently preferred over plasma.

Chemical Contamination

Sterile tubes are not necessary for collection of blood samples for routine chemical assays. However, the tubes must be chemically pure. Detergents must be completely rinsed from reusable tubes so that the detergents do not interfere with test results.

Improper Labeling

Serious errors may result if a tube containing the sample is not labeled immediately after the sample is collected. The tube should be labeled with the date, time of collection, patient's name, and clinic number. The veterinary technician should double check the sample identification with the request form, if one is used, as the sample is prepared and the test is run.

Improper Sample Handling

Ideally, all chemical measurements should be completed within an hour of sample collection, which is not always feasible. In this case, samples must be properly handled and stored so that levels of their chemical constituents approximate those in the patient's body at the time of collection. Samples must not be allowed to become too warm. Heat may be detrimental to a sample, destroying some chemicals and activating others, such as enzymes. If a serum or plasma sample has been frozen, it must be thoroughly mixed after thawing to avoid concentration gradients.

Patient Influences

If practical, a sample should be obtained from a fasting animal. The blood glucose level can be elevated and the inorganic phosphorus level decreased immediately after a meal. Also, postprandial (after-eating) lipemia results in a turbid or cloudy plasma or serum. Kidney assays are also affected due to the transient increase in GFR after eating. Water intake need not be restricted before obtaining a blood sample.

REFERENCE RANGES

Reference ranges are also known as normal values. The reference range for a particular blood constituent is a range of values derived when a laboratory has repeatedly assayed samples from a significant number of clinically normal animals of a given species by specific test methods. Numerous medicine and clinical pathology books list the reference ranges of blood constituents for domestic species. Alternatively, reference ranges may be formulated by local diagnostic laboratories or in individual practice laboratories.

Establishing reference range values for any laboratory is time-consuming and expensive. To establish a list of reference values for the laboratory, the veterinary technician would have to assay samples from a significant number of clinically normal animals. Some investigators recommend analysis of at least 20 animals and others recommend more than 100 animals with similar characteristics. Other considerations include the variety of breeds and species most often seen in the veterinary practice; the gender and sexual status, such as intact or neutered, of the tested animals; the environment, including husbandry and nutrition, of these animals; and climate. Climate is a consideration because drastic seasonal changes may also affect assay results.

PROTEIN ASSAYS

Plasma proteins are produced primarily by the liver and the immune system, consisting of reticuloendothelial tissues, lymphoid tissues, and plasma cells. Proteins have many functions in the body, and alterations in plasma protein concentrations occur in a variety of disease conditions, especially disease of the liver and kidneys. More than 200 plasma proteins exist. Some plasma protein concentrations change markedly during certain diseases and can be used as diagnostic aids. Other protein concentrations change little during disease. Age-related changes in plasma protein concentrations are also seen. Plasma protein functions include the following:

- Helping form the structural matrix of all cells, organs, and tissues
- Maintaining osmotic pressure
- Serving as enzymes for biochemical reactions
- Acting as buffers in acid-base balance
- Serving as hormones
- Functioning in blood coagulation
- Defending the body against pathogenic microorganisms
- Serving as transport/carrier molecules for most constituents of plasma

The plasma protein assays commonly performed in veterinary medicine include total protein, albumin, and fibrinogen.

Total Protein

Total plasma protein measurements include fibrinogen values, whereas total serum protein determinations measure all the protein fractions except fibrinogen, which is removed during the clotting process. The total protein concentration may be affected by altered hepatic synthesis, altered protein distribution, and altered protein breakdown or excretion, as well as dehydration and overhydration.

Total protein concentrations are especially valuable in determining an animal's state of hydration. A dehydrated animal usually has a relatively elevated total protein concentration (hyperproteinemia), whereas an overhydrated animal usually has a relatively decreased total protein concentration (hypoproteinemia). Total protein concentrations also are useful as initial screening tests for patients with edema, ascites, diarrhea, weight loss, hepatic and renal disease, and blood clotting problems.

Two methods are commonly used for determination of total protein levels: the refractometric method and the biuret photometric method. The refractometric method measures the refractive index of serum or plasma with a refractometer (see

Chapter 1). The refractive index of the sample is a function of the concentration of solid particles in the sample. In plasma, the primary solids are the proteins. This method is a good screening test because it is fast, inexpensive, and accurate. The biuret method measures the number of molecules containing more than three peptide bonds in serum or plasma. This method is commonly used in analytic instruments in the laboratory. It is a simple method and yields accurate results. Other chemical tests to measure protein include dye-binding methods, precipitation methods, and the Lowry method. These tests are not commonly performed in veterinary practice. They are usually used to measure a small amount of protein in urine and cerebrospinal fluid (CSF). Specialized tests to separate the various protein populations are performed in some reference laboratories and research facilities. These methods include salt fractionation, chromatography, and gel electrophoreses (see Chapter 8).

The aformentioned tests can be performed on samples other than serum and plasma (e.g., urine, CSF). Other tests also used include the sulfosalicylic acid test, Pandy test, and Nonne-Apelt test. For the Pandy test, 1 drop of CSF is added to 1 ml of saturated aqueous phenol. Turbidity is observed before and after the mixture is shaken. After shaking, the CSF disperses as small droplets in the phenol, which should not be confused with a positive reaction (i.e., development of turbidity). If the sample is normal, no appreciable immunoglobulin is present and the solution remains clear (at most, slightly turbid), which is considered a negative result. If immunoglobulin is present at a concentration of 25 mg/dl or more, the solution becomes cloudy white. The degree of turbidity may be subjectively graded from 11 to 41, corresponding to increasing immunoglobulin concentration. For the Nonne-Apelt test, 1 ml of saturated ammonium sulfate solution is overlaid carefully with 1 ml of CSF and allowed to stand undisturbed for 3 minutes. The junction between the two fluids remains clear with normal CSF. However, if CSF immunoglobulin concentration is increased, a white-gray zone forms at the junction. This reaction may be graded subjectively from 11 to 41, reflecting increasing immunoglobulin concentration. The sulfosalicylic acid test is described in Chapter 5.

Albumin

Albumin is one of the most important proteins in plasma or serum. It makes up 35% to 50% of the total plasma protein in most animals, and any significant state of hypoproteinemia is most likely caused by albumin loss. Hepatocytes synthesize albumin, and any diffuse liver disease may result in decreased albumin synthesis. Renal disease, dietary intake, and intestinal protein absorption also may influence the plasma albumin level. Albumin is the major binding and transport protein in the blood and is responsible for maintaining osmotic pressure of plasma. The primary photometric test for albumin is the bromcresol green dye-binding method.

Globulins

The globulins are a complex group of proteins. Alpha globulins are synthesized in the liver and primarily transport and bind proteins. Two important proteins in this fraction are high-density lipoproteins and very-low-density lipoproteins. Beta globulins include complement (C3, C4), transferrin, and ferritin. They are responsible for iron transport, heme binding, and fibrin formation and lysis. Gamma globulins (immunoglobulins) are synthesized by plasma cells and are responsible for antibody production (immunity). Immunoglobulins (Ig) identified in animals are IgG, IgD, IgE, IgA, and IgM.

Direct chemical measurements of globulin are rarely performed. Globulin concentration is normally estimated by determining the difference between the total protein and albumin concentrations.

Albumin/Globulin Ratio

An alteration in the normal ratio of albumin to globulin (A/G) is frequently the first indication of a protein abnormality. The ratio is analyzed in conjunction with a protein profile. The A/G can be used to detect increased or decreased albumin and globulin concentrations. Many pathologic conditions alter the A/G. However, if the albumin and globulin concentrations are reduced in equal proportions, such as with hemorrhage, no alteration in A/G will be present.

The A/G is determined by dividing the albumin concentration by the globulin concentration. In dogs, horses, sheep, and goats, the albumin concentration is usually greater than the globulin concentration (A/G is more than 1.00). In cattle, pigs, and cats, the albumin concentration is usually equal to or less than the globulin concentration (A/G is less than 1.00).

Fibrinogen

Fibrinogen is synthesized by hepatocytes. It is the precursor of fibrin, the insoluble protein that forms the matrix of blood clots, and is one of the factors necessary for clot formation. If fibrinogen levels are decreased, blood does not form a stable clot or does not clot at all. Fibrinogen makes up 3% to 6% of the total plasma protein content. Because it is removed from plasma by the clotting process, no fibrinogen is found in serum. Acute inflammation or tissue damage may elevate plasma fibrinogen levels. The most common method of fibrinogen evaluation is the heat precipitation test described in Chapter 2. The fibrinogen value is calculated by subtracting the total plasma protein value of the heated tubes from that of the unheated tubes. (This value should be lower because fibrinogen has been removed from the plasma.) Plasma is the only sample that may be used because serum does not contain fibrinogen. Plasma collected with ethylenedianine tetraacetic acid (EDTA) is preferred. Heparinized plasma may yield falsely low results.

HEPATOBILIARY ASSAYS

The liver is the largest internal organ and is complex in structure, function, and pathologic characteristics. It has many functions, including metabolism of amino acids, carbohydrates, and lipids; synthesis of albumin, cholesterol, plasma proteins, and clotting factors; digestion and absorption of nutrients related to bile formation; secretion

of bilirubin, or bile; and elimination, such as detoxification of toxins and catabolism of certain drugs. These functions are run by enzymatic reactions. The gallbladder is closely associated with the liver, both anatomically and functionally. Its primary function is as a storage site for bile. Malfunctions in the liver or gallbladder result in predictable clinical signs of jaundice, hypoalbuminemia, problems with hemostasis, hypoglycemia, hyperlipoproteinemia, and hepatoencephalopathy.

Hepatic cells exhibit extreme diversity of function and are capable of regeneration if damaged. As a result, more than 100 different types of tests are available to evaluate liver function. Usually liver disease is greatly progressed before clinical signs appear. Liver function tests are designed to measure substances that are produced by the liver, modified by the liver or released when hepatocytes are damaged or those enzymes with altered serum concentrations as a result of cholestasis. Liver cells also compartmentalize the work so that damage to one zone of the liver may not affect all liver functions. Liver function tests are usually performed with serial determinations and several different types of liver tests completed to assist in verifying the functional status of the organ. No single test is superior to any other for detecting hepatobiliary disease. New tests are being developed to allow detection of hepatic disease before the liver is severely damaged. The primary tests used in veterinary medicine for evaluation of the liver and gallbladder are summarized in Box 3-1.

Enzymes Released from Damaged Hepatocytes

With this type of liver disease, the hepatocytes are damaged and enzymes leak into the blood, causing a detectable rise in blood levels of enzymes associated with liver cells. These components, commonly referred to as the "leakage enzymes," include the transferase enzymes alanine aminotransferase (ALT) and aspartate aminotransferase (AST) and the dehydrogenase enzymes sorbitol dehydrogenase (SDH) and glutamate dehydrogenase (GLDH). Transferases catalyze the reactions that transfer amine groups from amino acids to keto acids in the

> **BOX 3-1**
> **Major Hepatobiliary Assays**
>
> **Enzymes Released from Damaged Hepatocytes**
> Alanine Aminotransferase
> Aspartate Aminotransferase
> Sorbitol Dehydrogenase
> Glutamate Dehydrogenase
>
> **Enzymes Associated with Cholestasis**
> Alkaline Phosphatase
> Gamma Glutamyltranspeptidase
>
> **Hepatocyte Function Tests**
> Bilirubin
> Bile Acids
> Dye Excretion

production of new amino acids. The enzymes are therefore found in tissues that have high rates of protein catabolism. Although other transferases are present in hepatocytes, the only readily available tests are for ALT and AST. Dehydrogenases catalyze the transfer of hydrogen groups, primarily during glycolysis. Transferases and dehydrogenases are found either free in the cytoplasm of hepatocytes or bound to the cell membrane. The serum levels of these enzymes vary in different species, and most also have nonhepatic sources.

Alanine Aminotransferase

ALT was formerly known as serum glutamic pyruvic transaminase (SGPT). In dogs, cats, and primates, the major source of ALT is the hepatocyte, where the enzyme is found free in the cytoplasm. ALT is considered a liver-specific enzyme in these species. Horses, ruminants, pigs, and birds do not have enough ALT in the hepatocytes for this enzyme to be considered liver specific. Other sources of ALT are renal cells, cardiac muscle, skeletal muscle, and the pancreas. Damage to these tissues may also result in increased serum ALT levels. Administration of corticosteroids or anticonvulsant medications may also lead to increases in serum ALT. ALT is used as a screening test for liver disease because it is not precise enough to identify specific liver diseases.

No correlation exists between the blood levels of the enzyme and the severity of hepatic damage. Increases in ALT are usually seen within 12 hours of hepatocyte damage and peak levels are seen in 24 to 48 hours. The serum levels will return to reference ranges within a few weeks unless a chronic liver insult is present.

Aspartate Aminotransferase

AST was formerly known as serum glutamic oxaloacetic transaminase (SGOT). AST is present in hepatocytes, both free in the cytoplasm and bound to the mitochondrial membrane. More severe liver damage is required to release the membrane-bound AST. AST levels tend to rise more slowly than do ALT levels and return to normal levels within a day, provided chronic liver insult is not present. AST is found in significant amounts in many other tissues, including erythrocytes, cardiac muscle, skeletal muscle, the kidneys, and the pancreas. An increased blood level of AST may indicate nonspecific liver damage or may be caused by strenuous exercise or intramuscular injection. The most common causes of increased blood levels of AST are hepatic disease, muscle inflammation or necrosis, and spontaneous or artifactual hemolysis. If the AST level is elevated, the serum or plasma sample should be examined for hemolysis. Creatine kinase activity should also be assessed to rule out muscle damage before attributing an AST increase to liver damage.

Sorbitol Dehydrogenase

The primary source of SDH is the hepatocyte. Smaller amounts of the enzyme are found in the kidney, small intestine, skeletal muscle, and erythrocytes. SDH is present in the hepatocytes of all common domestic species but is especially useful for evaluating liver damage in large animals such as sheep, goats, swine, horses, and cattle. Large animal hepatocytes do not contain diagnostic levels of ALT, so SDH offers a liver-specific diagnostic test. The plasma level of SDH rises quickly with hepatocellular damage or necrosis. SDH assay can be used in all species to detect hepatocellular damage or necrosis, thus eliminating the need for other tests, such as the ALT assay. The disadvantage of SDH analysis is that SDH is unstable in serum and its activity declines within a few hours. If testing is delayed, samples should be frozen. SDH tests are not readily available to the average veterinary laboratory. Samples sent to outside laboratories should be packed in ice for transport.

Glutamate Dehydrogenase

GLDH is a mitochondrial-bound enzyme found in high concentrations in the hepatocytes of cattle, sheep, and goats. An increase in this enzyme is indicative of hepatocyte damage or necrosis in cattle and sheep. GLDH could be the enzyme of choice for evaluating ruminant and avian liver function, but no standardized test method has been developed for use in a veterinary practice laboratory.

Enzymes Associated with Cholestasis

Blood levels of certain enzymes become elevated with cholestasis (bile duct obstruction), metabolic defects in liver cells, and administration of certain medications and also as a result of the action of certain hormones, especially those of the thyroid. These enzymes are primarily membrane bound. The exact mechanism that induces increased levels of these enzymes in cholestasis is not well documented.

Alkaline Phosphatase

Alkaline phosphatase (AP) is present as isoenzymes in many tissues, particularly osteoblasts in bone; chondroblasts in cartilage, intestine, and placenta; and cells of the hepatobiliary system in the liver. The isoenzymes of AP tend to remain in circulation for approximately 2 to 3 days, with the exception of the intestinal isoenzyme that circulates for just a few hours. A corticosteroid isoenzyme of AP has been identified in dogs with exposure to increased endogenous or exogenous glucocorticoids. Because AP occurs as isoenzymes in these various tissues, the source of an isoenzyme or location of the damaged tissue may be determined by electrophoresis and other tests performed in commercial or research laboratories.

In young animals, most AP comes from osteoblasts and chondroblasts because of active bone development. In older animals, nearly all circulating

AP comes from the liver as bone development stabilizes. The assays used for AP in a practice laboratory determines the total blood AP concentration. AP concentrations are most often used to detect cholestasis in adult dogs and cats. Because of wide fluctuations in normal blood AP levels in cattle and sheep, this test is not as useful for detecting cholestasis in these species.

Gamma Glutamyltranspeptidase

Gamma glutamyltransferase (GGT or γGT) is sometimes referred to as gamma glutamyltranspeptidase. GGT is found in many tissues, including renal epithelium, mammary epithelium (particularly during lactation), and biliary epithelium, but its primary source is the liver. Cattle, horses, sheep, goats, and birds have higher blood GGT activity than dogs and cats. Other sources of GGT include the kidneys, pancreas, intestine, and muscle cells. The blood GGT level is elevated with liver disease, especially with obstructive liver disease.

Hepatocyte Function Tests

Many substances are taken up, modified, produced, and/or secreted by the liver. Alteration in the ability to perform these specific functions provides an overview of liver function. Tests of hepatocyte function performed in veterinary practice include bilirubin and bile acids. Other substances produced by hepatocytes are less-sensitive indicators of liver function because test results may not show abnormalities until two thirds to three fourths of liver tissue is damaged. These less-sensitive tests include albumin, ammonia, and cholesterol.

Bilirubin

Bilirubin is an insoluble molecule derived from the breakdown of hemoglobin by macrophages in the spleen. The molecule is bound to albumin and transported to the liver. The hepatic cells metabolize and conjugate the bilirubin to the molecule bilirubin glucuronide. This molecule is then secreted from the hepatocytes and becomes a component of bile. Bacteria within the gastrointestinal system act on the bilirubin glucuronide and produce a group of compounds collectively referred to

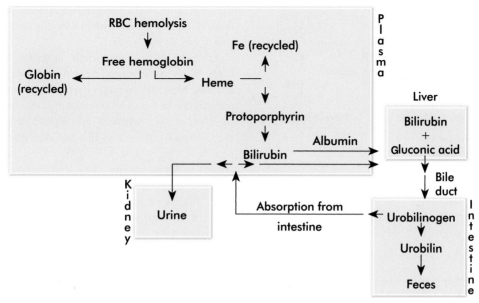

Figure 3-1. Bilirubin metabolism. (From Sirois M: *Principles and practice of veterinary technology,* ed 2, St Louis, 2004, Mosby.)

as urobilinogen. Urobilinogen is broken down to urobilin before being excreted in feces. Bilirubin glucuronide and urobilinogen may also be absorbed directly into the blood and excreted by the kidneys (Fig. 3-1).

Measurements of the circulating levels of these various populations of bilirubin can help pinpoint the cause of jaundice. Differences in the relative solubility of each of these molecules allow them to be individually quantified. In most animals, the prehepatic (bound to albumin) bilirubin comprises approximately two thirds of the total bilirubin in serum. Increases in this population indicate problems with uptake (hepatic damage). Increases in conjugated bilirubin indicate bile duct obstruction.

Assays can directly measure total bilirubin (conjugated bilirubin plus unconjugated bilirubin) and conjugated bilirubin. Conjugated bilirubin is sometimes referred to as direct bilirubin because test methods directly measure the amount of conjugated bilirubin in the sample. Unconjugated bilirubin is sometimes referred to as indirect bilirubin because its concentration is indirectly calculated by subtracting the conjugated bilirubin concentration from the total bilirubin concentration of the sample.

Bilirubin is assayed to determine the cause of jaundice, evaluate liver function, and check the patency of bile ducts. Blood levels of conjugated (direct) bilirubin are elevated with hepatocellular damage or bile duct injury or obstruction. Blood levels of unconjugated (indirect) bilirubin are elevated with excessive erythrocyte destruction or defects in the transport mechanism that allow bilirubin to enter hepatocytes for conjugation.

Bile Acids

Bile acids serve many functions. They aid in fat absorption (enabling the formation of micelles in the gastrointestinal system) and modulate cholesterol levels by bile acid synthesis. Bile acids are synthesized by hepatocytes from cholesterol and are conjugated with glycine or taurine. Conjugated bile acids are secreted across the canalicular membrane and reach the duodenum by way of the biliary system. The gallbladder stores bile acids (except in the horse) until contraction associated with feeding. When bile acids reach the ileum, they

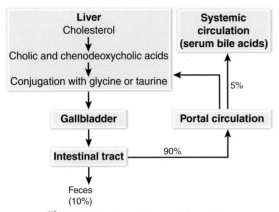

Figure 3-2. Circulation of bile acids.

are transported to the portal circulation and travel back to the liver. Ninety percent to 95% of the bile acids are actively resorbed in the ileum. The remaining 5% to 10% is excreted in the feces. The reabsorbed bile acids are carried to the liver where they are reconjugated and excreted as part of the enterohepatic circulation of bile acids (Fig. 3-2).

Spillover bile acids that escape from enterohepatic circulation may be detected in normal animals; serum concentrations of bile acids correlate portal concentrations. As a result, postprandial serum bile acid (SBA) concentrations are higher than fasting concentrations. Any process that impairs the hepatocellular, biliary, or portal enterohepatic circulation of bile acids results in elevated SBA levels. The great advantage of SBA determinations as a liver function test is that they evaluate the major anatomic component of the hepatobiliary system and are stable in vitro.

The SBA level is normally elevated after a meal because the gallbladder has contracted and released increased amounts of bile into the duodenum. Paired serum samples performed after 12 hours of fasting and 2 hours postprandial are needed to perform the test. The difference in the bile acid concentration of the samples is reported. In horses, a single sample is tested. Inadequate fasting or spontaneous gallbladder contraction can increase fasting bile acid levels. Exposing the patient to even the aroma of food can result in spontaneous gallbladder contraction. Prolonged fasting and diarrhea can decrease bile acids.

Elevated SBA levels usually indicate liver diseases such as congenital portosystemic shunts, chronic hepatitis, hepatic cirrhosis, cholestasis, or neoplasms. Bile acid levels are unspecific regarding the type of liver problem that exists and are therefore used as a screening test for liver disease. Bile acid levels may detect liver problems before an animal becomes icteric. They also may be used to follow the progress of liver disease during treatment. Increased bile acid concentrations can also result from extrahepatic diseases that secondarily affect the liver. Decreased bile acid concentration may be seen in intestinal malabsorptive diseases. In horses, increased bile acid concentrations can be the result of hepatobiliary disease or decreased feed intake. The reference ranges for bile acids in cows are widely variable. Bile acid testing is not a sensitive indicator of disease in cows.

Bile acids may be determined by several methods; the most commonly used is an enzymatic method. The 3-hydroxy bile acids react with 3-hydroxisteroid dehydrogenase and then with diformazan. Color generation is measured by end point spectrophotometry. Lipemic postprandial samples must be cleared by centrifugation to avoid interference with spectrophotometry. A bile acid test that uses immunologic methods (enzyme-linked immunosorbent assay) is now available for use in the veterinary clinic.

Cholesterol

Cholesterol is a plasma lipoprotein produced primarily in the liver, as well as ingested in food. Cholestasis caused an increase in serum cholesterol in some species. However, large differences exist in lipoprotein profiles of different species, and the clearance of lipoproteins is not well characterized in most veterinary species. A number of automated analyzers are available that provide cholesterol and other lipoprotein values. Hyperlipidemia is often secondary to other conditions (Box 3-2). Primary hyperlipidemia is rare and associated with inherited conditions in some breeds.

BOX 3-2
Causes of Secondary Hyperlipidemia

Cholestasis
Diabetes mellitus
Hepatic lipidosis
Hypothyroidism
Hyperadrenocorticism
Acute necrotizing pancreatitis
Nephrotic syndrome
Corticosteroid administration

Cholesterol assay is sometimes used as a screening test for hypothyroidism. Thyroid hormone controls synthesis and destruction of cholesterol in the body. Insufficient thyroid hormone, or hypothyroidism, results in hypercholesterolemia because the rate of cholesterol destruction is relatively slower than the rate of synthesis. Other diseases associated with hypercholesterolemia include hyperadrenocorticism, diabetes mellitus, and nephrotic syndrome. Dietary causes of hypercholesterolemia are rare but may include high-fat diets or postprandial lipemia.

Cholesterol by itself does not cause the grossly lipemic plasma seen after eating; triglycerides also are usually present. Administration of corticosteroids also may cause an elevated blood cholesterol concentration. Fluoride and oxalate anticoagulants may elevate enzymatic method results.

Other Tests of Liver Function
Although not commonly performed in the veterinary practice, several additional tests are available at reference laboratories and research facilities. The tests are based on the ability of the liver to excrete waste and foreign substances and include the dye excretion tests, ammonia tolerance test, and caffeine clearance test.

Dye Excretion
The two available dye excretion tests are the bromsulfophthalein (BSP) excretion and indocyanine green (ICG) excretion tests. Both require administration of a dye that binds to a protein in serum. The dyes are taken up by the hepatocytes and excreted into the bile. The disappearance of the dye from the plasma requires functional hepatocytes, adequate hepatic blood flow, and bile flow. The dye used for BSP is no longer used in human medicine, and its availability is limited. The overall complexity and expense of the testing have relegated their use primarily to research facilities.

Bromsulfophthalein Excretion
BSP excretion is a sensitive hepatic function test that is especially useful for detecting chronic lesions or portosystemic shunts with no leakage of liver enzymes. Coagulation defects and mysterious anemias sometimes may be explained by BSP test results. In horses, the test is handy to differentiate the jaundice of hepatic disease from that of simple anorexia, and hepatoencephalopathy from "wobbler syndrome." Specific indications in ruminants include fascioliasis, liver abscesses, ketosis, and photosensitization. BSP clearance may aid in diagnosis of aflatoxicosis in swine. Hepatic lesions delay BSP excretion. Delays caused by hepatocellular injury indicate a loss of at least 55% of the liver's functional mass. The magnitude of delay is poorly correlated to both the extent of hepatic lesions, when mild, and the clinical signs of liver dysfunction.

Delayed BSP clearance can be erroneous. Slowed BSP excretion results from perivascular dye injection (which can be painful), poor hepatic perfusion (shock, heart failure, dehydration), and fever. Ascites also interferes with BSP clearance because the dye lingers in pooled fluids. Certain inborn defects of BSP metabolism occur without liver disease, notably in some Southdown and Corriedale sheep. Obesity prolongs BSP retention because the amount of BSP per unit of body mass is relatively increased. In conclusion, bilirubin competes with BSP for excretion by the liver. For this reason, the BSP test should not be performed in animals with hyperbilirubinemia of 3 mg/dl or more. The results reveal nothing more than the already apparent jaundice.

Two conditions may disguise liver disease by speeding BSP clearance. Because albumin carries

BSP in the plasma, hypoalbuminemia (nephrotic syndrome, protein-losing gastroenteropathies, extreme liver disease) speeds clearance by increasing hepatic access to the free dye. Phenobarbital use also hastens BSP clearance. BSP clearance has no correlation with the extent of fatty infiltration of the liver.

Indocyanine Green Clearance

ICG is an organic dye similar to BSP. Introduced to human medicine because of occasional reactions to BSP, it is used to estimate hepatic blood flow.

Preinjection plasma is required to prepare a blank and a standard solution. This test can be used in both fed and fasted animals, but the latter is preferred. An intravenous dosage of 0.8 to 1.1 mg/kg body weight is recommended for horses, whereas 1 mg/kg body weight is recommended for dogs and 1.5 mg/kg body weight for cats. Usually five to six plasma samples are taken between 0, 5, 10, 15, and 30 minutes after injection. ICG concentration is measured photometrically at 805 nm, and the half-life is determined. Normal ICG clearances are as follows: dogs, 8.4 ± 2.3 minutes; horses (fed), 3.5 ± 0.67 minutes; and horses (fasted), 1.6 ± 0.57 minutes. Normal 30-minute retention is 14.7% ± 5% in dogs and 7.3% ± 2.9% in cats. Delayed ICG clearance has been reported in a variety of disorders, such as hyperbilirubinemia, hypoproteinemia, decreased hepatic blood flow, hepatic necrosis, and extrahepatic bile duct obstruction.

Ammonia Tolerance

Ammonia is produced by enteric microflora and during amino acid metabolism and transported to the liver through the portal circulation. Enzymes in the liver convert the ammonia to urea for excretion. Any condition that reduces the uptake of ammonia or conversion of ammonia to urea can lead to increased plasma ammonia concentration. However, normal compensatory mechanisms of the liver may result in normal fasting plasma ammonia concentrations. Impaired ammonia uptake is best identified with an ammonia tolerance test. A fasting sample is collected to provide baseline date. Patients identified with increased plasma ammonia

in fasting samples should not undergo the tolerance test because of the high risk of nervous system damage. After collection of the fasting sample, ammonium chloride is administered either rectally or orally by stomach tube or in a gelatin capsule. An additional sample is collected 30 minutes later. In patients with adequate hepatic function, the postadministration results may be the same as the fasting sample or moderately increased. Patients with urea cycle enzyme deficiencies (arginosuccinate synthetase) and abnormal portal blood flow, particularly congenital portovascular anomalies, often demonstrate a threefold to tenfold increase in plasma ammonia concentrations above the baseline. The test's chief limitation is in the handling of blood samples. Samples must be collected in ammonia-free heparin and the blood must be centrifuged immediately. The plasma should be placed on ice and analyzed within 30 minutes of collection or frozen at 220° C. Ammonia levels are stable in frozen plasma for a few days. Whole blood cannot be tested because its ammonia content increases with storage. Although the test can dramatically elevate the blood ammonia level, it does not cause nor worsen neurologic signs. Occasional vomiting with oral administration of the ammonia chloride is the only problem.

Caffeine Clearance

This is a specific assay of hepatic microsomal function. Demethylation of caffeine depends only on the specific P448 microsomal system of healthy hepatocytes; therefore it accurately reflects aberrations in hepatocellular function. This test is now used in human medicine; few experimental studies have been performed in canine species.

Caffeine sodium benzoate is dissolved in 2 ml sterile water (50:50 wt/wt), and 7 mg of caffeine/kg body weight are then injected intravenously. Plasma samples are collected from 15 to 480 minutes, and the caffeine concentration (in milligrams per milliliter) is measured by automated enzyme immunoassay. Plasma caffeine clearance and half-life are calculated from those values.

Normal half-life values in dogs are 6 ± 0.6 hours, and clearance is 1.7 ± 0.1 ml/min per kilogram of body weight. Elimination of caffeine is prolonged in hepatic insufficiency, with a clearance of 0.8 ± 0.1 ml/min per kilogram of body weight.

KIDNEY ASSAYS

The kidneys play a major role in maintaining homeostasis in animals. Their primary functions are to conserve water and electrolytes in times of a negative balance and increase water and electrolyte elimination in times of a positive balance; excrete or conserve hydrogen ions to maintain blood pH within normal limits; conserve nutrients, such as glucose and proteins; remove the end products of nitrogen metabolism, such as urea, creatinine, and allantoin, so that blood levels of these end products remain low; produce renin (an enzyme involved in controlling blood pressure), erythropoietin (a hormone necessary for erythrocyte production), and prostaglandins (fatty acids used to stimulate contractility of uterine and other smooth muscle, lower blood pressure, regulate acid secretion in the stomach, regulate body temperature and platelet aggregation, and control inflammation); and aid in vitamin D activation.

The kidneys receive blood from the renal arteries. The blood enters the glomerulus of the nephrons where nearly all water and small dissolved solutes pass into the collecting tubules. Each nephron contains sections that function to reabsorb or secrete specific solutes. Resorption of glucose occurs in the proximal convoluted tubule. Mineral salts secretion and reabsorption occurs in the ascending limb of the loop of Henle and distal convoluted tubule. The nephron has a specific resorptive capability for each substance called the renal threshold. Most water is reabsorbed as well. As a result of water reabsorption, the volume excreted is less than 1% of the volume that originally entered the kidney. Blood returns from the kidneys to the rest of the body through the renal veins, which connect to the caudal vena cava. Urine and blood may be analyzed to evaluate kidney function. Chapter 5 details urinalysis procedures. The primary serum chemistry tests for kidney function are urea nitrogen and creatinine. Other tests include various assays designed to evaluate the rate and efficiency of glomerular filtration.

Blood Urea Nitrogen

Some references use the term *serum urea nitrogen* (SUN) instead of *blood urea nitrogen* (BUN). Urea is the principal end product of amino acid breakdown in mammals. BUN levels are used to evaluate kidney function on the basis of the ability of the kidney to remove nitrogenous waste (urea) from blood. Under normal conditions, all urea passes through the glomerulus and enters the renal tubules. Approximately half of the urea is reabsorbed in the tubules and the remainder excreted in the urine. If the kidney is not functioning properly, sufficient urea is not removed from the plasma, leading to increased BUN levels.

Contamination of the blood sample with urease-producing bacteria (e.g., *Staphylococcus aureus, Proteus* spp., and *Klebsiella* spp.) may result in decomposition of urea and subsequently decreased BUN levels. To prevent this, analysis should be completed within several hours of collection or the sample should be refrigerated. A variety of photometric tests are available for measurement of urea nitrogen. All have an acceptable level of accuracy and precision. Chromatographic tests are also available and provide a semiquantitative serum urea nitrogen result. These methods tend to be less accurate and should be used only as quick screening tests.

Urea is an insoluble molecule and must be excreted in a high volume of water. Dehydration results in increased retention of urea in the blood (azotemia). High-protein diets and strenuous exercise may cause an elevated BUN level because of increased amino acid breakdown, not because of decreased glomerular filtration. Differences in rate of protein catabolism in male versus female animals, as well as young and older animals, will also affect BUN levels.

Serum Creatinine

Creatinine is formed from creatine, which is found in skeletal muscle, as part of muscle metabolism. Creatinine diffuses out of the muscle cell and into most body fluids, including blood. If physical activity remains constant, the amount of creatine metabolized to creatinine remains constant and the blood level of creatinine remains constant.

The total amount of creatinine is a function of the animal's total muscle mass. Under normal conditions, all serum creatinine is filtered through the glomeruli and eliminated in urine. Any condition that alters the glomerular filtration rate (GFR) will alter the serum creatinine levels. Creatinine also may be found in sweat, feces, and vomitus and may be decomposed by bacteria.

Blood creatinine levels are used to evaluate renal function on the basis of the ability of the glomeruli to filter creatinine from blood and eliminate it in urine. Like BUN, creatinine is not an accurate indicator of kidney function because nearly 75% of the kidney tissue must be nonfunctional before blood creatinine levels rise. Commonly used test methods for serum creatinine include the Jaffe method, as well as several enzymatic methods. Postprandial decreases in creatinine occur from transient increase in the GFR after a meal.

BUN/Creatinine Ratio

Because BUN and creatinine both have a wide range of reference intervals, their use as indicators of renal function is limited. The GFR may be decreased as much as four times below normal before changes are seen in the BUN or serum creatinine levels. In addition, healthy animals often have values below the reference ranges. In renal disease, hyperplasia of renal tissue may mask early signs of renal failure. The ratio of BUN to creatinine is used in human medicine for diagnosis of renal disease. Although this is not yet well established in veterinary species, it can be used to assess patient status during treatment.

BUN and creatinine have an inverse logarithmic relationship. The reciprocal of creatinine tracked over time can be used to track progress of disease and effectiveness of treatment. A disproportionate increase in BUN can indicate dehydration, dietary treatment failure, or owner noncompliance with treatment regimens.

Urine Protein/Creatinine Ratio

Quantitative assessment of renal proteinuria is of diagnostic significance in renal disease. In the absence of inflammatory cells in the urine, proteinuria indicates glomerular disease. For accurate determination of proteinuria, a 24-hour urinary protein value should be determined. This is a tedious task, and errors are common. A mathematical method that compares the urine protein level with the urine creatinine levels in a single urine sample is more accurate and comprehensive. This urine protein to creatinine (P/C) ratio is based on the concept that the tubular concentration of urine increases both the urinary protein and creatinine concentrations equally.

This method has been validated for the canine species. Usually 5 to 10 ml of urine are collected between 10 AM and 2 PM, preferably by cystocentesis. The urine sample should be kept at 4° C or stored at 20° C. The sample is centrifuged and the supernatant is used. The protein and creatinine concentrations for each sample can be determined by a variety of photometric methods. The urine P/C ratio for healthy dogs should be less than 1. A urine P/C between 1 and 5 may have prerenal (hyperglobulinemia, hemoglobinemia, myoglobinemia) or functional (exercise, fever, hypertension) origin, whereas urine P/C greater than 5 is caused by renal disease.

Uric Acid

Uric acid is a metabolic by-product of nitrogen catabolism and is found mainly in the liver. Uric acid is usually transported to the kidneys bound to albumin. In most mammals, the compound passes through the glomerulus and is largely reabsorbed by the tubule cells. It is then converted to allantoin and excreted in the urine. In Dalmatian dogs a defect in uric acid uptake into hepatocytes results in decreased conversion to allantoin. Therefore this breed excretes uric acid, and not allantoin, in urine.

Uric acid is the major end product of nitrogen metabolism in avian species. It constitutes approximately 60% to 80% of the total nitrogen excreted in avian urine and is secreted actively by the renal tubules. Measurement of plasma or serum uric acid is used as an index of renal function in birds. Uric acid can also be increased artifactually in samples from toenail clippings because of fecal urate contamination. Uric acid concentrations will increase after a meal in carnivorous birds. With renal disease, uric acid concentrations increase when the kidney has lost more than 70% of its functional capacity.

Tests of Glomerular Function

In patients with azotemia or those that are symptomatic for renal disease without azotemia, several additional tests can be performed to evaluate kidney function. These clearance studies require collection of timed, quantified urine samples along with concurrent plasma samples. Two primary types of clearance studies are performed: the effective renal plasma flow (ERPF) and GFR. The ERPF uses test substances eliminated by both glomerular filtration and renal secretion, typically the amide *p*-aminohippuric acid. The GFR uses test substances eliminated *only* by glomerular filtration, typically creatinine, inulin, or urea. The test substance is administered and urine and plasma samples collected. The ERPF or GFR are then calculated as follows:

$$\text{GFR or ERPF (ml/kg per minute) of substance} = Ux \times V/Px$$

where Ux represents substance present in urine (in milligrams per milliliter), V represents the amount of urine collected over a defined period (in milligrams per kilogram per minute), and Px represents the plasma concentration of substance.

Creatinine Clearance Tests
Endogenous Creatinine Clearance
Because creatinine appears in the glomerular filtrate with negligible tubular secretion, it is a natural tracer of glomerular filtration. Fortunately, its short-term blood concentrations are stable enough to satisfy the clearance formula used for steady infusion studies of inulin and p-aminohippuric acid. The test is relatively simple (Box 3-3). A measure of blood creatinine and an accurate, timed urine collection are required for this test. Precision is of the utmost importance. Sloppy bladder catheterization and sampling ruin the results, especially with the briefer methods. The bladder must be rinsed

---

BOX 3-3
Overview of Endogenous Creatinine Clearance Test

- A pretest blood sample is obtained for plasma creatinine analysis.
- The urinary bladder is catheterized and rinsed several times with saline
- All voided urine is collected over a specified time frame (most commonly 24 hours)
- The urinary bladder is catheterized at the end of the specified time and the remainder of the urine is collected
- Saline bladder rinse is repeated and the creatinine concentration of the urine rinse is determined
- Creatinine clearance is calculated with the following equation:

$$\text{Creatinine clearance} = \frac{[Uv \times Uc/Pc]}{\text{body weight (kg)}}$$

- Uv, urine volume (ml/min); Uc, urine creatinine concentration (mg/dl); Pc, plasma creatine concentration (mg/dl)
- Normal clearance in dogs is 2.8 ± 0.96 ml/min/kg.

---

before and after the test, saving the after-rinses with the urine for creatinine analysis. Clearance is calculated by dividing urinary creatinine excretion (urine creatinine concentration × urine volume) by plasma creatinine concentration. The estimate, if imprecise, is practical.

To avoid errors, plasma creatinine should be determined by the combination creatinine PAP test instead of the Jaffe method. The combination creatinine PAP test is an enzymatic chromogenic method to determine creatinine concentration. The Jaffe method also determines noncreatinine chromogens in plasma, which do not appear in urine. Excess serum ketones, glucose, and proteins all falsely elevate GFR estimates because of chromatic interference and cross-reactivity.

Exogenous Creatinine Clearance
Exogenous creatinine clearance is an accurate method to measure GFR in small animals. Plasma creatinine concentration increases, making plasma

---

BOX 3-4
Overview of the Exogenous Creatinine Clearance Test

- A subcutaneous injection of creatinine is administered
- A measured volume of water is administered *per os* by gastric intubation.
- The urinary bladder is catheterized and rinsed with saline after a specified time period (typically 40 minutes)
- A blood sample is obtained for plasma creatinine analysis
- All voided urine is collected for a specified time period and a second blood sample obtained
- Calculate creatinine clearance using the mean values of both samples.
- Normal values in the dog are 4.09 ± 0.52 ml/kg/min.
- A related procedure for evaluating GFR involves the use of an isohexol injection and does not require collection of urine samples

---

noncreatinine chromogens concentration negligible. This allows the application of the Jaffe method to determine creatinine concentrations (Box 3-4). Avoiding dehydration in the animal is critical in the performance of this test; free access to water must be ensured before any glomerular filtration tests.

Single-Injection Inulin Clearance

Inulin is excreted entirely by glomerular filtration, without tubular secretion, reabsorption, or catabolism. As a result, inulin clearance tests that use a constant infusion rate and quantitative urine sampling may be considered the best method to evaluate GFR. Single-injection inulin clearance is a simpler method that alternatively may be used. After a 12-hour fast (free access to water is permitted during the test), inulin is injected intravenously at a dosage of 100 mg/kg or 3 g/m^2 (body surface calculation gives more accurate results); serum samples are then obtained at 20, 40, 80, and 120 minutes. Total inulin clearance is calculated from the decrease of serum inulin concentration by using a two-compartment model. Normal dogs

present a GFR of 83.5 to 144.3 ml/min per square meter of body surface area.

Sodium Sulfanilate

Sodium sulfanilate is removed only by glomerular filtration in dogs; its disappearance from the plasma is an index of glomerular filtration. The test can detect unilateral nephrectomy and diminished renal function in dogs before azotemia develops. The half-life of sodium sulfanilate is prolonged up to five times in horses with glomerulonephritis. Although the test also is performed in cats, the mode of sodium sulfanilate excretion is not confirmed in this species. This test is no longer widely used.

Phenolsulfonphthalein Clearance

Phenolsulfonphthalein is an organic dye excreted by the renal tubules. Nonetheless, its clearance is accepted as a measure of renal blood flow because this usually limits its efflux more than tubular secretion rates. Phenolsulfonphthalein clearance is decreased only when more than two thirds of the nephrons are nonfunctional or when renal perfusion is compromised. This test is no longer widely used.

Other Estimates of Glomerular Filtration Rate and Effective Renal Plasma Flow

These methods are performed at reference and research centers and require specialized equipment. The double-isotope method involves injection of a tracer solution and uses a gamma camera for nuclear imaging of kidneys at serial time intervals. The nonisotope method is similar, but after injection of contrast media serial blood samples are collected and analyzed with x-ray fluorescent laboratory assays.

Water-Deprivation Tests

Polyuria or polydipsia may lead to suspicions about the kidney, which may be erroneous. Diuresis and subsequent polydipsia may mean failing nephrons or kidney function disrupted by hyperadrenocorticism (Cushing's disease), diabetes mellitus, or nephrogenic diabetes insipidus. The kidneys may be normal but not receive the signal to concentrate urine, as in neurogenic diabetes insipidus. Finally, the diuresis may be a totally appropriate renal compensation for pathologic water intake (psychogenic polydipsia).

Vasopressin or antidiuretic hormone (ADH), from the neurohypophysis, signals the kidneys to retain water by increasing the duct's permeability to water. Water in the urine passes out of the collecting duct and into the hypertonic renal medulla, concentrating the urine that remains behind in the collecting duct. If the system fails (e.g., inappropriate diuresis), either the neuroendocrine pathway that releases ADH in response to hypovolemia/plasma hyperosmolarity has been interrupted or the nephrons are unable to respond.

Water-Deprivation Test

This test is performed by observation of the response to endogenous or exogenous ADH. The basis for this test is to dehydrate the patient safely until a definite stimulus exists for endogenous ADH release (usually at approximately 5% body weight loss). That end point may vary. When denied water, patients dehydrate at different rates and must be monitored for weight loss, clinical signs of dehydration, and increased urine osmolarity or specific gravity. At the end point, the kidney should be under strictest endocrine orders to concentrate urine. Continued diuresis and dilute urine indicate lack of endogenous ADH or unresponsive nephrons. In dogs with kidney failure, this unresponsiveness precedes azotemia.

Contraindications to this test include dehydration and azotemia. Dehydrated patients risk hypovolemia and shock. They already should have maximal ADH release; if they could concentrate urine, they would. The test then is useless and dangerous, especially in animals with diabetes insipidus or neurogenic diabetes insipidus. Azotemia already attests to kidney dysfunction. Again, the test reveals nothing new and adds a prerenal component to the azotemia.

Vasopressin Response

When patients demonstrate the above-mentioned signs or a previous water-deprivation test has failed, a vasopressin response test is indicated. The vasopressin response test is simply a challenge with exogenous ADH; it focuses on the kidneys' abilities to respond. Urine osmolarity or specific gravity is the index of function. Normal kidneys should concentrate urine with this technique despite the patient's free access to water. Vasopressin must be handled carefully because it is a labile drug and settles out in oil suspensions. Test failures may result from use of old or poorly mixed solutions. Also, intramuscular vasopressin injection causes pain. Because of vasopressin's vasomotor activity, its use is theoretically contraindicated in pregnancy.

In both tests, even normal kidneys may be unable to concentrate urine to normal extremes. Diuresis quickly washes solutes from the renal medulla, weakening the osmotic gradient that draws water from the collecting ducts. Gradual water deprivation over a 3- to 5-day period before use of the water deprivation test is recommended to renew renal solutes and allow an evaluation of the impact of dehydration on the animal.

The basic water deprivation and vasopressin response tests may be combined in a single protocol that may differentiate several causes of polyuria/polydipsia (Box 3-5). The modified water-deprivation test is specifically contraindicated in patients with known renal disease, uremia resulting from prerenal or primary renal disorder, or suspected or obvious dehydration.

Fractional Clearance of Electrolytes

The fractional clearance (FC), also referred to as fractional excretion (FE), of electrolytes is a mathematical manipulation that describes the excretion of specific electrolytes (particularly sodium, potassium, and phosphorus) relative to the GFR. The most commonly used FE test is that of sodium. Bicarbonate and chloride FE testing is rarely performed. The tests can differentiate prerenal from postrenal azotemia. Random, concurrent blood and urine samples are required. The FE_X is calculated as follows:

$$FE_X = (U_X/P_X) \times (P_{CR}/U_{CR}) \times 100$$

where X is the electrolyte measurement used, which can be any of the four (sodium, potassium, phosphorus, and chloride); U_X and P_X are the urine and plasma concentrations, respectively, of that

---

BOX 3-5
Overview of Water Deprivation-Vasopressin Response

- Water intake is gradually reduced over a 72-hour period before initiation of the test
- All food and water are then withdrawn and the urinary bladder emptied at the start of the test
- An accurate exact body weight is obtained at the start of the test and repeated every 30 to 60 minutes
- Urine specific gravity, osmolality, and serum urea nitrogen are recorded and hydration and CNS status are evaluated at the start of the test and repeated every 30 to 60 minutes and at the conclusion of the test
- The test is ended when the animal is clinically dehydrated, appears ill, or has lost about 5% of its body weight
- A final blood sample is obtained for determination of the vasopressin concentration before the vasopressin response test.

Vasopressin Response
- Aqueous vasopressin is administered by IM injection
- At 30 minute intervals for a maximum of 2 hours, the urinary bladder is emptied and body weight, urine specific gravity, osmolality, and serum urea nitrogen are recorded and hydration and CNS status are evaluated

After Testing
- Small amounts of water are provided every 30 minutes for 2 hours.
- If the patient shows no evidence of vomiting, dehydration, or CNS abnormalities 2 hours after the test, water is provided ad lib.

---

specific electrolyte; and P_{CR} and U_{CR} are the urine and plasma concentrations of creatinine, respectively. Normal results are as follows:

- Dogs: sodium, 1; potassium, 20; chloride, 1; phosphorus, 39
- Cats: sodium, 1; potassium, 24; chloride, 1.3; phosphorus, 73

Urethral Pressure Profilometry

Urinary incontinence is a common complaint in canine medicine. Most cases are caused by sphincter mechanism incompetence. The specific functional test to explore the urethral sphincter mechanism is the urethral pressure profilometry. This test requires appropriate equipment and is restricted to referral institutions. A double-sensor microtip pressure transducer catheter is used. The catheter is inserted through the urethra into the urinary bladder. The tip sensor measures intravesical pressure at the same time as the other sensor records urethral resistance to perform a continuous comparison.

Inorganic Phosphorus

Serum inorganic phosphorus (Pi) is usually the reciprocal of serum calcium. Normally, serum Pi is reabsorbed in kidney tubules. This mechanism is under hormonal control (parathyroid hormone) and is affected by serum pH. Initially, renal damage that alters the GFR leads to decreased urinary Pi and increased serum Pi. Subsequent alteration in calcium and Pi leads to increase in serum calcium and decrease in serum Pi. See the electrolyte information later in this chapter for additional information on testing for Pi.

Enzymuria

Many of the chemical tests performed on serum or plasma can also be performed on urine samples. Enzymes that may be present in urine of patients with renal disease include urinary GGT and urinary N-acetyl-D-glucosaminidase (NAG). Urinary GGT and NAG are enzymes released from damaged tubule cells. Comparison of the units of GGT or NAG per milligram of creatinine can indicate the extent of renal damage. Both GGT and NAG increase rapidly with nephrotoxicity, and increases occur sooner than changes in serum creatinine, creatinine clearance, or fractional excretion of electrolytes.

PANCREAS ASSAYS

The pancreas is actually two organs, one exocrine and the other endocrine, held together in one stroma.

The exocrine portion, also referred to as the acinar pancreas, comprises the greatest portion of the organ. This portion secretes an enzyme-rich juice that contains enzymes necessary for digestion into the small intestine. The three primary pancreatic enzymes are trypsin, amylase, and lipase. These digestive enzymes are released into the lumen of other organs through a duct system. Trauma to pancreatic tissue is often associated with pancreatic duct inflammation that results in a backup of digestive enzymes into peripheral circulation.

Interspersed within the exocrine pancreatic tissue are arrangements of cells that, in a histologic section, take on the appearance of "islands" of lighter-staining tissue. These are called the islets of Langerhans. Four types of islet cells are present but they cannot be distinguished on the basis of their morphologic characteristics. The four cell types are designated α, β, δ, and PP cells. The δ and PP cells comprise less than 1% of the islet cells and secrete somatostatin and pancreatic polypeptide, respectively. β-Cells comprise approximately 80% of the islet and secrete insulin. The remaining area, nearly 20%, consists of α-cells that secrete glucagon and somatostatin. The pancreas has little regenerative ability. When pancreatic islets are damaged or destroyed, pancreatic tissue becomes firm and nodular with areas of hemorrhage and necrosis. These islets are no longer able to function. Diseases of the pancreas may result in inflammation and cellular damage that causes leakage of digestive enzymes or insufficient production or secretion of enzymes.

Exocrine Pancreas Tests

The tests commonly performed to evaluate the acinar functions of the pancreas include amylase and lipase. Trypsinlike immunoreactivity and serum pancreatic lipase immunoreactivity are also available as tests for pancreatic function. In cats, serum amylase and lipase activities have been shown to have limited clinical significance in the diagnosis of pancreatitis. In experimentally induced pancreatitis in cats, serum amylase actually decreases. Serum activities of both enzymes are frequently normal in cats with pancreatitis.

Amylase

The primary source of amylase is the pancreas, but it is also produced in the salivary glands and small intestine. Increases in serum amylase are nearly always caused by pancreatic disease, especially when accompanied by increased lipase levels. The rise in blood amylase level is not always directly proportional to the severity of pancreatitis. Serial determinations provide the most information.

Amylase functions to break down starches and glycogen in sugars, such as maltose and residual glucose. Increased levels of amylase appear in blood during acute pancreatitis, flare-ups of chronic pancreatitis, or obstruction of the pancreatic ducts. Enteritis, intestinal obstruction, or intestinal perforation may also result in increased serum amylase from increased absorption of intestinal amylase into the bloodstream. In addition, because amylase is excreted by the kidneys, a decrease in GFR for any reason can lead to increased serum amylase. Serum amylase activity greater than three times the reference range usually suggests pancreatitis.

Two amylase test methods are available: the saccharogenic method and the amyloclastic method. The saccharogenic method measures production of reducing sugars as amylase catalyzes the breakdown of starch. The amyloclastic method measures the disappearance of starch as it is broken down to reduce sugars through amylase activity. Calcium-binding anticoagulants, such as EDTA, should not be used because amylase requires the presence of calcium for activity. The presence of lipemia may reduce amylase activity. The saccharogenic method is not ideal for canine samples because maltase in canine samples may artificially elevate assay results. Normal canine and feline amylase values can be up to 10 times higher than those in human beings. Therefore samples may have to be diluted if tests designed for human samples are used.

Lipase

Nearly all serum lipase is derived from the pancreas. The function of lipase is to break down the long-chain fatty acids of lipids. Excess lipase is normally filtered through the kidneys, so lipase levels tend to remain normal in the early stages of pancreatic disease. Gradual increases are seen as disease progresses. With chronic, progressive pancreatic disease, damaged pancreatic cells are replaced with connective tissue that cannot produce enzyme. As this occurs, a gradual decrease in both amylase and lipase levels are seen.

Test methods for determination of lipase levels usually are based on hydrolysis of an olive oil emulsion into fatty acids using the lipase present in patient serum. The quantity of sodium hydroxide required to neutralize the fatty acids is directly proportional to lipase activity in the sample. Newer tests for lipase are available from some reference laboratories capable of detecting canine lipase by using immunologic methods.

Lipase assay may be more sensitive for detecting pancreatitis than is amylase assay. The degree of lipase activity, like amylase activity, is not directly proportional to the severity of pancreatitis. Determinations of blood lipase and amylase activities usually are requested at the same time to evaluate the pancreas.

Increased lipase activity is also seen with renal and hepatic dysfunction, although the exact mechanisms for this are unclear. Steroid administration is correlated with increased lipase activity with no concurrent change in amylase activity.

Amylase and Lipase in Peritoneal Fluid

Comparison of amylase and lipase activity in peritoneal fluid with serum may provide additional diagnostic information. A finding of higher amylase and lipase activity in peritoneal fluid than in serum strongly suggest pancreatitis provided intestinal perforation has first been ruled out.

Trypsin

Trypsin is a proteolytic enzyme that aids digestion by catalyzing the reaction that breaks down the proteins of ingested food. Trypsin activity is more readily detectable in feces than in blood. For this reason, most trypsin analyses are done on fecal samples. Trypsin is normally found in feces, and its absence is abnormal.

Two fecal test methods are used in the laboratory: the test tube method and the x-ray film test. The test tube method involves mixing fresh feces with a gelatin solution. The test solution does not become a gel if trypsin is present in the sample to break down the protein (gelatin). If trypsin is absent, the solution becomes a gel. The x-ray film test uses the gelatin coating on undeveloped x-ray film to test for the presence of trypsin. A strip of x-ray film is placed in a slurry of feces and bicarbonate solution. If trypsin is present in the fecal sample, the gelatin coating is removed from the film upon rinsing with water. If no trypsin is present, the gelatin coating remains on the film after rinsing. The test tube method is considered more accurate than the x-ray film test in evaluating fecal trypsin proteolytic activity.

Only fresh feces should be used. Fecal trypsin activity may be decreased if the patient has recently eaten raw egg whites, soybeans, lima beans, heavy metals, citrate, fluoride, or some organic phosphorous compounds. Calcium, magnesium, cobalt, and manganese in the feces may increase trypsin activity. Proteolytic bacteria in the fecal sample may result in false-positive or apparently normal results, especially in older samples.

Serum Trypsinlike Immunoreactivity

Serum trypsinlike immunoreactivity (TLI) is a radioimmunoassay that uses antibodies to trypsin. The test can detect both trypsinogen and trypsin. The antibodies are species specific. Trypsin and trypsinogen are produced only in the pancreas. With pancreatic injury, trypsinogen is released into the extracellular space and converted to trypsin, which diffuses into the bloodstream. The test is available only for the dog and cat.

TLI provides a sensitive and specific test for diagnosis of exocrine pancreatic insufficiency in dogs. Dogs with exocrine pancreatic insufficiency (EPI) have a serum TLI of less than 2.5 mg/L. Normal dogs have a range of 5 to 35 mg/L. Dogs with other causes of malassimilation may have normal serum TLI. Dogs with chronic pancreatitis may have normal TLI values or between 2.5 and 5 mg/L. Normal cats have 14 to 82 mg/L TLI, whereas cats with EPI have less than 8.5 mg/L.

Serum TLI decreases in parallel with functional pancreatic mass. The inflammation associated with acute and probably chronic pancreatitis may enhance leakage of trypsinogen and trypsin from the pancreas and increase TLI. Also, decreased GFR increases TLI (trypsinogen is a small molecule that easily passes into the glomerular filter). Serum TLI is an important indicator of functional pancreatic mass. It is most informative if coupled with N-benzoyl-L-tyrosyl-p-aminobenzoic acid (BTPABA) and fecal fat results to characterize and diagnose malassimilation.

Serum TLI increases after eating (especially proteins) but values remain within reference intervals. In addition, pancreatic enzyme (exogenous) supplementation does not alter TLI. Therefore food should be withheld for at least 3 hours and preferably 12 hours before taking a blood sample. The blood is coagulated at room temperature and the serum stored at 20° C until assay.

Serum Pancreatic Lipase Immunoreactivity

Serum feline pancreatic lipase immunoreactivity (fPLI) is specific for pancreatitis, and its use is now recommended instead of the previously validated serum feline trypsinlike immunoreactivity test as a serum test to diagnose cats with symptoms of pancreatitis.

Endocrine Pancreas Tests

A variety of tests are available to evaluate the endocrine functions of the pancreas. In addition to the traditional blood glucose tests, other tests now available include fructosamine, β-hydroxybutyrate, and glycosylated hemoglobin. Urinalysis, serum cholesterol, and triglyceride tests also provide information on the function of the pancreas.

Glucose

Regulation of blood glucose levels is complex. Glucagon, thyroxine, growth hormone, epinephrine, and glucocorticoids are all agents favoring hyperglycemia. They boost blood glucose levels by encouraging glycogenolysis, gluconeogenesis, and/or lipolysis while discouraging glucose entry into cells. Insulin is the hypoglycemic hormone. Promoting glucose flux into its target cells, it also triggers anabolism, a process that converts glucose to other substances. This regulatory effect prevents the blood glucose concentration from exceeding the renal threshold and the spilling of glucose into the urine.

The pancreatic islets respond directly to blood glucose concentrations and release insulin (from the beta cells) or glucagon (from the alpha cells) as needed. Glucagon release also directly stimulates insulin release. Epinephrine is under direct sympathetic neural control; hyperglycemia is one aspect of the classic "flight or fight" state. The other hormones mentioned respond to hypothalamic/pituitary command. At any point in time, most of these agents are acting, shifting the blood glucose concentration up or down.

Because only insulin lowers blood glucose levels, aberrations of insulin action have the most obvious clinical effects. Hypofunction (diabetes mellitus) or hyperfunction (hyperinsulinism) can occur.

The blood glucose level is used as an indicator of carbohydrate metabolism in the body and may also be used as a measure of endocrine function of the pancreas. The blood glucose level reflects the net balance between glucose production, such as dietary intake and conversion from other carbohydrates, and glucose utilization, which is expended energy and conversion to other products. It also may reflect the balance between blood insulin and glucagon levels.

Glucose utilization depends on the amount of insulin and glucagon produced by the pancreas. As the insulin level increases, so does the rate of glucose utilization, resulting in decreased blood glucose levels. Glucagon acts as a stabilizer to prevent blood glucose levels from becoming too low. As the insulin level decreases (as in diabetes mellitus), so does glucose utilization, resulting in increased blood glucose concentration.

Many tests are available for blood glucose. Some of these react only with glucose, whereas others may quantitate all sugars in the blood. End point and kinetic assays are available. The kinetic enzymatic assays tend to be the most accurate and precise. Samples must be taken from a properly fasted animal. Serum and plasma for glucose testing must be separated from the erythrocytes immediately after blood collection. Glucose levels may drop 10% an hour if the sample of plasma is left in contact with erythrocytes at room temperature. Even the use of an SST may not be adequate to prevent this. Mature erythrocytes use glucose for energy and, in a blood sample, they may decrease the glucose level enough to give false-normal results if the original sample had an elevated glucose level. If the sample originally had a normal glucose level, erythrocytes may use enough glucose to decrease the level to below normal or to zero. If the plasma cannot be removed immediately, the anticoagulant of choice is sodium fluoride at 6 to 10 mg/ml of blood. Sodium fluoride may be used as a glucose preservative with EDTA at 2.5 mg/ml of blood. Refrigeration slows glucose utilization by erythrocytes.

Fructosamine

Glucose can bind a variety of structures, including proteins. Fructosamine represents the irreversible reaction of glucose bound to protein, particularly albumin. When glucose concentrations are persistently elevated in blood as in diabetes mellitus, increased binding of glucose to serum proteins occurs. The finding of increased fructosamine indicates a persistent hyperglycemia. Because the half-life of albumin in dogs and cats is 1 to 2 weeks, fructosamine provides an indication of the average serum glucose over that period. Fructosamine levels respond more rapidly to alterations in serum glucose than does glycosylated hemoglobin. However, serum fructosamine may be artifactually reduced in patients with hypoproteinemia.

Glycosylated Hemoglobin

Glycosylated hemoglobin represents the irreversible reaction of hemoglobin bound to glucose. The finding of increased glycosylated hemoglobin indicates a persistent hyperglycemia. The test result is a reflection of the average glucose concentration over the lifespan of an erythrocyte—3 to 4 months in dogs and 2 to 3 months in cats. Patients that are anemic may have artifactually reduced levels of glycosylated hemoglobin.

β-Hydroxybutyrate

Ketone bodies can also be detected in plasma. The ketone produced in greatest abundance in ketoacidotic patients is β-hydroxybutyrate. However, many tests for serum ketones only detect acetone. Tests for β-hydroxybutyrate that use enzymatic, colorimetric methods are now becoming available for use in the veterinary clinic.

Glucose Tolerance

Glucose tolerance tests directly challenge the pancreas with a glucose load and measure insulin's effect by evaluation of blood or urine glucose concentrations. If adequate insulin is released and its target cells have healthy receptors, the artificially elevated blood glucose level peaks 30 minutes after ingestion and begins to drop, reaching normal value within 2 hours, and no glucose appears in the urine. A normal glucose blood level at 2 hours postprandial may rule out diabetes mellitus. Prolonged hyperglycemia and glucosuria are consistent with diabetes mellitus. Profound hypoglycemia after challenge may indicate a glucose-responsive, hyperactive beta-cell tumor of the pancreas. This test may be simplified by determining a single 2-hour postprandial glucose.

Oral glucose tolerance is affected by abnormal intestinal function, such as enteritis or hypermotility, and excitement (as from gastric intubation); an intravenous glucose tolerance test is preferred. The intravenous test is the only practical option for ruminants. With the intravenous glucose tolerance test (Procedure 3-3), a challenge glucose load is injected after a 12- to 16-hour fast (except in ruminants). Blood glucose is subsequently checked and its progress mapped as a tolerance curve. Results are standardized as disappearance half-lives or glucose turnover rates expressed as percent per minute:

$$\text{Turnover rate} = (0.693/\text{half-life}) \times 100$$

PROCEDURE 3-3

Intravenous Glucose Tolerance Test

1. Evaluate the animal's diet. For patients on low carbohydrate diets, feed a high-carbohydrate diet (100 to 200 g/day for dogs) for 3 days before the test.
2. Fast the animal for 12 to 16 hours to lower the blood glucose level to 70 mg/dl in patients with suspected hyperinsulinism (do not fast ruminants or dogs with insulinoma)
3. Obtain a preinjection blood sample in a sodium fluoride tube for a baseline blood glucose determination.
4. Begin timing the trial at the start of infusion of glucose solution IV at 1.0 g/kg administered over a 30 second period.
5. Obtain blood samples at 5, 15, 25, 35, 45, and 60 minutes after glucose infusion, using sodium fluoride as an anticoagulant, and submit all blood samples for glucose assay. An additional blood sample is collected after 120 minutes for feline patients
6. Plot glucose values on a semilogarithmic graph paper and determine the time required for glucose levels to decrease by 50% (glucose half-life)
7. Results: The postinfusion blood glucose level should fall to approximately 160mg/dl in 30 to 60 minutes and return to baseline values in 120-180 minutes.

Decreased glucose tolerance (increased half-life, decreased turnover rate) occurs in diabetes mellitus and less consistently in hyperthyroidism, hyperadrenocorticism, hyperpituitarism, and severe liver disease. Increased glucose tolerance (decreased half-life, increased turnover rate) is observed with hypothyroidism, hypoadrenocorticism, hypopituitarism, and hyperinsulinism. However, results may be erroneous. Normal animals on low-carbohydrate diets may manifest "diabetic curves." The effect of this can be minimized by providing the animal with 2 to 3 days of high-carbohydrate meals before testing. The intravenous glucose tolerance test

results are so variable in normal horses, depending on diet and fasting, that they are not useful.

Glucose tolerance tests are usually unnecessary to obtain a diagnosis of diabetes mellitus. Persistent hyperglycemia and glucosuria, frequently with a history of polyuria, polydipsia, polyphagia, and weight loss, are sufficient to diagnose diabetes mellitus. The test may be of value in detecting hyperinsulinism because most beta-cell tumors of the pancreas are not rapidly responsive to glucose. They may even cause diabetic glucose tolerance curves because insulin-antagonist hormones are released as a result of the initial hypoglycemia. Patient stress and chemical restraint also affect glucose tolerance test results. Serum glucose measurements themselves may be erroneously low if blood samples are not subjected to anticoagulants and are allowed to sit at room temperature. However, the test is still used.

The best use for the glucose tolerance test is in animals with borderline hyperglycemia without persistent glucosuria. However, this test is not cost-effective for the owner and may not result in significant therapeutic change. This dilemma is most often seen in cats in which high renal thresholds for glucose and stress-induced hyperglycemia are common and misleading. Extra information may be obtained from the intravenous glucose tolerance test if immunoreactive insulin concentrations are followed simultaneously. This protocol may differentiate diabetes mellitus resulting from absolute lack of insulin (type 1) from that resulting from target-cell insensitivity (type 2) or inappropriate slow insulin release (type 3).

Insulin Tolerance

The insulin tolerance test also probes the causes of diabetes mellitus. Specifically, it checks the responsiveness of target cells to challenge with regular crystalline (short-acting) insulin 0.1 IU/kg subcutaneously or intramuscularly. Serum glucose levels are measured in blood samples obtained before insulin injection (fasting blood glucose) and every 30 minutes after injection for 3 hours. If the serum glucose level fails to drop to 50% of the fasting concentration within 30 minutes of insulin injection (insulin resistance), the insulin receptors are unresponsive or insulin action is being severely antagonized. The latter may occur in hyperadreno-corticism and acromegaly. Insulin resistance profoundly influences prognostic and therapeutic decisions. If the insulin-induced hypoglycemia persists for 2 hours (hypoglycemia unresponsiveness), hyperinsulinism, hypopituitarism, or hypoadrenocorticism should be suspected. Because the test may cause this hypoglycemia, with possible weakness and convulsions, a glucose solution should always be on hand for rapid intravenous administration.

Glucagon Tolerance

The main indications for the glucagon tolerance test are repeated normal or borderline results with the amended insulin/glucose ratio test (see subsequent discussion) or lack of an insulin assay. The glucagon tolerance test gives another assessment of hyperinsulinism. Glucagon stimulates the pancreatic beta cells directly and indirectly to increase the blood insulin level. In normal animals, glucagon injection (0.03 mg/kg intravenously up to a total of 1.0 mg in dogs and 0.5 mg in cats) transiently elevates the blood glucose level to greater than 135 mg/dl. In normal animals, this concentration level is greater than 135 mg/dl. In normal animals, this concentration returns to fasting concentrations. In normal cats, peak insulin occurs at 15 minutes, declining to basal concentration at 60 minutes. Type 1 diabetic cats present a flat insulin response. If the animal has a pancreatic beta-cell tumor, the serum glucose level peak is lower than normal and is followed within 1 hour by hypoglycemia (serum glucose is less than 60 mg/dl) because excessive insulin is secreted by the stimulated neoplasm.

To perform the test, the patient is fasted until the serum glucose level dips below 90 mg/dl (usually less than 10 hours). Glucagon is injected, and sodium fluoride anticoagulated blood samples are obtained before glucagon injection and 1, 3, 5, 15, 30, 45, 60, and 120 minutes after injection to monitor the glucose response. Unfortunately, the test is insensitive and may cause hypoglycemia convulsions up to 4 hours later. Patients must be fed immediately after the test and observed for hours.

Insulin/Glucose Ratio

The cause of hyperinsulinism may be assessed by taking simultaneous measurements of serum glucose and insulin levels in a fasting animal. Hypoglycemia normally inhibits insulin secretion. Pancreatic beta-cell tumors, hyperactive and unresponsive to glucose, secrete an abundance of insulin inappropriate to the prevailing blood glucose concentration. Although fasting serum insulin concentrations are often normal in hyperinsulinism, ratios of insulin to glucose concentrations are usually aberrant.

The absolute ratio of insulin to glucose can be amended to increase diagnostic accuracy. The amended insulin/glucose ratio (AIGR) subtracts 30 from the serum glucose concentration. At a serum glucose level of 30 mg/dl or less, insulin is normally undetectable, so this discriminant puts the zero of both the glucose and insulin scale at the same physiologic place. Because abnormally high insulin concentrations are more obvious at low serum glucose concentrations, the AIGR is most valuable in animals with a confirmed hypoglycemia of less than 60 mg/dl. Insulin and glucose have to be measured from the same serum sample. Then serial determinations may be performed to select an insulin concentration in hypoglycemia. However, the test is not totally dependable. If the results are unconvincing, the procedure should be repeated or other tests tried. Specifically, diagnostic imaging and insulinlike growth factor tests should be tried to rule out or confirm paraneoplastic hypoglycemia.

Miscellaneous Tests of Insulin Release

When results of a glucagon response test or AIGR are equivocal, glucose, epinephrine, leucine, tolbutamide, or calcium challenges may be attempted. These substances, like glucagon, may provoke a hyperinsulinemic response from pancreatic islet cell tumors, resulting in decreased serum glucose levels. However, tumors vary in their sensitivity to these agents and false-negative results (no response) can occur. These tests are also dangerous because they can precipitate severe, prolonged hypoglycemia.

OTHER ENDOCRINE SYSTEM ASSAYS

In addition to the pancreas, a variety of organs and tissues release hormones that function in the endocrine system. The primary organs of the endocrine system are the adrenal glands, thyroid and parathyroid glands, and the pituitary gland. These glands produce and secrete hormones directly into capillaries and have a variety of target organs and effects.

Adrenocortical Function Tests

Adrenocortical function tests are commonly performed. Adrenal dysfunction is increasingly common, too often because of misuse of corticosteroids. The adrenal axis starts with the hypothalamus. Stimuli originating in the brain, such as from stress, cause the hypothalamus to secrete corticotropin-releasing factor (CRF). Under the influence of CRF, the adenohypophysis secretes adrenocorticotrophic hormone (ACTH), the hormone that stimulates adrenocortical growth and secretion, particularly of glucocorticoid-synthesizing tissue. Cortisol is the major hormone released in domestic mammals. It, in turn, feeds back to inhibit both CRF and ACTH release, completing a balanced system.

True or mimicked hyperfunction of the system is the common complaint. Brain or pituitary tumors leading to secondary bilateral adrenal hyperplasia, idiopathic adrenal hyperplasia, or neoplasia (one or both glands) may cause excessive cortisol release and hyperadrenocorticism. Overenthusiastic glucocorticoid therapy is the most common cause of cortisol excess. Because exogenous, like endogenous, glucocorticoids inhibit adrenotrophic hormones, iatrogenic hyperadrenocorticism is accompanied by the paradox of atrophied adrenal glands. Sudden withdrawal of exogenous glucocorticoids leads to adrenal hypofunction. However, hypoadrenocorticism (Addison's disease) by definition includes mineralocorticoid deficiency, which does not occur in iatrogenic disease from rapid withdrawal of glucocorticoids. Addison's disease also may result from overuse of mitotane (Lysodren; for adrenal hyperplasia) or from idiopathic causes.

Screening tests for hyperadrenocorticism must be carefully interpreted because many dogs with nonadrenal disease such as diabetes mellitus, liver disease, or renal disease may have false-positive results. Thereafter, final diagnosis of hyperadrenocorticism is made on the basis of clinical signs in conjunction with several of the various laboratory tests. Conversely, if negative laboratory testing occurs with consistent clinical evidence, the animal should be retested 1 or 2 months later (if clinical signs persist).

ACTH and cortisol concentrations may be a helpful diagnostic aid in differentiation of primary (adrenal-dependent) from secondary (pituitary-dependent) hypoadrenocorticism. However, a single measurement has limited usefulness because levels can fluctuate on a diurnal cycle. More often, these measurements are taken as baseline data and compared with data obtained from challenge to the adrenal gland with ACTH or dexamethasone. Animals with functioning adrenocortical tumors have low concentrations from the negative feedback effect. Animals with pituitary-dependent hypoadrenocorticism should have higher concentrations. Low to undetectable ACTH concentrations occur in secondary Addison's disease, whereas normal (or increased) concentrations are expected in primary Addison's disease. ACTH is a labile protein and requires special handling of the plasma sample. Aprotinin (protease inhibitor) within the EDTA tube and/or immediate freezing of the plasma may be required. Tests for cortisol and ACTH are immunoassays and some are available to the veterinary practice laboratory. Some tests are performed on serum; others can be performed only on plasma samples. A few tests can also be performed on urine samples. Urine cortisol/creatinine ratios have also been used as screening tests for adrenal function.

ACTH Stimulation Test

Animals with suspected hypoadrenocorticism (Addison's disease) or hyperadrenocorticism (Cushing's disease) may be evaluated with an ACTH

PROCEDURE 3-4

ACTH Stimulation Test

1. Collect a plasma sample for determination of baseline plasma cortisol concentration.
2. Administer synthetic ACTH (Cosyntropin) by intravenous injection
   a. Dosage varies by species; 125 µg (cats); 250 µg (dog) or 1 mg (horse)
3. Collect a second plasma sample for cortisol determination at 30 minutes post ACTH administration in dogs and cats and 2 hours post administration in horses.
4. Collect a third plasma sample for cortisol determination one hour post ACTH administration in dogs and cats and 4 hours post administration in horses.
5. Results:
   a. Normal pretest cortisol concentration:
      Dog: 0.5 to 4 µg/dl or 14 to 110 nmol/L
      Cat: 0.3 to 5 µg/dl or 8.3 to 138 nmol/L
   b. Normal post-ACTH cortisol concentration:
      Dog: 8 to 20 µg/dl or 220 to 552 nmol/L
      Cat: 5 to 15 µg/dl or 138 to 414 nmol/L

6. Interpretation:
   a. Exaggerated post-ACTH cortisol concentration is observed in most dogs (80%) and 51% cats (borderline increased in 16%) with hyperadrenocorticism. Cats may have increased only one of the post-ACTH cortisol determinations.
   b. Reduced post-ACTH cortisol concentration is observed, consistent, in both Addison's disease, iatrogenic Cushing's disease and, mitotane, ketoconazole, or metyrapone therapy.
   c. Normal post-ACTH cortisol concentration does not rule out Cushing's disease (occurs in 50% of dogs with adrenal-dependent Cushing's disease).

response test. In addition, the test is indicated to distinguish among iatrogenic and spontaneous hyperadrenocorticism (Procedure 3-4). It also may test the efficacy of mitotane, ketoconazole, or metyrapone therapy. The ACTH stimulation test evaluates the degree of adrenal gland response to administration of exogenous ACTH. Degree of response to stimulation by glucocorticoid should be in proportion to the glands' size and development. Hyperplastic adrenal glands have exaggerated responses, whereas hypoplastic adrenal glands show diminished responses. The test can detect these abnormalities but not reveal their ultimate cause. The ACTH response test is a screening test. Adrenal glands that are hyperactive from neoplasia may be insensitive to ACTH. Nonetheless, current figures indicate that the test is more than 80% accurate in diagnosing adrenocortical hyperfunction in the dog and more than 50% in the cat.

Dexamethasone Suppression

Dexamethasone suppression tests evaluate the adrenal glands differently by using the adrenal feedback loops. The low-dosage test confirms or replaces the ACTH response test for hyperadrenocorticism (Cushing's disease). The high-dosage test goes further, differentiating pituitary from adrenal causes of hyperadrenocorticism (Procedure 3-5). In cats, only a high-dose dexamethasone suppression test is suitable.

Dexamethasone, a potent glucocorticoid, suppresses ACTH release from the normal pituitary gland, resulting in a drop in plasma cortisol concentration. Hyperadrenocorticism of any etiology

PROCEDURE 3-5

Dexamethasone Suppression Tests

Low Dosage

1. Obtain a blood sample for baseline plasma cortisol determination at 8 am. (Some clinicians also do a 2- or 3-hour test as well.)
2. Immediately administer intravenous dexamethasone at 0.01 mg/kg for dogs and 0.1 mg/kg for cats
3. Obtain a second plasma sample for cortisol determination 8 hours after dexamethason injection
4. Results:

Adrenal condition	Pretest cortisol level	Posttest cortisol level
Normal	1.1–8.0 µg/dl	0.1–0.9 µg/dl (<1.4)
Hyperadrenal	2.5–10.8 µg/dl	1.8–5.2 µg/dl (>1.4)

High Dosage

1. Use the same protocol as above, except the dexamethasone dosage is 0.1 mg/kg for dogs and 1.0mg/kg for cats

2. Results:
   Pituitary-dependent hyperadrenocorticism: Normal values as above
   Adrenal-dependent hyperadrenocorticism: As for hyperadrenal values above

NOTE: Successful suppression is defined as a 50% decrease in the plasma cortisol concentration from the baseline value. In 15% of dogs with pituitary-dependent hyperadrenocorticism, the plasma cortisol level is not suppressed by 50%. About 20% of dogs with adrenal-dependent hyperadrenocorticism have suppression of the plasma cortisol level by less than 50%, but all values remain above these considered adequate for suppression (greater than 1.5 µg/dl).

is usually resistant to suppression from small dexamethasone doses because a diseased pituitary gland is abnormally insensitive to the drug and continues elaborating excessive ACTH, although 35% of dogs with pituitary-dependent hyperadrenocorticism have a 4-hour post-dexamethasone cortisol level lower than 1mg/dl or 50% of the baseline concentration. Neoplastic adrenal glands are autonomously secreting cortisol independent of endogenous ACTH control. The excessive cortisol production suppresses secretion of ACTH by the normal pituitary gland through negative feedback inhibition. Small doses of dexamethasone do not affect plasma cortisol measurements. However, such doses may complicate test results and may differentiate only normal animals from those with hyperadrenocorticism.

With larger dexamethasone doses, more differences appear. The sensitivity of a diseased pituitary gland to dexamethasone is incomplete; large dexamethasone doses overcome it and the abnormally high plasma ACTH and cortisol concentrations fall. Abnormal adrenal glands, however, continue to secrete cortisol autonomously. Thus plasma cortisol concentrations unresponsive to all dexamethasone doses are probably caused by primary adrenal gland disease. Suppression by large but not small doses suggests pituitary gland disease. The test has 73% accuracy in differentiating pituitary from adrenal causes in dogs and 75% sensitivity to diagnose hyperadrenocorticism in cats.

A dual high-dosage dexamethasone test and ACTH response test are described in Procedure 3-6. Although combined protocol is a step saver,

PROCEDURE 3-6

Protocol for Combined Dexamethasone Suppression and ACTH Corticotropin Stimulation Test

1. Collect a plasma sample for cortisol determination.
2. Administer dexamethasone 0.1 mg/kg IV.
3. Collect a plasma sample for cortisol determination 4 hours post injection.
4. Immediately administer synthetic ACTH IV at a dose of 125 µg (cats); 250 µg (dog)
5. Collect a third plasma sample for cortisol determination at 30 minutes post ACTH administration in dogs and cats and 2 hours post administration in horses.
6. Collect a fourth plasma sample for cortisol determination one hour post ACTH administration in dogs and cats and 4 hours post administration in horses.
7. Results:
   a. Normal pretest cortisol concentration:
      Dog:0.5–4 µg/dl or 14–110 nmol/L
      Cat: 0.3–5 µg/dl or 8.3–138 nmol/L
   b. Normal post-dexamethasone cortisol concentration:
      1–1.4 µg/dl or 28–39 nmol/L
   c. Normal post-ACTH cortisol concentration:
      Dog: 8–20 µg/dl or 220–552 nmol/L
      Cat: 5–15 µg/dl or 138–414 nmol/L
8. Interpretation:
   a. Elevated post-dexamethasone and elevated post-ACTH cortisol concentration indicates hyperadrenocorticism.
   b. Elevated post-dexamethasone and normal post-ACTH cortisol concentration indicates hyperadrenocorticism.
   c. Normal post-dexamethasone and exaggerated post-ACTH cortisol concentration indicates pituitary-dependent hyperadrenocorticism.

possibly ambiguous results necessitate more tests and expense. The ACTH response segment of the test is particularly prone to error. Because dexamethasone alters the adrenal responsiveness to ACTH (enhances or inhibits, depending on the duration of activity), the timing of the test is crucial. Normal standards must be newly established for any changes in protocol.

Corticotropin-Releasing Hormone Stimulation

This test may be indicated to differentiate among pituitary-dependent and primary hyperadrenocorticism. Plasma cortisol concentration and ACTH should not be elevated after corticotropin-releasing hormone (CRH) stimulation in dogs with adrenal-dependent Cushing's disease.

The protocol of this test consists of obtaining a pretest sample to determine cortisol and ACTH, administering 1 mg/kg of CRH, and obtaining blood samples again 15 and 30 minutes later to evaluate cortisol and ACTH.

Thyroid Assays

Thyroid hormones have pervasive effects, influencing the metabolic rate, growth, and differentiation of all body cells. Because the clinical signs of thyroid malfunction are numerous and confusing, function tests are valuable. The thyroid glands are governed like the adrenal cortices. Thyrotropin-releasing factor (TRF) from the hypothalamus encourages the anterior pituitary to release thyrotropin or thyroid-stimulating hormone (TSH). TSH enhances thyroid growth, function, and thyroxine release. Thyroxine is really composed of two varieties of hormones, triiodothyronine (T_3) and thyroxine (T_4), varying in their extent of iodination. T_4 also is converted to the more active T_3 in tissues.

Thyroxine completes the regulatory cycle by inhibiting TRF and TSH release.

Thyroid disease is manifested primarily as hypofunction in dogs, horses, ruminants, and swine and as hyperfunction in cats. The cause may be dietary iodine deficiency or excess or goitrogens, most common in large animals. Primary glandular disease (neoplasia, autoimmune disease, idiopathic atrophy) comprises most cases, whereas pituitary (secondary thyroid disease) comprises 5% of hypothyroid dogs. In food animals, diagnosis is based on clinical signs (e.g., abortion, stillbirths, alopecia, and goiter in fetuses and neonates), serum T_4 concentrations, serum protein-bound iodine concentrations, and pasture iodine analyses. Feeds may be examined for goitrogenic plants (*Brassicae* spp.) or excess calcium, which decreases iodine uptake.

Baseline thyroxine concentrations are used diagnostically, but normal values vary dramatically. Semiquantitative immunologic tests are available to measure T_4 concentrations. Their diagnostic inadequacy mirrors that of plasma cortisol determinations. Some drugs, such as insulin or estrogens, may increase T_4 concentrations; others, such as glucocorticoids, anticonvulsants, antithyroid drugs, penicillins, trimethoprim sulfamides, diazepam, androgens, and sulfonylureas, may decrease T_4 concentrations. In addition, total T_4 (TT_4) may be increased in hypothyroid dogs as a result of the presence of anti-T_4 antibodies. Specific determination of the active form of thyroxine non–protein-bound or free T_4 (FT_4) by equilibrium dialysis is a more accurate approach to thyroid function. Thereafter, determination of both endogenous TSH and T_4 (TT_4 or FT_4) are suitable to diagnose canine hypothyroidism.

TSH Response

This test is used on small animals (except in cats with hyperthyroidism) and horses and provides a reliable diagnostic separation of patients with normal versus abnormal thyroid function (Box 3-6). Exogenous TSH challenge may sort out borderline cases and separate real hypothyroid patients from those with other illness or drug-depressed thyroxine concentrations and also may pinpoint the site of the lesions.

BOX 3-6
Overview of TSH response test

- A pretest blood sample is collected for baseline serum T_4 determination.
- TSH is administered and T_4 determination made on a second blood sample is collected 4 to 6 hours after injection
- Results: T_4 post-TSH stimulation in normal dogs should be approximately twice the baseline value or should exceed 2.0 µg/dl or 25 nmol/L

The test usually is used to explore canine hypothyroidism. After TSH is injected, thyroid response (usually serum T_4 levels, the most reliable index) is followed. An increase in the serum T_4 level occurs in normal animals. Primarily exhausted or insensitive thyroids do not respond to exogenous TSH. Indeed, endogenous TSH concentrations are already high from failing T_4 inhibition. Therefore serum T_4 level is not increased in these animals. With pituitary or brain disease, however, the thyroid glands remain responsive. Such lesions result in too little endogenous thyrotropin. Although an increase in the serum T_4 level is expected in animals with pituitary lesions, 2 to 3 days of TSH challenge may be necessary before increased serum T_4 levels are seen. The extra TSH is required to overcome chronic glandular atrophy, similar to "priming the pump."

Glucocorticoids seem to inhibit both TSH and T_4 secretion, so euthyroidism with low serum T_3 levels only often accompanies Cushing's disease or vigorous glucocorticoid therapy. Fortunately, the TSH and ACTH response tests may be performed simultaneously. In such animals, the glands remain responsive to TSH but the absolute values of prechallenge and postchallenge serum T_4 are low or low resting with normal post-TSH values. Feline hyperthyroidism is usually caused by functional thyroid adenomas. Oddly, with exogenous TSH challenge, little or no increase occurs in the serum T_4 level, as in canine primary hypothyroidism. This phenomenon suggests that the neoplasm either functions independently of the trophic hormone or is already manufacturing and leaking T_4 at maximum capacity. A lack of TSH responsiveness, appropriate clinical manifestations, and high baseline plasma T_4 concentrations all attest to feline hyperthyroidism.

In horses, iodine-deficiency hypothyroidism is rare because iodized salt usually is offered free choice or in feeds. Overzealous iodine supplementation with kelp meal or vitamin-mineral mixes, however, provokes hypothyroidism and goiter. Excessive use of iodine inhibits thyroid function. In the assessment of thyroid function in horses, the normal serum T_4 values are 1 to 3 mg/dl, which is lower than in other species. Hypothyroidism should be suspected only with serum T_4 concentrations of less than 0.5 mg/dl.

Rare tumors of the pars intermedia of the pituitary, compressing the anterior pituitary, may cause secondary hypothyroidism in older horses. Because pituitary damage induces a plethora of signs, the TSH response test may be especially helpful.

Thyrotropin-Releasing Hormone (TRH) Response

TRH response is used on small animals and provides a reliable diagnostic separation of patients with normal versus abnormal thyroid function. FT_4 is the fraction of thyroxine that is not bound to protein. FT_4 levels are less influenced by nonthyroidal diseases or drugs that total T_4 concentrations. Exogenous TRH challenge may sort out borderline cases and separate real hypothyroid and hyperthyroid patients from those with other illness or drug-depressed thyroxine concentrations. The test usually is used to explore canine hypothyroidism when TSH is not available. Baseline serum TT_4 and FT_4 concentrations are determined. Four hours after 0.1 mg/kg or 0.2 mg (total dose) of TRH are injected intravenously, thyroid response (serum TT_4 and FT_4 levels) is followed. An increase of the serum TT_4 concentration of 50% or 1 µg/dl (13 nmol/L) and FT_4 (1.9 times) concentration, compared with baseline concentrations, occurs in normal animals. The evaluation of FT_4 levels allows a clearer distinction between euthyroid and hypothyroid dogs when TT_4 results are equivocal. TRH response test may be used to diagnose mild to moderate feline hyperthyroidism. Baseline serum TT_4 and FT_4 concentrations are determined. Approximately 4 hours after 0.1 mg/kg of TRH are injected intravenously, serum TT_4 and FT_4 levels are determined. An increase of the serum TT_4 less than 50%, compared with baseline concentrations, occurs in hyperthyroid cats. Increases between 50% and 60% are borderline, and increases more than 60% rule out hyperthyroidism.

Triiodothyronine Suppression Test

Hyperthyroidism is common in middle-age to old cats in the United States and Great Britain. Diagnosis may be based on resting thyroid hormone concentrations. Determination of both TT_4 and FT_4 may help distinguish a nonthyroidal disease. The combination of high FT_4 value with low TT_4 is indicative of nonthyroidal illness, whereas a high FT_4 concentration and high-normal TT_4 concentration indicates hyperthyroidism. However, some cases may require a functional test to confirm or rule out the disease.

Thyroid suppression testing is based on the expected negative feedback regulation of TSH, induced by high concentrations of circulating thyroid hormone. Hyperthyroid cats should not have a normal pituitary-thyroid regulation. As a result, administration of exogenous T_3 must induce a decrease on endogenous T_4 unless feedback TSH regulation is altered.

To perform the test, a basal T_3 and T_4 determination is required. Seven T_3 doses of 25 µg orally every 8 hours are administered at home. Approximately 2 to 4 hours after the seventh dose, a blood sample is obtained for T_3 and T_4 determination. Cats with hyperthyroidism have serum T_4 concentrations higher than 1.5 µg/dl or 20 nmol/L, whereas nonhyperthyroid cats have lower values. Low posttest T_3 concentrations indicate an invalid test resulting from failure of exogenous T_3 administration.

Pituitary Function Tests

Diagnosis of canine acromegaly may be based on documentation of elevated growth hormone (GH). Serial GH determinations (three to five samples taken at 10-minute intervals) are performed because affected dogs have constant levels of GH instead of fluctuating GH concentrations. In addition, affected dogs do not respond to stimulation with GH-releasing hormone (GHRH). This test requires intravenous administration of 1μg/kg GHRH or 10 μg clonidine. Posttest plasma GH in normal dogs increases 5 to 15 μg/L or 13 to 25 μg/L, respectively.

ELECTROLYTE ASSAYS

Electrolytes are the negative ions, or anions, and positive ions, or cations, of elements found in all body fluids of all organisms. Some of the functions of electrolytes are maintenance of water balance, fluid osmotic pressure, and normal muscular and nervous functions. They also function in the maintenance and activation of several enzyme systems and in acid-base regulation. Acid-base status depends on electrolytes, so these should be interpreted together. The major electrolytes in plasma are calcium, inorganic phosphorus, magnesium, sodium, potassium, chloride, and bicarbonate. Evaluation of electrolytes, such as sodium and potassium, was at one time not commonly performed in practice laboratories because of the special analytic instrumentation needed. The most common techniques for measurement of electrolytes use ion-specific electrochemical methods. Ion-specific methods require special instrumentation. Automated ion-specific instruments are now readily available and reasonably priced, so many veterinary practices have the ability to perform electrolyte testing. More information on electrochemical testing can be found in Chapter 1.

Volume displacement by lipid typically affects electrolyte measurement, although this is method dependent. An increased concentration of lipid results in plasma volume with decreased water content. Electrolytes are distributed in the aqueous portion of plasma and are not found in the lipid portion. Therefore procedures that measure electrolytes in total plasma volume (per unit of plasma), such as flame photometry or indirect potentiometry, will result in artifactually decreased electrolyte values. This will occur only in very lipemic samples

(e.g., triglyceride concentrations greater than 1500 mg/dl). Procedures that measure electrolytes in the aqueous phase only (per unit of plasma water), such as direct potentiometry, will result in accurate electrolyte concentrations.

Calcium

More than 99% of the calcium in the body is found in bones. The remaining 1% or less has major functions in the body, which include maintenance of neuromuscular excitability and tone (decreased calcium can result in muscular tetany), maintenance of activity of many enzymes, facilitation of blood coagulation, and maintenance of inorganic ion transfer across cell membranes. Calcium in whole blood is almost entirely in plasma or serum. Erythrocytes contain little calcium.

Calcium concentrations are usually inversely related to inorganic phosphorus concentrations. As a general rule, if the calcium concentration rises, the inorganic phosphorus concentration falls. Hypercalcemia is an elevated blood calcium concentration. Hypocalcemia is a decreased blood calcium concentration.

Samples for calcium testing should not be collected using EDTA or oxalate or citrate anticoagulants because they bind with calcium and make it unavailable for assay. Hemolysis results in a slight decrease in calcium concentration in samples as the fluid from the ruptured erythrocytes dilutes the plasma.

Inorganic Phosphorus

More than 80% of the phosphorus in the body is found in bones. The remaining 20% or less has major functions, such as energy storage, release, and transfer; involvement in carbohydrate metabolism; and composition of many physiologically important substances, such as nucleic acids and phospholipids.

Most of the phosphorus in whole blood is found within the erythrocytes as organic phosphorus. The phosphorus in plasma and serum is inorganic phosphorus and is the phosphorus assayed in the laboratory. Inorganic phosphorus levels in plasma and serum provide a good indication of the total phosphorus in an animal. Plasma or serum phosphorus and calcium concentrations are inversely related. As phosphorus concentrations decrease, calcium concentrations increase.

Hyperphosphatemia is an increased serum or plasma phosphorus concentration. Hypophosphatemia is a decreased serum or plasma phosphorous concentration. Hemolyzed samples should not be used. The organic phosphorus liberated from the ruptured erythrocytes may be hydrolyzed to inorganic phosphorus, which results in a falsely elevated inorganic phosphorus concentration. The serum or plasma should be separated from the blood cells as soon as possible after blood collection and before the sample is stored.

Sodium

Sodium is the major cation of plasma and interstitial, or extracellular, fluid. It plays an important role in water distribution and body fluid osmotic pressure maintenance. In the kidney, sodium is filtered through the glomeruli and resorbed back into the body through the tubules in exchange, as needed, for hydrogen ions. In this manner, sodium plays a vital role in pH regulation of urine and acid-base balance. Sodium concentrations are measured by flame photometry, which is usually not available in practice laboratories, or by dry reagent testing. Hypernatremia refers to an elevated blood level of sodium. Hyponatremia is a decreased blood level of sodium. The sodium salt of heparin should not be used as an anticoagulant because it can falsely elevate the results. Hemolysis does not significantly alter results, but it may dilute the sample with erythrocyte fluid, causing falsely lower results.

Potassium

Potassium is the major intracellular cation and is important for normal muscular function, respiration, cardiac function, nerve impulse transmission, and carbohydrate metabolism. In acidotic animals, potassium ions leave the intracellular fluid as they are replaced by hydrogen ions, resulting in elevated plasma potassium levels, or hyperkalemia. The plasma potassium level also may be elevated in the presence of cellular damage or necrosis, which causes release of potassium ions into the blood. Decreased plasma potassium levels, or hypokalemia, may be associated with inadequate potassium intake, alkalosis, or fluid loss resulting from vomiting or diarrhea.

Plasma is the preferred sample because platelets may release potassium during the clotting process, causing artificially elevated potassium levels. Hemolysis should be avoided because the concentration of potassium within erythrocytes is higher than the concentration in plasma. Hemolysis releases potassium into the plasma, resulting in artificially elevated potassium levels. The sample should not be refrigerated until the plasma has been separated from the cells because cooler temperatures promote loss of potassium from the cells without evidence of hemolysis. Samples should not be frozen without first separating the blood cells because the resulting hemolysis makes the sample unsuitable for testing.

Magnesium

Magnesium is the fourth most common cation in the body and the second most common intracellular cation. Magnesium is found in all body tissues. More than 50% of the magnesium in the body is found in bones, closely related to calcium and phosphorus. Magnesium activates enzyme systems and is involved in production and decomposition of acetylcholine. Imbalance of the magnesium/calcium ratio can result in muscular tetany from release of acetylcholine. Cattle and sheep are the only domestic animals that show clinical signs related to magnesium deficiencies. Hypermagnesemia refers to an elevated blood magnesium level. Hypomagnesemia is a decreased blood magnesium level. Anticoagulants other than heparin may artificially decrease the results. Hemolysis may elevate the results through liberation of magnesium from erythrocytes.

Chloride

Chloride is the predominant extracellular anion. It plays an important role in maintenance of water distribution, osmotic pressure, and the normal anion/cation ratio. Chloride is usually included in electrolyte profiles because of its close relationship to sodium and bicarbonate levels. Hyperchloremia is an elevated blood chloride level. Hypochloremia is a decreased blood chloride level. Hemolysis may affect test results by diluting the sample with erythrocyte fluid. Prolonged storage without first separating out the blood cells may cause slightly low results.

Bicarbonate

Bicarbonate is the second most common anion of plasma. It is an important part of the bicarbonate/carbonic acid buffer system and aids in transport of carbon dioxide from the tissues to the lungs. These functions help keep the body pH in balance as acids and bases are continually introduced into the body. The kidney regulates bicarbonate levels in the body by excreting excesses after it has resorbed all that is needed. Bicarbonate levels are frequently estimated from blood carbon dioxide levels. The bicarbonate level is approximately 95% of the total carbon dioxide measured. Arterial blood is the sample of choice for bicarbonate determinations. If plasma is used, lithium heparinate is the anticoagulant of choice. The sample should be chilled in ice water to prevent glycolysis from altering the acid-base composition. Freezing the sample results in hemolysis. Most test methods require incubation at 37° C.

MISCELLANEOUS CHEMISTRY ASSAYS

Creatine Kinase

Creatine kinase (CK) was previously known as creatine phosphokinase (CPK). It is produced primarily in striated muscle cells and, to some extent, in the brain. CK is considered one of the most organ-specific enzymes available for clinical evaluation. When skeletal muscle, including cardiac muscle, is damaged or destroyed, CK leaks out of the cells and produces an elevated blood CK level. Although the brain produces some CK, how much

CK from the brain actually enters the peripheral circulation is uncertain. CK is frequently assayed if an animal has an elevated blood AST level but shows no clinical signs of liver disease. CK is also evaluated in CSF because its measurement in CSF has been suggested as an ancillary diagnostic test for nonspecific damage to neural tissue (e.g., neural hypoxia, trauma, inflammation, or compression by a space-occupying lesion, such as a tumor). The CSF CK value therefore may be a useful guide to prognosis in canine neurologic cases and in premature foals. Increased values also may be observed after seizures.

Although the CK assay is an organ-specific assay, it cannot determine which muscle has been damaged or indicate the severity of the muscle damage. Anything that damages the muscle cell membrane can cause an increased blood CK level. This damage may stem from intramuscular injections, persistent recumbency, surgery, vigorous exercise, electric shock, laceration, bruising, and hypothermia. Myositis and other myopathies also cause elevated blood CK levels. CK levels in samples may be artificially increased by oxidizing agents such as bleach, EDTA, citrate, fluoride, exposure to sunlight, or delay in assay.

Lactate

Lactate (lactic acid) is produced by anaerobic cellular metabolism. Its presence does not indicate any specific disease. However, increased lactate levels indicate hypoxia or hypoperfusion. Lactate levels may be measured in plasma, peritoneal fluid, and CSF. Hypoxia of a section of bowel wall results in increased lactate production, much of which diffuses into the peritoneal cavity before entering the circulation to be removed by the liver. Use of paired blood and peritoneal fluid lactate measurements has been advocated as a diagnostic aid in equine colic cases. The blood lactate concentration of normal horses is always greater than that of peritoneal fluid. Horses with gastrointestinal disorders generally have peritoneal fluid lactate concentrations greater than corresponding blood values. Less severe gastrointestinal disorders, such as impactions, tend to cause a smaller difference between peritoneal fluid and blood lactate concentrations than do serious ones, such as intestinal torsion (a twisted section of bowel). Peritonitis also increases peritoneal fluid lactate values.

The sample for lactate measurement (blood or peritoneal fluid) should be collected in a fluoride oxalate or lithium heparin anticoagulant tube. The fluoride stops cellular metabolism of glucose and consequent production of lactate, and the oxalate prevents sample clotting.

Chemical Tests of Gastrointestinal Function

The principal functions of the gastrointestinal (GI) tract are the assimilation of nutrients (digestion and/or absorption) and excretion of waste products. Most nutrients are ingested in a form either too complex or insoluble for absorption. Within the GI tract these substances are solubilized and degraded enzymatically to simple molecules that may be absorbed across the mucosal epithelium.

Gastrointestinal diseases are common in veterinary practice. Specific diagnosis is essential, especially when the disease is chronic. In cases of malabsorption, intestinal biopsy tends to be required to obtain a definitive diagnosis. However, function tests are performed previously to rule out other diseases and confirm the need for more invasive diagnostic procedures. Therefore function tests are useful in guiding treatment.

Malassimilation may be classified by pathophysiologic process into maldigestive or malabsorptive forms. Maldigestion results from altered gastric secretion and lack of or decreased amounts of digestive enzymes, usually secreted by the pancreas and, less often, the intestinal mucosa. Malabsorption most often is caused by an acquired disease of the small intestinal wall or by bacterial overgrowth syndromes. Before clinical signs of maldigestion are seen, approximately 90% of the pancreas must be either nonfunctional or destroyed. The small intestine of a dog can function well with up to 85% loss, but greater than 50% loss may result in "short bowel syndrome" that cannot be compensated for by adaptive mechanisms.

Laboratory tests may evaluate gastric hydrochloric acid secretion, but most of them are directed to detect malassimilation and its origin. Gastric acid secretion also may be indirectly estimated by determining gastric juice pH; normal dogs have a fasting gastric pH from 0.9 to 2.5. Gastric juice pH may be continuously monitored by radiotelemetric technique.

Malassimilation tests are based on examination of feces for fecal dietary nutrients, fecal enzyme activities, and serum for concentrations of orally administered substrates or metabolites and specific tests for endogenous substances.

Gastrin Secretion

The diagnosis of Zollinger-Ellison syndrome (gastrinoma) may be required after identification of gastrointestinal ulceration and amine precursor uptake and decarboxylation, neoplasia (prevalently located in the pancreas), and the assessment of high serum gastrin concentrations. However, some cases may require provocative tests to document the excessive gastrin secretion. Stimulation of gastrin secretion may be accomplished by test meal, intravenous calcium infusion, or intravenous secretin infusion. Serum samples for gastrin determination must be obtained before, 2, 5, 15, and 30 minutes after intravenous administration of 2 to 4 IU/kg of secretin. A positive test is considered if twofold increase gastrin concentration occurs 2 and/or 5 minutes after administration.

Fecal Occult Blood

Blood loss into the gut is another cause of protein-losing gastroenteropathy. Dramatic bleeding is evident as black feces (melena) or frank fecal blood (hematochezia). Less-obvious, subtle bleeding is a significant sign of GI ulcers, neoplasia, or parasitism. Chronic, low-level bleeding may lead to iron-deficiency anemia.

Useful reagents to detect insidious bleeding include orthotoluidine (Occultest, Ames, Iowa) and benzidine (Hemoccult, Beckman Coulter Inc., Fullerton, Calif.). Impregnated strips or tablets are oxidized to a colored product by hemoglobin peroxidase activity in the feces. Both reagents are so sensitive that they respond to dietary hemoglobin and myoglobin; therefore the patient's diet must be meat free for 3 days before the test. A cottage cheese and rice diet, 50% of each, is recommended for the patient before the test is performed. This precaution is less pertinent to herbivores, but the technician must check that the diet has not been supplemented with meat or bone meal. Another test for fecal occult blood is the guaiac test. The test is less sensitive but also less affected by diet. However, the reagents used for the test are not commonly found in the veterinary clinic.

Fecal Proteolytic Activity

The assay for fecal proteolytic activity was found to be effective for the evaluation of exocrine pancreatic insufficiency in cats and other species. Fecal proteolytic activity can be determined colorimetrically by using an azocasein or azoalbumin substrate or the radial enzyme diffusion method. Dogs with EPI may seldom have normal fecal proteolytic activity. A reliable radial enzyme diffusion requires fecal samples of three different days. Normal values of diameter of digestion halo are 10.7 ± 2.7 mm in dogs and 9.6 ± 3.4 mm in cats.

Fecal α_1-Protease Inhibitor (α_1-Antitrypsin)

This plasma protease resists intraluminal proteolytic degradation. Detection of α_1-protease inhibitor may be accomplished by radial immunodiffusion or enzyme-linked immunosorbent assay in dogs. The assay is species specific. Documentation of protein-losing enteropathy or gastrointestinal hemorrhage is appropriate.

The best method for diagnosing protein-losing enteropathy is quantitative loss of chromium-52–labeled albumin. The test is based on intravenous administration of radioactive chromium, which links to circulating plasma albumin; albumin loss is proportional to radioisotope quantity (radioactivity) in feces.

Lipid Absorption

Lipid absorption relies on bile, pancreatic lipase, and a healthy intestinal mucosa. Associated lesions cause steatorrhea and prevent the normal hyperlipemia that follows a fatty meal. Lipemia, as judged by plasma turbidity, is then a gauge of GI function.

The patient must be fasted for 12 hours and a baseline blood sample must be drawn and cen-trifuged. If fasting lipemia is encountered (e.g., in diabetes mellitus, starvation, feline steatitis, hypothyroidism, hyperadrenocorticism, liver/biliary disease, familial hyperlipemia of Schnauzers, white muscle disease of sheep, or hyperlipemia of ponies, among others), the test must be abandoned. If the plasma is clear, either corn oil (3 ml/kg) or peanut oil (2 ml/kg) is administered orally. Blood samples are drawn at hourly intervals for 4 hours. This plasma should be cloudy. Clear follow-up samples indicate disturbed absorptive function, but the site of disturbance may not be known. Some argue that this test reveals nothing more than the simple discovery of steatorrhea.

A variation of this method may better define the lesion. The test is repeated on another day; however, the oil is preincubated at room temperature for 20 minutes with pancreatic enzymes. A cloudy postchallenge plasma implies a pancreatic enzyme deficiency. If it is clear, inadequate bile production or intestinal malassimilation must be considered. The fat absorption test may yield false-negative results (no fat absorption) with delayed gastric emptying (fat induces this), gastric inactivation of added pancreatic enzymes, or enteritis.

Slight lipemia before oil administration indicates increased levels of low lipoproteins (mainly triglycerides and cholesterol). The enzyme lipoprotein lipase usually clears plasma of triglycerides; the activity of this enzyme is enhanced by insulin, thyroid hormones, glucagon, and heparin. Determination of triglyceride concentrations of slightly lipemic plasma may reveal increased triglyceride concentration, which could be attributed to disease of hepatic, pancreatic, renal, or endocrine origin. Slight postprandial lipemia also may be seen in some canine patients with malabsorptive syndromes.

Monosaccharide Absorption Tests

These tests more specifically probe intestinal function. Again, the agent is given orally; blood concentrations are the measure of absorption.

d-Xylose Absorption

d-xylose is a five-carbon sugar absorbed passively in the jejunum and excreted rapidly by the kidneys.

Because xylose absorption is simple and the agent is not metabolized, its fate is readily traced. Xylose absorption is inefficient and often affected by some intestinal diseases. Nonetheless, the test is relatively insensitive because control values are variable.

The test is performed in dogs and horses, as described in Box 3-7. Interference from rumen flora precludes use of the oral test in cattle and sheep; the alternative injection of monosaccharides into the abomasum is difficult enough to make its use rare.

Abnormal xylose absorption indicates intestinal malassimilation, specifically malabsorption. How-

ever, only slight differences separate normal and abnormal ranges; diseased animals may have normal results. Animals with lymphangiectasia still may have normal results because the lymphatics do not participate in xylose absorption. The rate of xylose absorption depends only on the amount given, the size of the absorptive area, intestinal blood circulation, and gastric emptying. The latter may be delayed by cold or hypertonic solutions, pain, apprehension, or feeding. Fasting or radiographs to confirm an empty stomach are required. Vomiting, however, falsely lowers blood values, as does ascites (xylose enters pooled fluids). Bacteria have the ability to metabolize xylose; therefore bacterial overgrowth may be monitored by this test. If bacterial overgrowth is suspected (in cases of intestinal stasis or pancreatic enzyme deficiency), the test should be repeated after 24 hours' use of oral tetracycline. Finally, renal disease falsely elevates blood xylose concentrations.

The fate of xylose also has been followed in dogs by collecting a 5-hour urine sample after a 25-g oral dose and determining the total xylose excreted. This method is more laborious but requires only one xylose assay.

Cats were thought to have plasma concentrations and kinetics similar to dogs. Other studies found xylose uptake to be variable in cats; plasma concentration did not increase to the levels found in dogs. Peak plasma concentration of xylose in normal cats ranged between 12 and 42 mg/dl when a dosage of 500 mg/kg body weight was used.

False-negative results may be caused by delayed gastric emptying, abnormal intestinal motility, reduced intestinal blood flow, bacterial overgrowth, and sequestration of xylose in ascitic fluid. False-positive results may be caused by decreased GFR; therefore ensuring the patient is fully hydrated and not azotemic at the time of testing is important.

Of the oral dose of xylose, 18% is excreted through the kidneys within 5 hours. This test has been improved by performing d-xylose and 3-*O*-methyl-d-glucose (3MG) absorption test comparing the differential absorption of two sugars to eliminate the nonmucosal effects of d-xylose absorption.

BOX 3-7

Overview of monosaccharide absorption test in dogs and horses

Oral Xylose Absorption in Dogs
- The patient is fasted and baseline xylose measurement determined.
- Xylose solution is administered via stomach tube and xylose measurements obtained from post administration blood samples collected 30, 60, 90, 120, 180, and 240 minutes after xylose administration.
- Blood xylose concentration are graphed over time
- A peak of less than 45 mg/dl between 30 and 90 minutes is abnormal. Peak values of 45 to 50 mg/dl are possibly abnormal. A peak above 50 mg/dl is probably normal.

Glucose and Xylose Absorption in Horses
- Glucose and xylose tests are performed separately with the same general protocol
- The patient is fasted for 12 to 18 hours and water is then withheld
- Baseline xylose (or glucose) concentrations are obtained
- The Xylose (or glucose) solution is administered via stomach tube and blood samples collected at 30-minute intervals for 4 to 5 hours.
- Maximum blood xylose level of 20.6 ± 4.8 mg/dl is expected at 60 minutes. The preadministration blood glucose concentration should be doubled by 120 minutes.

Serum Folate and Cobalamin

Serum concentrations of folate and cobalamin may be assessed by radioimmunoassay. Both concentrations tend to be decreased in malabsorption. Folate is absorbed in the proximal intestine, whereas cobalamin is absorbed in the ileum. Bacterial overgrowth also may alter these concentrations; folate synthesis is increased in bacterial overgrowth, whereas some bacteria may decrease the cobalamin availability.

Mucin Clot Test

Synovial fluid mucin forms a clot when added to acetic acid. The nature of the resultant clot reflects the quality and concentration of hyaluronic acid. The following is one method. To perform the test, 1 ml nonanticoagulated synovial fluid is added to a 7-N glacial acetic acid diluted 0.1:4. The synovial fluid/acetic acid solution is gently mixed and allowed to stand at room temperature for 1 hour before evaluating for the presence of a clot. The mucin clot generally is graded as good (large, compact, ropy clot in a clear solution), fair (soft clot in a slightly turbid solution), fair-poor (friable clot in a cloudy solution), or poor (no actual clot, but some large flecks in a turbid solution). Clot assessment is enhanced by gently shaking the tube. Good clots remain ropy, whereas poor clots fragment. If only a few drops of synovial fluid are obtained at arthrocentesis, an abbreviated mucin clot test may be performed. If available after preparation of a cytologic smear (and possibly total nucleated cell count), a drop of non–EDTA-preserved fluid is placed on a clean microscope slide. Three drops of diluted acetic acid are added and mixed. The resultant clot is graded after approximately 1 minute. Assessment may be easier against a dark background.

TOXICOLOGY

Numerous agents may be involved in common poisonings of dogs, cats, horses, and food animals, including herbicides, fungicides, insecticides, rodenticides, heavy metals (especially lead), household products (including phenols), automotive products (especially ethylene glycol), drugs (including medications), and various poisonous plants and animals. Often a presumptive diagnosis may be attained from an accurate history, including environmental factors, and a thorough clinical examination followed by response to therapy or by necropsy. However, establishing a specific etiologic diagnosis may be difficult in some cases.

A few simple tests may be performed in the veterinary practice laboratory. In such situations, personnel must be familiar and competent with the test procedure, reagents must not be outdated, and special equipment may be required. These requirements, together with a sporadic demand for such tests, frequently dictate that practitioners send all toxicologic specimens to a specially equipped laboratory for analysis.

Toxicologic Specimens

Suggestions on appropriate specimens and preferred methods of handling, packaging, and transport can be obtained by consultation with the toxicology laboratory. Such contact also ensures that the laboratory offers the procedures requested. Submitted specimens should be free from contamination by extraneous environmental compounds or debris. Specimens should not be washed, which may remove toxic residues. Samples of different fluids, tissues, and feeds must be submitted in separate leak-proof (airtight), clean plastic or glass containers. All containers should be individually identified by the owner's and veterinarian's names, animal's name or identification number, and the nature of the specimen before packaging into a large container for submission to the laboratory.

Samples of whole blood (at least 10 ml, usually heparinized), serum (at least 10 ml), vomitus, gastric lavage fluid, feces, and urine (approximately 50 ml) may be submitted from live animals. Samples of feed (portions of at least 200 g), water, and suspected baits also may be helpful in some cases. In fatal poisoning, samples collected during a thorough necropsy should include whole blood or serum; urine; gut (especially stomach) contents (at least 200 g, noting site of collection); and organ or tissue samples, especially liver and kidney, but sometimes brain, bone, spleen, or fat (generally, where practical, at least 100 g of each tissue). Sending too large a sample is always better than not sending enough because excess can be discarded.

In general, serum or blood samples are best submitted refrigerated, whereas gut contents and tissues are best frozen. Preservatives are usually not required. An exception would be tissue samples submitted for histopathologic examination, which require fixation in 10% formalin and must not be frozen. If a preservative is used on a specimen submitted for chemical analysis, it is probably worthwhile also to submit an aliquot of preservative for reference analysis. Frozen samples should be insulated from other specimens and should arrive at the laboratory while still frozen. Dispatch to the laboratory by courier is recommended.

Because litigation may result from poisoning cases, accurate and detailed records should be kept from the outset of the case. Establishment of a good working relationship with the toxicology laboratory, including provision of a good case history (and necropsy findings in fatal poisonings) when samples are submitted, helps ensure the best results.

The main advantages of the following tests are that they can be performed reasonably quickly in the practice laboratory. Results are therefore available more rapidly than if the sample were sent to a toxicology laboratory. However, they are best viewed as screening procedures, suggesting appropriate avenues of investigation and treatment. Verification of findings (especially positive ones) by a reputable toxicology laboratory is advisable, especially if subsequent legal action by the client is a possibility.

Lead Poisoning

Lead is a fairly common environmental pollutant, in the air of cities and in old lead-based paints, lead shot (ammunition), linoleum, car batteries, solder, roofing materials, and petroleum products. Lead poisoning (plumbism) can occur in all species. Clinical signs vary with the species and are related chiefly to the gastrointestinal tract and nervous system. Hematologic examination of blood from an animal with lead poisoning may reveal basophilic stippling of some erythrocytes and increased numbers of circulating nucleated red blood cells (metarubricytosis) (see Chapter 2). Such findings in an animal that is not anemic and has clinical signs consistent with lead poisoning strongly suggest plumbism.

No simple, reliable in-house tests exist to detect lead in blood, feces, urine, milk, or tissues. Blood lead levels can be determined readily (by atomic absorption spectrophotometry) at a toxicology laboratory on whole blood, collected in EDTA, heparin, or citrate blood tubes. Tissue samples (especially liver and kidney) and feces also may be tested. Histopathologic examination of liver, kidney, or bone, stained by the Ziehl-Neelsen technique, may reveal characteristic eosinophilic, acid-fast intranuclear inclusion bodies in hepatocytes, renal tubular cells, and osteoclasts, respectively.

Nitrate or Nitrite Poisoning

Nitrate or nitrite poisoning may occur in ruminants, pigs, and horses ingesting feeds with high concentrations of these compounds. Such may be the case in cereals, grasses, and root crops heavily fertilized with nitrogenous compounds. Water, especially from deep wells filled with seepage from heavily fertilized ground, may contain large quantities of nitrate. Nitrates are converted to nitrites in the feed or in the intestinal tract. Nitrites absorbed from the gut decrease the oxygen-carrying capacity of the blood by degrading hemoglobin to methemoglobin in erythrocytes. Consequently, the animal's blood becomes dark-red to brown. The severity of clinical signs is related to the quantity ingested. Death can be acute and many animals can be affected.

A rapid, fairly specific, semiqualitative test uses diphenylamine, which is converted to quinoidal compounds with an intensely blue color by nitrates and nitrites. Diphenylamine (0.5 g) is dissolved in 20 ml distilled water and the solution made up to 100 ml with concentrated sulfuric acid. This stock solution may be used undiluted or diluted 1:1 with 80% sulfuric acid. The solution is applied to the inner portion of the plant's stem. An intense blue color within 10 seconds of application of the undiluted solution suggests greater than 1% nitrate is present (and the feed is potentially toxic). False-positive results may occur with numerous substances, the most significant of which is iron. Such iron is generally on the outside of the stalk; therefore careful application circumvents this problem.

A more dilute diphenylamine solution (the previous stock solution diluted 1:7 with concentrated sulfuric acid) may be used to test for nitrates/nitrites in serum or plasma, other body fluids, and urine. Three drops of the diluted diphenylamine are added to 1 drop of the sample on a glass slide over a white background. Nitrate/nitrite produces an intense blue color immediately. Hemolysis may mask the color change.

Anticoagulant Rodenticides

Anticoagulant rodenticides (e.g., warfarin, diphacinone, pindone) act by inhibiting metabolism of vitamin K in the body. The latter is required for production of factors II, VII, IX, and X in the liver. Anticoagulant rodenticide poisoning initially prolongs the prothrombin time (PT) because factor VII is the first to be depleted. Subsequently, the partial thromboplastin time (PTT) and activated coagulation time (ACT) are prolonged as the other factors also become depleted. When an animal is bleeding as a result of such poisoning, both the PT and PTT (or ACT) are usually prolonged. Diagnosis of anticoagulant rodenticide poisoning is often based on these screening tests and the response to treatment with vitamin K.

Chemicals that Denature Hemoglobin

A variety of compounds, when ingested, may result in damage to (oxidative denaturation of) hemoglobin in erythrocytes with the formation of Heinz bodies (see Chapter 2). Such substances include paracetamol and methylene blue (cats), onions (dogs), red maple leaves (horses), and onions and brassicas (ruminants). Demonstration of Heinz bodies on a blood film is diagnostic of such poisoning.

Selenium-deficient animals are more prone to such oxidative injury because of a deficiency of glutathione peroxidase (an enzyme in erythrocytes that helps protect them against such damage).

Ethylene Glycol

Ethylene glycol is the major constituent of most antifreeze solutions. Accidental ingestion can cause serious or fatal toxicosis, usually in dogs and cats. Ethylene glycol and its metabolites can be detected in whole blood or serum samples by a toxicology laboratory. Its presence is strongly suggested when urine sediments from poisoned dogs or cats contain masses of calcium oxalate monohydrate crystals (see Chapter 5). Histopathologic examination of the kidney of fatally affected animals reveals renal tubular nephrosis and numerous oxalate crystals.

Recommended Reading

Karselis I: *The pocket guide to clinical laboratory instrumentation,* Philadelphia, 1994, FA Davis.

Meyer DJ, Harvey JW: *Veterinary laboratory medicine: interpretation and diagnosis,* St Louis, 2004, Elsevier.

Sodikoff C: *Laboratory profiles of small animal diseases: a guide to laboratory diagnosis,* St. Louis, 2001, Elsevier.

Thrall MA, Baker DC, Lassen ED: *Veterinary hematology & clinical chemistry,* Baltimore, 2004, Lippincott Williams & Wilkins.

Willard MD, Tvedten H: *Small animal clinical diagnosis by laboratory methods,* St Louis, 2003, Elsevier.

CHAPTER 4

Diagnostic Microbiology

Margi Sirois

KEY POINTS

- Bacterial morphologic characteristics are described on the basis of the shape and arrangement of the cells.
- Bacteria vary in their requirements for oxygen, temperature, and nutrients.
- Some bacteria contain specialized structures (e.g., capsules, spores) that can aid in their identification.
- Equipment and supplies needed to perform microbiology testing in the practice laboratory include an incubator, sample collection materials, culture media, and staining supplies.
- Culture media can be obtained in tubes or plates. Tube media can be solid or liquid.
- A variety of culture media are available, but most veterinary practice laboratories require only a few types.
- Primary identification of bacteria requires inoculation of culture media and observation of bacterial growth characteristics.

- Additional biochemical tests (e.g., catalase, oxidase) may be needed to confirm identity of bacteria in samples.
- Antibiotic sensitivity testing is performed to determine the resistance or susceptibility of bacteria to specific antimicrobials.
- Fungal samples are routinely collected from animals and require no specialized equipment.
- The primary test performed on fungal samples in the veterinary practice laboratory is the dermatophyte test.
- Dermatophyte test media contains a color indicator to aid in identification of fungal organisms.
- Identification of dermatophytes must be confirmed by microscopic examination.

Microbiology refers to the study of microbes. Microbes are organisms that are too small to be seen with the unaided eye. Bacteria, fungi and viruses are all microbes. The study of these organisms is referred to as bacteriology, mycology, and virology, respectively. Virology evaluations in the veterinary clinical laboratory are usually performed with immunologic methods. Bacteria and fungi can be evaluated with a number of routine microbiology procedures. Although some practices send all microbiology work to a reference laboratory, most practices do some testing in-house. Bacterial and fungal samples can be collected quickly, easily, and inexpensively, and tests do not require much in the way of specialized equipment. Careful attention to quality control is vital to ensuring the diagnostic value of results.

Most microbes found on and in the body are nonpathogenic (i.e., normal flora). The intestinal and respiratory tracts, skin, and parts of the urinary and reproductive tracts all have known normal flora. Samples collected from some locations, such as the spinal column, blood, and the urinary bladder, should be free of normal flora. Microbes that are considered normal flora and nonpathogenic when found in one location can produce significant disease if in a site where they should not reside.

BACTERIAL CELL MORPHOLOGY

Identification of bacterial pathogens is the primary purpose of microbiology examinations. Bacteria are small prokaryotic cells that range in size from 0.2 to 2.0 μm. The bacteria most frequently studied in the laboratory range from 0.5 to 1 μm in width and 2 to 5 μm in length. Most cellular organelles are absent except cell walls, plasma membranes, and ribosomes. Some contain capsules and flagella and can develop endospores. Bacteria have specific requirements for temperature, pH, oxygen tension, and nutrition. These requirements must be considered when collecting and preparing microbiology samples. In addition, identification of some bacteria can be aided by using these characteristics. The majority of clinically significant bacterial species require a pH in the range of 6.5 to 7.5. Bacteria that

require oxygen to survive are referred to as obligate aerobes. Bacteria that are killed in the presence of oxygen or whose growth is inhibited in the presence of oxygen are obligate anaerobes. Organisms referred to as facultative anaerobes can survive in the absence of oxygen but their growth is limited. Microaerophilic bacteria prefer reduced oxygen tension, and capnophilic bacteria require high levels of carbon dioxide.

Nutritional requirements vary among bacteria, and culture media types are chosen on the basis of these requirements. Some bacteria have strict requirements; these are referred to as fastidious microbes.

Temperature requirements also vary among different bacteria. However, nearly all bacteria that are pathogenic to animals grow best at 20° to 40° C and are referred to as mesophiles. Bacteria with lower and higher temperature requirements are referred to as psychrophiles and thermophiles, respectively.

Methods of identification are directed toward characterizing bacteria on the basis of a variety of criteria. These criteria include size, shape, arrangement, and chemical reactivity. These characteristics are often used in the differentiation of specific bacterial pathogens.

Bacteria may be organized into the following three groups according to their shape (Fig. 4-1):

1. Coccus (pl. cocci): spherical cells, such as *Staphylococcus aureus,* the causative agent of mastitis in animals.
2. Bacillus (pl. bacilli): shaped like rods or cylinders, such as *Bacillus anthracis,* the causative agent of anthrax in animals and human beings.
3. Spiral: usually occur singly and can be subdivided into loose spirals, such as *Borrelia anserina,* which causes avian borreliosis; tight spirals, such as *Leptospira pomona,* which causes red water disease in cattle; and comma-shaped spirals, such as *Campylobacter fetus,* a cause of abortion in cattle.
4. Pleomorphic: shape ranging from cocci to rods.

Bacteria are found in a variety of arrangements. Some grow as single cells and others remain

Bacilli   Cocci   Spirals

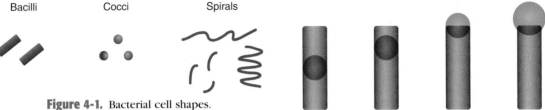

Figure 4-1. Bacterial cell shapes.

Figure 4-3. Bacterial endospores.

attached after dividing and form chains or clusters. Many exhibit patterns of arrangement, such as the following, that are important for their identification (Fig. 4-2):

1. Single. Some bacteria occur singly, such as spirilla (singular, spirillum) and most bacilli (singular, bacillus).
2. Pairs. Some bacteria occur in pairs, such as *Streptococcus pneumoniae* (diplococcus).
3. Clusters or bunches. Some bacteria occur in clusters, bunches, or groups. For example, *Staphylococcus aureus* forms grapelike clusters.
4. Chains. Some organisms grow in short or long chains, such as the *Streptococcus* species.
5. Palisades. Some organisms can be arranged in a palisade or "Chinese letter" pattern, such as *Corynebacterium* species.

With pleomorphic organisms, such as *Corynebacterium* species, judging whether the organism is a coccus or a bacillus may be difficult. If the Gram-stained smear was made from a pure culture and any of the cells present are definitely rod shaped, the organism must be regarded as a bacillus for purposes of identification.

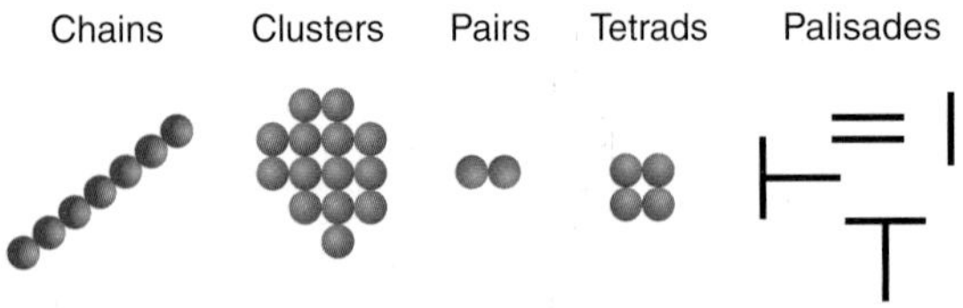

Spores

When cultured, a few genera of bacteria form intracellular refractile bodies called endospores or, more commonly, spores. Organisms in the genera *Bacillus* and *Clostridium* are spore formers. Bacterial spores are resistant to heat, desiccation, chemicals, and radiation.

Spores vary in size, shape, and location in the cell and may be classified as follows (Fig. 4-3):

- Central: present in the center of the cell, such as *Bacillus anthracis*
- Subterminal: present near the end of the cell, such as *Clostridium chauvoei*
- Terminal: present at the end or pole of the cell, such as *Clostridium tetani*

Performing a special spore stain may not be necessary because the endospores can usually be visualized as nonstaining bodies in Gram stained samples.

BACTERIAL GROWTH

Bacterial cells contain a single DNA strand and reproduce primarily by binary fission. When bacteria colonize any media, such as living tissue or a culture plate in a laboratory, bacteria growth proceeds through four distinct phases (Fig. 4-4). The initial phase, referred to as the lag phase, represents the time during which the bacteria are adapting their metabolism to use the resources on their new media. Assuming the media contains the appropriate growth factors and conditions for the particular bacterial species, the lag phase is followed by the exponential growth phase. The rate

Chains   Clusters   Pairs   Tetrads   Palisades

Figure 4-2. Bacterial cell arrangements.

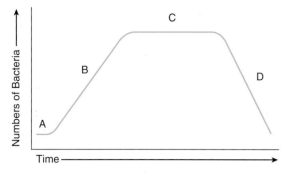

A – Lag phase
B – Exponential growth phase
C – Stationary phase
D – Log decline phase

Figure 4-4. Generalized bacterial growth curve.

of growth during this phase is often referred to as the doubling time or generation time. The generation time is variable with different species and under different environmental conditions. The exponential growth phase continues until essential nutrients are depleted, toxic waste products accumulate, and/or space becomes limiting. The colony then enters the stationary phase, representing the time during which the total numbers of cells show no net increase or decrease. The length of this phase is also variable among different bacterial species. The final phase is the logarithmic decline phase, or death phase. The rate of death is not necessarily the same as the rate of initial growth. Spore formation usually occurs during this phase.

EQUIPMENT AND SUPPLIES

The Laboratory

Ideally the practice facility should have a separate room away from the main traffic areas of the clinic for microbiologic procedures. The room must have adequate lighting and ventilation; a washable floor and limited traffic; at least two work areas, one for processing the samples and one for culture work, with smooth surfaces that are easily disinfected; electrical outlets; ample storage space; and easy access to an incubator and a refrigerator.

Laboratory Safety

Most of the microorganisms encountered in the microbiology laboratory are potentially pathogenic. All specimens should be treated as potentially zoonotic. The safety of every person working in the laboratory depends on strict observance of rules. Aseptic technique is always observed when transferring or working with infectious agents or specimens.

Veterinary technicians must wear personal protective equipment when handling patient specimens, including a clean, long-sleeved, knee-length, white laboratory coat to prevent contamination of street clothes and dissemination of pathogens to the general public. Disposable gloves are always worn in the microbiology laboratory, and face masks may be needed if production of aerosol particles is likely. Laboratory coats should be washed at least weekly in hot water and strong bleach. If the coat becomes soiled during daily diagnostic procedures, it is removed immediately and placed in the receptacle designated for dirty linens. All laboratory coats should be washed together. At no time should laboratory coats be mixed with other laundry from the veterinary clinic or with laundry from outside the laboratory. All personal protective equipment should be removed before leaving the laboratory. The veterinary technician must wash his or her hands thoroughly before leaving the laboratory.

Materials contaminated with potentially infectious agents must be decontaminated before disposal.

Scissors, forceps, and scalpel blade holders can be sterilized in an autoclave. Potentially hazardous materials (plates, test tubes, slides, pipettes, and broken glass) are placed in appropriate containers for disposal. If these materials must be discarded in the trash receptacles, they must first be autoclaved to eliminate any infectious agents. Bench tops are cleaned with disinfectant (70% ethanol or dilute bleach solution) at the beginning and end of the work period. Spilled cultures are treated with disinfectant and allowed contact for 20 minutes before they are cleaned up. The surfaces of all other equipment, such as incubators and refrigerators, should be wiped down with disinfectant on a daily basis. Nondisposable wire loops contaminated with microbes must be flamed immediately after use.

Eating, drinking, smoking, handling contact lenses, and applying cosmetics are not permitted in the laboratory. Appropriate signage should state this rule. Persons who wear contact lenses in the laboratory also should wear goggles or a face shield. Long hair must be tied back or tucked inside the laboratory coat. Labels should be moistened with water, not with the technician's tongue. No food is stored in the laboratory; instead it is stored outside the laboratory in designated cabinets or refrigerators.

All accidents must be reported promptly to the laboratory supervisor or to the veterinarian.

Equipment and Supplies Needed for the Microbiology Laboratory

A good-quality incubator capable of maintaining constant temperature and humidity is the primary equipment needed in the microbiology laboratory. More information on incubators is available in Chapter 1. Supplies needed for collecting and preparing bacterial and fungal samples include the following:

- Sterile cotton-tipped swabs
- Dull scalpel blades
- 3- to 20-ml syringes and 21- to 25-gauge needles
- Sterile endotracheal tube or jugular or urinary catheter
- Collection tubes and preservatives
- Rayon swab in transport media, such as Culturette (BD, Franklin Lakes, NJ) (Fig. 4-5)
- High-quality glass slides and cover slips
- Inoculating loops or wires, reusable metal or single-use disposable plastic (Fig. 4-6) and 10-µl calibrated loops
- Bunsen burner (natural gas or propane gas) or alcohol lamp (Fig. 4-7)
- Candle jar or anaerobe jar
- A variety of culture media, including plates and broth
- Antibiotic disks
- Gram stain and other stains as needed

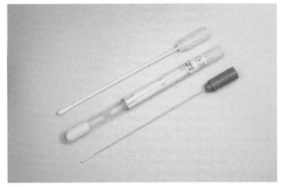

Figure 4-5. The Culturette consists of a rayon swab in transport media. (Courtesy of B. Mitzner, DVM.)

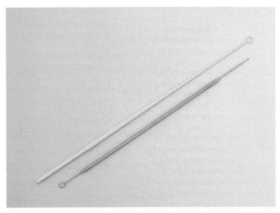

Figure 4-6. Disposable plastic inoculating loops. (Courtesy of B. Mitzner, DVM.)

- Scissors, forceps, scalpel with blades (stored in 70% alcohol and flamed to sterilize)
- "Discard jar" containing disinfectant for contaminated instruments
- Wooden tongue depressors for handling fecal specimens
- Racks to hold tubes and bottles
- Refrigerator "cold packs" and polystyrene shipping containers for samples that must be sent to reference laboratories

Staining of Microbiology Samples

Two commonly used stains are Gram stain and acid-fast stain. Samples taken directly from patients are

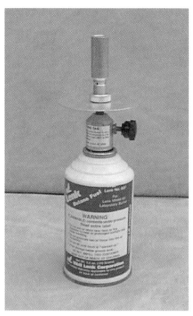

Figure 4-7. Propane burner for sterilizing metal inoculating loops. (Courtesy of B. Mitzner, DVM.)

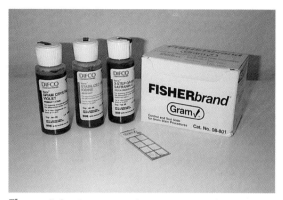

Figure 4-8. Gram stain kit. (Courtesy of B. Mitzner, DVM.)

often Gram stained before the sample is cultured. Information obtained from a direct smear may help determine the suitability of the specimen for identification, the predominant organism in a mixed specimen, the appropriate medium for culture, and the appropriate antibacterials for sensitivity testing. Staining kits for Gram and Ziehl-Neelsen (acid-fast) stains are available commercially (Fig. 4-8). Commercially prepared staining solutions may require filtering if a precipitate forms. Simple stains, such as crystal violet or methylene blue, are typically used for yeasts. Lactophenol cotton blue stain is used to confirm the identity of fungal organisms. Many other types of stains are available for microbiology but most are performed only in large reference or research laboratories.

Gram Stain

Gram staining is used to categorize bacteria as gram positive or gram negative on the basis of cell wall structure. Gram stain kits contain solutions of crystal violet, Gram's iodine, a decolorizer, and basic fuchsin or safranin.

Procedure

The sample should be applied thinly on the slide. Swab specimens may be rolled lightly onto the slide. Touching the sterile wire to one colony on the plate is usually sufficient to obtain enough bacteria for application to the slide. The colonies should be young (24-hour culture) because older colonies may not yield proper results, and the stained bacteria often become excessively decolorized.

Bacterial samples from plates are gently mixed in a drop of water or saline on the slide. If the sample is obtained from inoculated broth, two to three loopfuls are spread onto the slide. A sample also may be smeared directly onto a slide, such as from tissue or an abscess. Regardless of how the specimen is transferred onto the slide (swab, pipette, wire), care must be taken not to destroy the organisms.

The sample droplet on the slide may be encircled by using a wax pencil to help find the area after staining. After the material has dried on the slide, it is heat fixed by passing the slide through a flame two or three times, specimen side up. The technician should be careful to not overheat the slide. The temperature may be tested on the back of the hand. The slide should feel warm but not hot. Heat fixing prevents the sample from washing off, helps preserve cell morphology, and kills the bacteria and renders them permeable to stain.

The Gram staining procedure is as follows:

- The slide is placed on a staining rack over a sink.
- Crystal violet solution is poured onto the smear and allowed to sit 30 seconds.
- The slide is rinsed gently with water (tap water is acceptable).
- Iodine solution is poured onto the smear and allowed to stand for 30 seconds.
- The slide is rinsed gently with water.
- The smear is washed with decolorizer until no more purple color washes off (usually 10 seconds or less).
- The slide is rinsed with water and replaced on the rack.
- Basic fuchsin or safranin is poured onto the smear and allowed to stand for 30 seconds.
- The smear is rinsed with water.
- The smear is air dried or blotted between sheets of paper towel.
- The smear is examined microscopically with the 100× oil-immersion lens.

Interpretation

Bacteria that retain the crystal violet–iodine complex and stain purple are termed gram positive (Fig. 4-9). Those that lose the crystal violet or purple color and stain red by safranin or basic

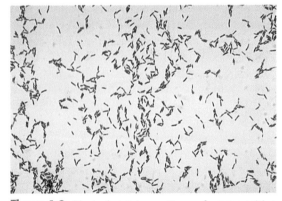

Figure 4-9. Typical staining pattern of gram-positive *Actinomyces* bacteria. (Courtesy Public Health Image Library, PHIL#6711, William A. Clark, Atlanta, 1977, Centers for Disease Control and Prevention.)

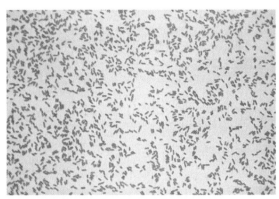

Figure 4-10. Typical staining pattern of gram-negative *Yersinia* bacteria. (Courtesy Public Health Image Library, PHIL#6711, Atlanta, 1980, Centers for Disease Control and Prevention.)

fuchsin are classified as gram negative (Fig. 4-10). The morphology of the bacteria on the smear also is important to note.

Determining the Gram stain reaction is an important step in the identification process. Performing the procedure properly and interpreting the results correctly require practice. To ensure proper staining quality, known (control) gram-positive and gram-negative organisms should be stained at least once a week and with each new batch of stain. These control organisms may be kept growing in the laboratory.

Potassium Hydroxide Test

Sometimes an organism may stain both gram positive and negative, which is called a gram-variable reaction. This may occur as a result of excessive decolorization, an overly thick smear, excessive heat fixation, old cultures, or poor quality of stain.

If a gram-variable reaction occurs, a quick way to check the reaction is with the potassium hydroxide (KOH) test. The procedure is as follows:

1. A loopful (or two, if necessary) of 3% KOH solution is placed on a slide.
2. A generous quantity of surface growth is removed from the culture and transferred to the drop of KOH.

3. The specimen is stirred into the KOH drop with a loop; the loop is then lifted slowly and gently. After a maximum of 2 minutes of stirring (usually 30 seconds), gram-negative organisms develop a mucoid appearance and produce a sticky strand when the drop is lifted with the loop. If the organisms are gram positive, the mixture stays homogeneous and does not form a strand on lifting.

4. The reaction is recorded as gram negative (sticky strand and mucoid mass formed) or gram positive (no sticky strand or mucoid mass formed).

Acid-Fast Stain

This stain is primarily used to detect *Mycobacterium* and *Nocardia* species. Numerous types of acid-fast stains are available, and some are not configured for easy use in the veterinary practice laboratory. Acid-fast stains contain several solutions, including a primary stain, typically dimethyl sulfoxide (DMSO) and carbol fuchsin; an acid-alcohol decolorizer; and a counterstain such as methylene blue. The slide is air dried and heat fixed by passing the slide, specimen side up, through a flame. The primary stain is used to flood the slide. The slide is then heated over the flame until the stain steams. The slide is cooled for 5 minutes and then rinsed with tap water. Acid alcohol is used to decolorize the slide for 1 to 2 minutes until the red color is gone, and the slide is rinsed again. The counterstain is added and then the slide rinsed with water and dried. Agents such as DMSO included in the initial staining procedure allow the stain to penetrate stain-resistant cells such as *Mycobacterium*. Subsequent addition of acid alcohol removes the stain. If the stain is not removed, the organism is "acid-fast" and appears red, whereas non–acid-fast microorganisms stain blue (Fig. 4-11).

Giemsa Stain

Giemsa stain is used to detect spirochetes and rickettsiae and demonstrate the capsule of *Bacillus anthracis* and the morphology of *Dermatophilus congolensis*. The smear is fixed in absolute methanol for 3 to 5 minutes and air dried. It is then dipped in diluted stain for 20 to 30 minutes. The

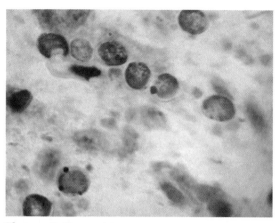

Figure 4-11. Acid-fast stain of *Mycobacterium*. (Courtesy of Marc Kramer, DVM, Avian and Exotic Animal Medical Center, Miami, FL.)

staining time may be extended as indicated by results. For *Borrelia anserina,* the smear is gently heated while it is covered with Giemsa stain and stained for 4 to 5 minutes. The smear is then rinsed, air dried, and examined for the purplish-blue–stained bacteria.

Specialized Stains

Flagella stains, capsule stains, endospore stains, and fluorescent stains are also available but have limited application in the average veterinary practice laboratory. Fluorescent stains tend to be quite expensive and are used primarily for the identification of *Legionella* and *Pseudomonas*. Flagella stains usually contain crystal violet and are used to detect and characterize bacterial motility. These tend to be somewhat expensive for the small veterinary practice laboratory. Other methods that can be used to test motility include the hanging drop preparation and the use of motility test media. Capsule stains are used for detection of pathogenic bacteria. All bacteria that contain capsules are pathogenic. However, not all pathogenic bacteria contain capsules. Capsule stains often require the use of a bright-field phase contrast microscopy.

Bacterial spores contain protein coats of keratin that are resistant to most normal staining procedures. Endospore stains detect the presence, location, and shape of spores and can aid in

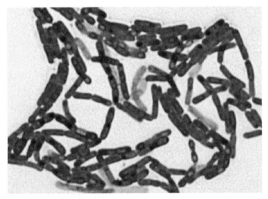

Figure 4-12. Malachite green endospore stain of *Bacillus anthracis.* (From Songer JG, Post KW: *Veterinary microbiology: bacterial and fungal agents of animal disease,* St Louis, 2005, Saunders.)

differentiation of bacteria. Endospore staining is done on an older culture (more than 48 hours) because spore formation occurs during the log-arithmic decline phase. The procedure involves addition of malachite green to the specimen on the slide and then heating the slide. The slide is washed and counterstained with safranin or basic fuchsin. Spores appear dark blue/green, with the remainder of the bacterial cell pink or red (Fig 4-12). Spores may also be found free from cells.

Quality Control

Each time a clinical specimen is stained, a sample from the control cultures should also be stained. This verifies the quality of the staining procedures and materials.

CULTURE MEDIA

Culture medium (pl. media) is any material, solid or liquid, that can support the growth of micro-organisms. For bacteriology, culture media may be purchased as dehydrated powder or as prepared agar plates or ready-to-use liquid media for biochemical tests. All the commonly used media may be obtained already prepared from supply houses. Large reference and research laboratories may prepare and sterilize their own media from dehydrated powder. Solidifying agents used in pre-paring solid media include agar and gelatin. Agar is a dried extract of sea algae known as agaraphytes. Gelatin is a protein obtained from animal tissues.

For maximum life, agar plates should be kept refrigerated at 5° to 10° C. Plates must be kept away from the internal walls of the refrigerator because contact with the jacket can freeze and ruin the media.

Types of Media

Six general types of culture media are available: transport media, general purpose media, enriched media, selective media, differential media, and enrichment media. Some culture media contain characteristics of more than one type. General purpose media, sometimes referred to as nutrient media, is not commonly used in veterinary practice. Enriched media are formulated to meet the requirements of the most fastidious pathogens. They are basic nutrient media with extra nutrients added, such as blood, serum, or egg. Examples include blood agar and chocolate agar. Selective media contain antibacterial substances, such as bile salts or antimicrobials, which inhibit or kill all but a few types of bacteria. They facilitate isolation of a particular genus from a mixed inoculum. MacConkey agar is a type of selective media. Differential media allow bacteria to be differen-tiated into groups by biochemical reactions on the medium. Simmons citrate is a differential medium. Enrichment media are liquid media that favor growth of a particular group of organisms. They contain nutrients that either encourage growth of the desired organisms or contain inhibitory substances that suppress competitors. Examples include tetrathionate broth and selenite broth. Transport media are designed keep microbes alive while not encouraging growth and reproduction. The Culturette used for specimen collection contains prepared transport media. More specific details on some of the commonly used culture media are presented next. This is not meant to be an all-inclusive list; dozens of additional types of media are available. However, many of those not included subsequently are found only in large reference or research laboratories.

Blood Agar

This enriched medium supports the growth of most bacterial pathogens. Although several types of blood agars are available, trypticase soy agar with sheep blood is the most commonly used type. Blood agar acts as an enrichment medium and a differential medium because four distinct types of hemolysis can be detected on blood agar, as follows:

- Alpha hemolysis: partial hemolysis that creates a narrow band of greenish or slimy discoloration around the bacterial colony (Fig. 4-13)
- Beta hemolysis: complete hemolysis that creates a clear zone around the bacterial colony
- Gamma hemolysis: hemolysis that produces no change in the appearance of the medium and no hemolysis around colonies
- Delta hemolysis: also called double-zone hemolysis, a zone of hemolysis surrounded by a narrow zone of hemolysis around a bacterial colony

MacConkey Agar and Eosin-Methylene Blue Agar

MacConkey and eosin-methylene blue (EMB) agars are selective and differential media. MacConkey agar contains crystal violet (which suppresses growth of gram-positive bacteria), bile salts that are selective for lactose-fermenting *Enterobacteriaceae*,

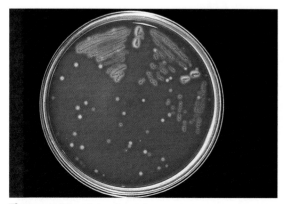

Figure 4-13. Alpha hemolysis of *Streptococcus* on blood agar. (Courtesy Public Health Image Library, PHIL#8170. Richard R. Facklam, Atlanta, 1977, Centers for Disease Control and Prevention.)

and a few other bile salt–tolerant gram-negative bacteria. Growth or no growth on MacConkey agar may be used as a test for primary identification of gram-negative genera. EMB media performs the same function and may also be used to identify lactose-fermenting organisms.

The indicators in MacConkey agar are lactose and neutral red. Lactose-fermenting organisms, such as *Escherichia coli* and *Enterobacter* and *Klebsiella* species produce acid from lactose and grow as pinkish-red colonies on this medium. Bacteria that cannot ferment lactose attack the peptone in MacConkey agar, producing an alkaline reaction and colorless colonies. Clinical specimens for routine isolation usually are cultured separately on both blood and MacConkey agars. Examination of both blood and MacConkey agar cultures, inoculated with the same clinical specimen, can yield considerable information. For example, no growth on the MacConkey agar plate but good growth on the blood agar plate suggests that the isolated pathogen is probably gram positive.

Thioglycollate Broth

Thioglycollate is a liquid medium used to culture anaerobic bacteria to determine the oxygen tolerance of microbes. The medium contains a stable oxygen gradient, with high concentrations of oxygen near the surface of the agar and anaerobic conditions near the bottom.

Obligate aerobes will grow only in the oxygen-rich top layer, whereas obligate anaerobes will grow only in the lower part of the tube. Facultative anaerobes can grow throughout the medium but will primarily grow in the middle of the tube, between the oxygen-rich and oxygen-free zones. The primary use of thioglycollate broth in veterinary practice is as an enrichment media and for blood cultures.

Urea Tubes

Urea slants are streaked with inoculum and incubated overnight at 37° C. Urea medium is a peach color. If the bacteria hydrolyze the urea in the medium, ammonia production turns the medium to a pink color. A negative result produces no color change (Fig. 4-14).

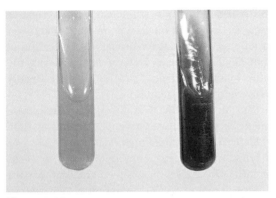

Figure 4-14. Urea tubes. The pink coloration indicates a positive reaction, (urea hydrolysis). Yellow indicates a negative reaction. (Courtesy Public Health Image Library, PHIL#6711, Atlanta, 1976, Centers for Disease Control and Prevention.)

Sulfide-Indole Motility Tubes

The tube of sulfide-indole motility (SIM) medium is inoculated with a straight stab to a depth of approximately 1 inch. Care is taken to withdraw the wire out along the same line as on entry. Hydrogen sulfide production is indicated by blackening of the medium. Indole production requires the addition of 5 drops of Kovac's reagent to the top of the medium. If tryptophan has been broken down to indole by the bacteria in the tube, a red ring immediately forms on top of the medium.

Simmons Citrate Tubes

Simmons citrate medium differentiates bacteria according to their use of citrate. Only the slant surface is inoculated. If bacteria use the citrate in the medium, a deep blue color develops. The unchanged medium is green.

Triple Sugar Iron Agar

Triple sugar iron agar medium is used for presumptive identification of salmonellae and initial differentiation of enteric bacteria. The media contain an indicator system for hydrogen sulfide production and a pH indicator, phenol red, that colors the uninoculated medium red. All *Enterobacteriaceae* ferment glucose, and the small amount (0.1%) is attacked preferentially and rapidly. At an early stage of incubation, both slant and butt turn yellow as a result of acid production. However, after the glucose is metabolized under aerobic conditions, and if the organism cannot ferment lactose or sucrose, the slope reverts to the red (alkaline) condition. The butt, under anaerobic conditions, remains yellow (acidic) (Fig. 4-15). To allow this reaction, the triple sugar iron agar always must be used in tubes with loose caps or plugged with sterile cotton.

If the organism can ferment lactose and/or sucrose in addition to the glucose, the lactose and sucrose are then attacked with resulting acid production, and the medium turns yellow (acidic) throughout. Lactose and sucrose are present in 1% quantities to maintain acidic conditions in the slant, which remains yellow. With organisms that produce hydrogen sulfide, blackening of the medium is partly superimposed on the other reactions. The triple sugar iron slants should be read after about 16 hours' incubation at 37° C. After longer incubation, the blackening tends to reach the bottom of the tube and obscures the yellow butt.

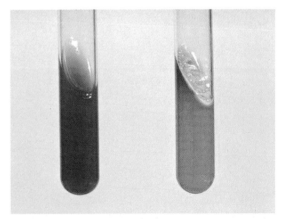

Figure 4-15. Triple sugar iron agar is used to classify bacteria according to their ability to ferment glucose, lactose, or sucrose, as well as produce hydrogen sulfide. A yellow result indicates fermentation; the reddish result indicates no fermentation. (Courtesy Public Health Image Library, PHIL#6710, Atlanta, 1976, Centers for Disease Control and Prevention.)

The following summarizes the reactions of *Salmonella* species in triple sugar iron agar:

- Alkaline (red) slant and alkaline (red) butt: none of the sugars attacked
- Alkaline (red) slant and acidic (yellow) butt: glucose fermentation only
- Acidic (yellow) slant and acidic (yellow) butt: glucose attacked in addition to lactose and/or sucrose
- Blackening along stab line and through medium: hydrogen sulfide production

The triple sugar iron slant is stab inoculated with a single colony from the selective medium with a straight inoculating wire. The wire is pushed down to the bottom of the agar and, on withdrawing the wire, the agar slant is streaked. The inoculating wire still contains enough bacteria to inoculate a tube of lysine decarboxylase broth. During the search for salmonellae, at least two suspicious colonies should be individually tested in triple sugar iron agar per brilliant green plate. The triple sugar iron tubes should be incubated, with loose caps, at 37° C for 16 to 24 hours.

Brain-Heart Infusion Broth

Brain-heart infusion broth is a useful, general-purpose broth used to increase the number of organisms (preenrichment) before they are plated on solid medium. The broth is inoculated with the patient sample and subcultures taken as needed for additional testing.

For culture of blood samples, approximately 1 ml of the patient's blood sample is added to nutrient broth or a special blood culture medium, which can be obtained commercially. Because a patient's blood contains many substances inhibitory to bacteria, adding the blood sample directly to broth dilutes the effect of these natural inhibitors.

Mannitol Salt Agar

Mannitol salt agar is not routinely used but is a highly selective medium for staphylococci and could be used to isolate *Staphylococcus aureus* from contaminated specimens. The medium has a high salt content (7.5%) and contains mannitol and the pH indicator phenol red. Staphylococci are salt tolerant. *S. aureus,* but usually not *S. epidermidis,* ferments mannitol. The resulting acid turns *S. aureus* colonies and the surrounding medium yellow.

Bismuth Sulfite Agar

In this selective medium, freshly precipitated bismuth sulfite acts with brilliant green to suppress growth of coliforms while permitting growth of salmonellae. Sulfur compounds provide a substrate for hydrogen sulfide production. The metallic salts in the medium stain the colony and surrounding medium black or brown in the presence of hydrogen sulfide.

Atypical colonies may appear if the medium is heavily inoculated with organic matter. This situation may be prevented by suspension of the sample in sterile saline and use of the supernatant for inoculation.

The freshly prepared medium has a strong inhibitory action and is suitable for heavily contaminated samples. Storing the poured plates at 4° C for 3 days causes the medium to change color to green, making it less selective with small numbers of salmonellae being recovered.

The following summarizes the typical appearance of the more important bacterial organisms on bismuth sulfite agar and the appearance of their colonies:

- Salmonella typhi: black "rabbit eye" colonies, with surrounding black zone and metallic sheen after 18 hours; uniformly black after 48 hours' incubation
- Other Salmonella species: variable colony appearance after 18 hours (black, green, or clear and mucoid); uniformly black colonies seen after 48 hours, often with widespread staining of the medium and a pronounced metallic sheen
- Other organisms (coliforms, *Serratia, Proteus* species): usually inhibited but occasionally dull green or brown colonies with no metallic sheen or staining of surrounding medium

Mueller-Hinton

Mueller-Hinton is a general purpose media primarily used for the performance of the agar diffusion antimicrobial sensitivity test. The chemical composition of the media does not interfere with the diffusion of the antimicrobials through the agar.

Sabouraud Dextrose and Bismuth-Glucose-Glycine-Yeast Media

Both of these media are used specifically for the culture of fungi and yeasts. Bismuth-glucose-glycine-yeast agar is commonly referred to as "biggy." Dermatophyte test media found in most veterinary clinics is composed of Sabouraud dextrose agar and is commonly found in the veterinary practice.

Combination and Modular Culture Media

Several modular culture systems are available for use in the veterinary practice laboratory. The Bulls Eye (HealthLink, Jacksonville, FL) (Fig. 4-16) and Target (Troy Biologicals, Troy, MI) systems are five-chambered agar plates containing both selective and nonselective media plus a central area with Mueller-Hinton agar for sensitivity testing. "Dipslides" or "paddle" media such as Uri-Dip (Troy Biologicals) or Solar-Cult (Solar Biologicals, Ogdensburg, NY) (Fig. 4-17) are useful tools for urinary tract infection (UTI) screening. They consist

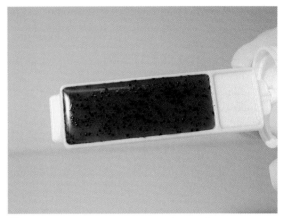

Figure 4-17. Solar-Cult media used for screening patients for urinary tract infections. (Courtesy Solar Biologicals, Ogdensburg, NY.)

of a two-sided agar paddle attached to the cap of a screw-top plastic tube. They are made with a variety of media combinations, although the most common ones have either MacConkey or EMB and cystine lactose electrolyte–deficient (CLED) agar. After incubation, a colony count is performed and the color of the CLED agar is compared with a chart for presumptive identification. Positive cultures that meet quantitation criteria for UTI should be sent to an outside laboratory for confirmation and susceptibility testing.

Enterotubes (BD, Franklin Lakes, NJ) (Fig. 4-18) are one type of commercially available microbiology test kits that incorporate multiple types of media designed to provide differentiation of enteric bacteria on the basis of their biochemical reactions on the media. These tend to be relatively expensive and may not be financially justified unless large numbers of microbiology tests are performed on a variety of species.

Quality Control Cultures

Some cultures are required in a laboratory for quality control purposes. Various procedures and supplies must be monitored for quality and accuracy, including antibacterial susceptibility tests, media, biochemical tests, and certain tests for identification, such as the zone of beta hemolysis around

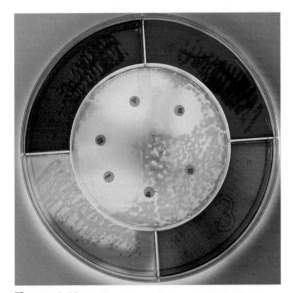

Figure 4-16. Bull's Eye culture media. (Courtesy Healthlink, Jacksonville, FL.)

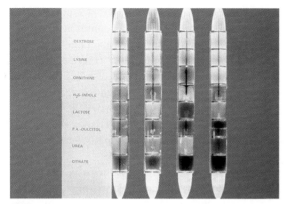

Figure 4-18. The Enterotube is a multitest system containing eight different agar preparations. (Courtesy Public Health Image Library, PHIL#5421, Theo Hawkins, Atlanta, 1977, Centers for Disease Control and Prevention.)

S. aureus for the cyclic adenosine monophosphate test. A selection of control organisms can be obtained on disks. Media not containing fermentable sugars, such as trypticase soy agar, are suitable for maintaining fewer fastidious organisms, such as *S. aureus* and *Enterobacteriaceae*. The bacteria can be stab inoculated into a tube of medium and subcultured approximately every 2 months.

Streptococcus, Pasteurella, and *Actinobacillus* species die quickly on culture plates. Streptococci may be kept in a tube of cooked meat broth and subcultured approximately every 4 weeks. *Pasteurella* and *Actinobacillus* species remain viable if mixed with approximately 0.5 ml of sterile whole blood in a small tube and stored in a deep freeze at −10° C or lower. Otherwise these two genera should be subcultured on blood agar approximately every 3 days. Control cultures may be kept at room temperature in screw-capped tubes but preferably in a refrigerator at 4° C, which reduces the metabolic rate of the organisms.

SPECIMEN COLLECTION

Samples for microbiologic evaluation can be collected quickly, and most do not require specialized materials or equipment for proper evaluation. Specimens are collected by various methods,

including aspiration, swabbing, and scraping. The specific techniques used depend on the type of lesion and its location on the animal's body. Careful attention to aseptic technique is critical to achieving diagnostic-quality results. More details on sample collection techniques by aspiration, swabbing, and scraping can be found in Chapter 9.

The specific choice of collection method depends on the location of the lesion on the animal's body, as well as the specific type of testing desired. Samples that are to be immediately processed can usually be collected by using sterile cotton swabs. However, this is the least suitable method of collection because contamination risk is high and cotton can inhibit microbial growth. Oxygen can also be trapped in the fibers, making recovery of anaerobic bacteria less likely. If delays in processing the sample are expected, a rayon swab in transport media (e.g., Culturette) must be used to preserve the quality of the sample. Aspirated samples can be collected by fine-needle biopsy.

The specimen selected must contain the organism causing the problem. Normal flora and contaminants may complicate sample collection and subsequent interpretation of results. Better results will be obtained if specimens are collected from sites that would normally be sterile because infections are likely to be caused by a single predominant organism. Good examples are urine (collected by cystocentesis) or intact skin pustules. Ears and fecal samples do not lend themselves well to in-house microbiology testing because of the number of commensal and secondary organisms that typically populate such exposed areas.

The following guidelines apply to proper specimen collection:

1. A complete history and sufficient clinical data must be obtained to help select procedures most appropriate to isolate organisms that may be present. Required data include the owner's name, clinic name, address, and phone number. Species, name, age, sex, number of animals affected or dead, duration of the problem, and major signs observed also should be included. The tentative diagnosis, organism suspected, any treatment given, and

type of laboratory investigation required should be included in the record.

2. The specimen must be collected aseptically. Specimen contamination is the most common cause of diagnostic failure. The importance of aseptic collection of microbiologic specimens cannot be overemphasized. Samples should be collected as soon as possible after the onset of clinical signs.

3. Multiple specimens must be kept separate to avoid cross-contamination. This practice is essential for intestinal specimens because of the flora normally present there.

4. The specimen container is labeled, especially if a zoonotic condition is suspected, such as anthrax, rabies, leptospirosis, brucellosis, or equine encephalitis. Tissues in suspected zoonoses should be submitted in a sealed, leak-proof, unbreakable container.

5. Adequate time should be taken. Obtaining results quickly at the expense of accuracy is counterproductive.

Table 4-1 summarizes sample collection guidelines for microbiology specimens.

PRIMARY IDENTIFICATION OF BACTERIA

Procedure 4-1 shows the typical sequences used in processing microbiologic specimens.

A systematic approach is needed in the identification of pathogenic bacteria. The practice laboratory should develop flow charts for use in the clinic that represent the bacteria seen most often and the tests used to differentiate those bacteria. Figure 4-19 is an example of a flow chart that can be used for differentiation of microbes. Specimens are first streaked onto a primary medium, such as blood agar and MacConkey agar. The plates are incubated for 18 to 24 hours and then examined for growth. Suspected pathogens on the incubated plate should be further identified regarding their genus and/or species by using the flow chart. With comparatively few tests, an organism may be identified to the genus level with

a fair degree of certainty. Table 4-2 summarizes identifying characteristics of common bacterial pathogens in veterinary species. Table 4-3 summarizes bacterial pathogens of veterinary importance, species affected, resultant diseases or lesions, and specimens required for diagnosis. Appendix B, Bacterial Pathogens of Veterinary Importance, contains a summary of characteristics of and diseases produced by microbial pathogens seen in mammals and birds.

Most gram-positive and gram-negative organisms grow on blood agar. gram-positive organisms usually do not grow on MacConkey agar, but this agar supports growth of most gram-negative organisms. Selection of the colony from the routine blood agar plate is preferable rather than from MacConkey agar. The danger in subculturing from a selective medium such as MacConkey agar is that inhibited organisms may be present as microcolonies on the plate. One of these could inadvertently be the colony of interest.

Inoculation of Culture Media

Care must be taken to prevent contamination when inoculating media and handling the specimen. Aseptic (sterile) technique must be used at all times. Before obtaining samples from a cadaver or excised organs, sear the surface of the organ or tissue with a flamed spatula before it is cut open for sample collection. Culture plates are kept closed unless inoculating or removing colony specimens for testing. When transferring samples from or to a tube, pass the tube neck through a flame before and after transfer of material and avoid putting down the cap. Instead, the cap is held between the last two fingers. When flaming an inoculation loop or wire, place the near portion of the wire in the flame first and then work toward the contaminated end. Placing the contaminated end into the flame first could result in splattering of bacteria, causing aerosol contamination. When the specimen collected is a liquid, a small quantity of well-mixed samples is inoculated at the edge of the plate with a sterile swab or bacteriologic loop. Some laboratories use presterilized glass rods for streaking samples because Bunsen burners are not always

TABLE 4-1

Sample Collection Guidelines for Microbiology Specimens

Site	Acceptable Specimen	Transport Device	Comments
Central nervous system	Spinal fluid	Blood culture medium	Hold, ship at RT
Blood	Whole, unclotted blood Minimum of 3 ml	Blood culture medium	Hold, ship at RT Submit ≤3 samples per 24 hr collected during febrile spike
Eye	Conjunctival swab Corneal scrapings Ocular fluid	Amies or semisolid reducing medium Syringe	Hold, ship at RT Inoculate plated media directly with corneal scrapings if fungal keratitis suspected
Bone and joints	Joint aspirate Bone marrow aspirate, bone	Blood culture medium Sterile tube	Hold, ship at RT
Urinary tract	Urine by cystocentesis Catheterized urine Midstream urine	Sterile tube	Hold, ship under refrigeration
Upper respiratory tract	Nasopharyngeal swab Sinus washings Biopsy specimen	Semisolid reducing medium Sterile tube	Ship refrigerated except washings, biopsies (RT)
Lower respiratory tract	Transtracheal wash Lung aspirate or biopsy	Sterile tube Semisolid reducing medium	Hold, ship at RT
Gastrointestinal tract	Feces Rectal swab	Sterile cup or bag Cary-Blair or semisolid reducing medium	Feces: hold, ship at RT; refrigerate *Campylobacter, Brachyspira* suspects
Skin	Aspirate or swab, if superficial Deep swab of draining tract Tissue biopsy Scabs, hairs, scrapings	Sterile syringe semisolid reducing medium Sterile tube with saline Paper envelope	Anaerobe suspects not refrigerated
Milk	Remove milk from teat cistern; collect 5-10 mL aseptically	Sterile tube	Freeze
Necropsy tissue	Lesions, including adjacent, normal tissue Minimum of 1 cm³ to maximum of 35 cm³ Include one serosal or capsular surface intact	Whirl-Pak bags Screw-cap jars	Individual containers to prevent cross-contamination; ship refrigerated
Reproductive tract	Prostatic fluid, raw semen Uterus Vagina Abortion	Sterile tube Biopsy or swab Swab Fetal lung, liver, kidney, stomach contents, placenta in separate Whirl-Pak bags or screw-capped containers	Guarded swabbing for uterine cultures; hold, ship at RT Ship refrigerated

RT, Room temperature.
Reprinted from Songer JG, Post KW: *Veterinary microbiology: bacterial and fungal agents of animal disease,* St Louis, 2005, Saunders.

PROCEDURE 4-1

Typical Sequence of Testing of Microbiology Specimens

1. Collection specimen
2. Direct Gram stain of specimen
3. Inoculate culture media
4. Incubate 18–24 hours
5. Check for growth
   a. Negative (no growth)
      1) Reincubate
      2) Recheck
      3) If no growth, report as "no growth"
   b. Positive (colonies on media)
      1) Select representative colonies
      2) Gram stain
      3) Continue with identification procedures (additional media, biochemical testing, etc.)

available and glass rods are can be autoclaved. Disposable inoculating loops and wires are also available. If the specimen has been initially collected on a sterile swab, this is streaked directly onto the plate.

Streaking Culture Plates

The preferred method of streaking an agar plate is the "quadrant" streak method (Procedure 4-2 and Fig. 4-20). In Figure 4-20, area **A** is the primary streak or "well" of the plate. The bacteriologic loop may or may not be flamed and cooled before making streaks **B, C,** and **D.** This depends on the estimated number of bacteria present in the specimen. The use of two loops, one of which is flamed and cooling while the other is being used, is a practical technique.

Each streaked area is overlapped only once or twice to avoid depositing excessive numbers of bacteria in an area. Otherwise, the resultant colonies are not discrete and isolated. Isolated colonies typically grow in area **D** of the plate. The use of the entire plate is important, keeping the streak lines close together to include as many streaks as

possible and taking care not to overlap the other streak lines. If several types of colonies grow on the plate, each colony is subcultured onto separate plates and the procedure repeated until a pure culture is obtained.

Inoculation of Slants

If agar slants are used, only the surface of the slant may be inoculated, or the butt and the surface may be inoculated. To inoculate only the surface of the slant, a straight flamed wire is used to obtain a colony of bacteria from the primary isolation plate. The surface of the slant is streaked in an S shape. To inoculate both the butt and slant, the butt of the slant is stabbed with the tip of the inoculating wire and then carefully withdrawn up the same insertion path. The surface of the slant is then streaked in an S shape (Procedure 4-3 and Fig. 4-21). Enough bacteria should be on the wire to inoculate the surface even after stabbing the butt. The tube's cap should be replaced loosely.

Incubation of Cultures

For pathogens that can invade the internal organs of an animal, the optimal growth temperature is usually near 37° C. For some fish pathogens, skin pathogens (such as dermatophytes), and environmental organisms, the optimal growth temperature is lower. Care should be taken to maintain the incubator temperature at 37° C, which is the optimal temperature, because bacterial growth cannot occur above this temperature.

Incubation time depends on the generation time of individual bacterial species and the type of medium on which they are growing. For routine cultures, plates should be incubated for 48 hours, with plates examined after 18 to 24 hours of incubation. Organisms such as *Nocardia* species may take 72 hours before colonies are visible. The culture plates should be inverted during incubation so that moisture does not collect on the surface of the agar, which may cause clumping of colonies.

Some pathogens require carbon dioxide for growth in the culture atmosphere. A candle jar may be used for this purpose. The plates are placed in a

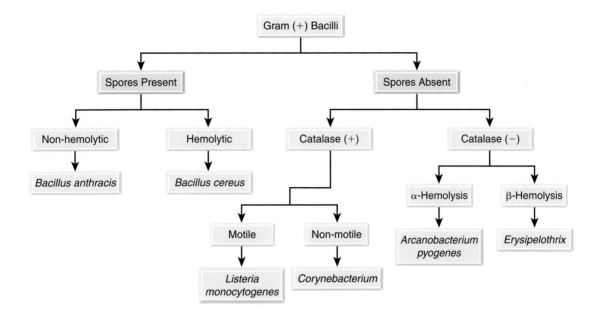

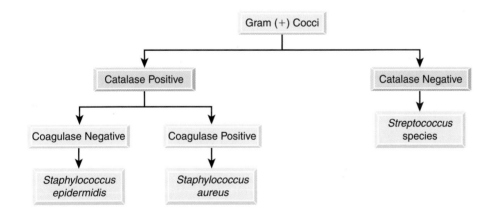

Figure 4-19. Examples of flow charts used for differentiation of bacteria.

TABLE 4-2

Common Bacterial Pathogens in Veterinary Specimens

	Blood Agar	MacConkey Agar	Other Characteristics
Gram-Positive			
Staphylococcus	Smooth, glistening, white to yellow pigmented colonies	No growth	Catalase-positive glucose fermenter; double-zone hemolysis usually indicates coagulase positive; coagulase activity is a useful differential test
Streptococcus	Small, glistening colonies; hemolysis	No growth except some enterococci	Catalase negative, usually identified by type of hemolysis; beta-hemolytic strains more likely to be pathogens; others are often part of flora; *Streptococcus agalactiae* cAMP positive
Arcanobacterium pyogenes	Small, hemolytic, streplike colonies	No growth	Catalase negative; slow growth, often requiring 48 hr for distinct colonies; growth enhanced in candle jar
Corynebacterium pseudotuberculosis	Slow-growing, opaque, dry, crumbly colonies; usually hemolytic	No growth	Catalase positive; weak urease positive
Corynebacterium renale	Small, smooth, glistening colonies (24 hr); become opaque and dry later	No growth	Catalase positive; urease positive
Rhodococcus equi	Small, moist, white (24 hr); become large, pink colonies; no hemolysis	No growth	Catalase positive; delayed urease positive
Listeria monocytogenes	Small, hemolytic, glistening colonies	No growth	Catalase positive; motile at room temperature
Erysipelothrix rhusiopathiae	Small colonies after 48 hr; greenish (alpha) hemolysis	No growth	Catalase negative; hydrogen sulfide positive
Nocardia	Slow-growing, small, dry, granular, white to orange colonies	No growth	Partially acid fast; colonies tenaciously adhere to media
Actinomyces	Slow-growing, small, rough, nodular white colonies	No growth	Require increased carbon dioxide or anaerobic incubation; not acid fast
Clostridium	Variable, round, ill-defined, irregular colonies; usually hemolytic	No growth	Obligate anaerobes
Bacillus	Variable, large, rough, dry, or mucoid colonies	No growth	Usually hemolytic; large rods with endospores

cAMP, cyclic adenosine monophosphate.

TABLE 4-2

Common Bacterial Pathogens in Veterinary Specimens—cont'd

	Blood Agar	MacConkey Agar	Other Characteristics
Gram-Negative			
Escherichia coli	Large, gray, smooth, mucoid colonies; hemolysis variable	Hot pink to red colonies; red cloudiness in media	Hemolysis frequently associated with virulence
Klebsiella pneumoniae	Large, mucoid, sticky, whitish colonies; not hemolytic	Large, mucoid, pink colonies	Nonmotile; require biochemical tests to differentiate from *Enterobacter*
Proteus	Frequently swarming without distinct colonies	Colorless; limited swarming	
Other enterics	Gray to white, smooth, mucoid colonies	Colorless colonies	Biochemical tests for identification; serotyping indicated for *Salmonella*
Pseudomonas	Irregular, spreading, grayish colonies: variable hemolysis; may show a metallic sheen	Colorless, irregular colonies	Oxidase positive; fruity odor; may produce yellow to greenish soluble pigment in clear media
Bordetella bronchiseptica	Very small, circular dew-drop colonies; variable hemolysis	Small, colorless colonies	May require 48 hr for distinct colonies; oxidase positive; rapid urease positive; citrate positive
Brucella canis	Very small, circular, pin-point colonies after 48-72 hr; not hemolytic	No growth	Oxidase positive; catalase positive; urease positive
Moraxella	Round, translucent, grayish-white colonies; variable hemolysis	No growth	Oxidase and catalase positive; often nonreactive in routine biochemical tests; colonies may pit media
Antinobacillus	Round, translucent colonies; variable hemolysis	Variable growth; colorless colonies	Glucose fermenter, nonmotile; urease positive; sticky colonies
Mannheimia haemolytica	Round, gray, smooth colonies; hemolysis under the colony	Variable growth; colorless colonies	Glucose fermenter in TSI; weak oxidase positive
Pasteurella multocida	Gray, mucoid, round to coalescing colonies; no hemolysis	No growth	Glucose fermenter in TSI; weak oxidase and indole positive

TSI, Triple sugar iron (agar).

large jar, a lit candle is put on top of the plates, and the jar is sealed. The candle flame soon dies, leaving a decreased amount of oxygen and increased carbon dioxide in the jar's atmosphere. (This does not create an anaerobic condition.) The plates are incubated for 18 to 24 hours and then checked for growth. If no growth occurs, the plates are reincubated in the candle jar for another 18 to 24 hours and rechecked for growth. Larger laboratories may have incubators that automatically monitor temperature, carbon dioxide and oxygen levels, and humidity.

TABLE 4-3

Bacterial Pathogens of Veterinary Importance

Group	Genera	
Spirochetes	*Leptospira*	*Borrelia*
	Treponema	*Brachyspira*
Spiral and curved bacteria	*Campylobacter* *Helicobacter*	
Gram-negative aerobic bacilli	*Pseudomonas* *Brucella* *Bordatella*	*Francisella* *Neisseria*
Gram-negative facultative bacilli	*Escherichia* *Shigella* *Salmonella* *Klebsiella* *Enterobacter* *Serratia*	*Proteus* *Yersinia* *Citrobacter* *Aeromonas* *Actinobacillus* *Haemophilus* *Pasteurella*
Gram-negative anaerobic bacilli	*Bacteroides* *Fusobacterium*	
Gram-positive bacilli	*Bacillus* *Clostridium* *Lactobacillus*	*Listeria* *Erysipelothrix*
Gram-negative pleomorphic	*Rickettsia* *Ehrlichia* *Anaplasma* *Mycoplasma*	*Haemobartonella* *Eperythrozzon* *Chlamydia*
Gram-positive cocci	*Staphylococcus* *Streptococcus* *Enterococcus*	

Colony Characteristics

An experienced technician can recognize several bacteria on the basis of gross observation of the colonies. Various colony characteristics, including the following, may help identify the bacterium involved (Fig. 4-22):

- Size (in millimeters or described as pinpoint, medium, or large)
- Pigment
- Density (opaque, transparent)
- Elevation (raised, flat, convex, droplike)
- Form (circular, irregular, rhizoid, filamentous, undulate)

PROCEDURE 4-2

Quadrant Streak Method for Isolating Bacteria

1. Use a sterile bacteriologic loop to remove a small amount of the bacterial colony from the culture plate or a loopful from a broth culture
2. *Optional* Divide a plate into 4 quadrants by marking the bottom of the Petri dish with a black marker
3. Hold the loop horizontally against the surface of the agar to avoid digging into the agar when streaking the inoculum
4. Lightly streak the inoculating loop over one quarter (Quadrant A) of the plate using a back-and-forth motion; keep each streak separate
5. Pass the loop through a flame and allow it to cool
6. Place the inoculating loop on the edge of Quadrant A and extend the streaks into Quadrant B using a back-and-forth motion
7. Pass the loop through a flame and allow it to cool
8. Place the inoculating loop on the edge of Quadrant B and extend the streaks into Quadrant C using a back-and-forth motion
9. Pass the loop through a flame and allow it to cool
10. Place the inoculating loop on the edge of Quadrant C and extend the streaks into Quadrant D using a back-and-forth motion

- Texture (glassy, smooth, mucoid, buttery, brittle, sticky)
- Odor (pungent, sweet, etc.)
- Any hemolysis (alpha, beta, gamma)

Culture of Anaerobes

Because most anaerobes survive exposure to air for less than 20 minutes, collection of samples for anaerobic culture on swabs is not acceptable.

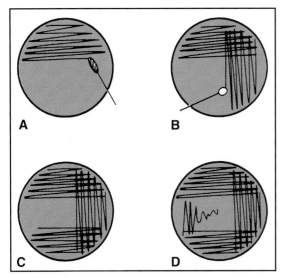

Figure 4-20. Quadrant streak method for isolation of bacteria. (From McCurnin DM, Bassert JM: *Clinical textbook for veterinary technicians,* ed 6, St Louis, 2006, Saunders.)

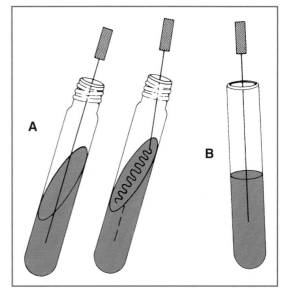

Figure 4-21. Inoculation procedure for tube media. **A,** Inoculation of agar slant and butt, such as triple sugar iron. **B,** Inoculation of motility test media. (From McCurnin DM, Bassert JM: *Clinical textbook for veterinary technicians,* ed 6, St Louis, 2006, Saunders.)

PROCEDURE 4-3

Inoculating Agar Slant and Butt

1. Use a sterile bacteriologic needle to remove a small amount of the bacterial colony from the culture plate or a loopful from a broth culture
2. Stab the needle directly into the center of the agar, pushing the needle all the way down to the bottom of the tube
3. Withdraw the inoculating needle through the same path in the agar
4. Streak the slant using a back-and-forth motion starting at the bottom of the slant

Preferred anaerobic specimens include blocks of tissue (2-inch-cube minimum) in a closed, sterile container, and pus and exudate collected in a sterile syringe, with the air expelled and the needle plugged with a rubber stopper or bent backward on itself. Specialized anaerobic specimen collection systems are also available.

Specimens should be cultured as soon as possible after collection. The specimen is inoculated onto a blood agar plate and into thioglycollate broth. The blood agar plates are put into an anaerobe jar, which provides an anaerobic environment during incubation. A self-contained system, such as a Gas Pack (Oxoid, Columbia, MD.) may be used.

Conditions in which isolation of anaerobes may be significant include soft-tissue abscesses, postoperative wounds, peritonitis, septicemia, endocarditis, endometritis, gangrene, pulmonary infection, and foot rot in cattle, sheep, and swine. The isolated anaerobe may be the sole etiologic agent or a partner in a synergistic relationship with another bacterium. For example, liver abscesses seen at slaughter in otherwise healthy feedlot cattle commonly yield the anaerobe *Fusobacterium necrophorum* and the aerobe *Actinomyces pyogenes*. For conditions involving *Clostridium chauvoei, C. septicum, C. novyi,* and *C. sordellii,* most laboratories use the fluorescent antibody technique in

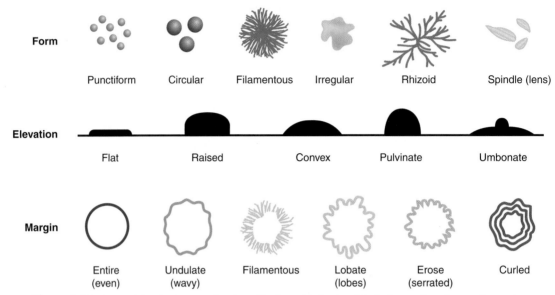

Figure 4-22. Bacterial colonies may be described on the basis of their form, elevation, and margins.

diagnosis. Specimens include affected muscle and a rib containing bone marrow.

Additional Bacterial Testing

Determining the genus of a pathogenic organism is often possible by using just the staining and culture characteristics. This is referred to as a presumptive or tentative identification. Often the presumptive identification gives the veterinarian enough information to develop a diagnostic and treatment plan. However, some organisms must be further differentiated to the species level and require additional testing for positive identification. A partial list of commonly performed tests follows.

Motility

Several methods are commonly used to test motility: the hanging drop prep, the wet prep, and motility media. For a wet prep, a young broth culture is used. A moderately heavy suspension of the bacterial sample is made in a few milliliters of nutrient broth incubated for 2 to 3 hours at room temperature. A loopful of this culture is placed on a microscope slide under a cover slip and examined with the high dry objective. If the bacteria are

obviously motile, with individual cells moving backward or forward among other cells, the answer has been obtained. Brownian movement should not be mistaken for true motility. Brownian movement is the shifting of cells or particles, with little movement relative to each other.

Wet preps tend to evaporate rapidly under the microscope and some bacteria may not appear obviously motile unless provided with additional liquid. The hanging drop prep can eliminate these problems. Special slides are available that contain concave depressions in the center. The slide should be cleaned with alcohol and wiped dry. A small ring of petroleum jelly is placed around the concave area of the slide just before use. To prepare a hanging drop prep, place a drop of bacterial suspension on a cover slip and invert the cover slip onto the concave area of the slide. Press the cover slip down slightly so the petroleum jelly seals the concavity. The suspension will be left hanging upside down into the well of the concave slide. This preparation does not tend to dry out quickly and can be observed for a fairly long period.

If the organisms are nonmotile on microscopic examination, motility media should be used. Two tubes of a motility medium, such as SIM medium, are stab inoculated. One tube is incubated at 37° C and the other at room temperature for 24 to 48 hours. If growth is restricted to the stab inoculation line, the organism is nonmotile. Diffuse growth throughout the medium means the bacterium is motile. To interpret the results, the tubes are held against a good light and the inoculated tubes compared with an uninoculated one. The SIM medium is unsuitable for motility testing of organisms that produce hydrogen sulfide in this medium because the blackening that results may make the motility test difficult to read.

Catalase Test

The catalase test is performed on gram-positive cocci and small gram-positive bacilli. It tests for the enzyme catalase, which acts on hydrogen peroxide to produce water and oxygen. A small amount of a colony from a blood agar plate is placed on a microscope slide and a drop of catalase reagent (3% hydrogen peroxide) is added. If the colony is catalase positive, gas bubbles are produced. No bubble production indicates a negative result.

No blood agar should be transferred with the colony because blood agar can produce a slightly positive reaction. A positive reaction also may occur if a mixed colony is sampled, that is, one with both catalase-positive and catalase-negative organisms growing together. The plate must be carefully streaked to obtain isolated colonies. Staphylococci can be used as catalase-positive controls and streptococci as catalase-negative controls.

Coagulase Test

The coagulase test is performed on catalase-positive, gram-positive cocci. *S. aureus* produces coagulase, an enzyme that coagulates plasma. Two versions of the test are available: the slide coagulase test and the tube coagulase test. The coagulase test is used to differentiate between coagulase-positive *S. aureus, S. intermedius,* and coagulase-negative *Staphylococcus,* such as *S. epidermidis* or *S. saprophyticus.*

The tube coagulase test uses lyophilized plasma (purchased from a medical supply house) diluted according to the manufacturer's directions. Approximately 0.5 ml is placed in a test tube and

inoculated with a loopful of the organism cultured on a noninhibitory medium, such as blood agar. The tube is incubated at 37° C and read hourly for 4 hours. A negative reaction is indicated by no clot formation, whereas a positive reaction is indicated by clots. If the test result remains negative, the sample is incubated again for 24 hours and then read.

The slide coagulase test is a commercially available, rapid screening test that detects surface-bound coagulase or clumping factor. More than 95% of coagulase-producing staphylococci possess clumping factor. A loopful of staphylococci from a colony is first emulsified in a drop of water or saline solution to yield a thick suspension. A drop of fresh rabbit or human plasma is then added and stirred with a sterile loop. A positive reaction is indicated by clumping within 5 to 20 seconds.

Oxidase Activity

This test depends on the presence of cytochrome C oxidase in bacteria. A drop of 1% tetramethyl-*p*-phenylenediamine is added to a piece of filter paper in a Petri dish. The filter paper must be damp but not saturated. Prepared dry reagent slides are also available for performing the oxidase test and eliminate the need for reagent handling. A short streak of the sample is made on the filter paper or prepared slide using a glass rod or the end of a Pasteur pipette that has been bent into a hook. The sample should be applied with a gentle rubbing action. A nickel-chromium wire bacteriologic loop should not be used because any traces of iron may give a false-positive result.

In a positive test, the reagent is reduced to a deep purple color within 60 seconds. If the color-change reaction takes longer than this, the result should be regarded as negative. Oxidase reagent tends to be unstable and becomes discolored with time. It should be discarded if it becomes dark purple. *Pseudomonas aeruginosa* can be used as an oxidase-positive control and *E. coli* as an oxidase-negative control.

Acid Production from Glucose

A tube of 1% glucose in peptone broth, containing a pH indicator, is inoculated and incubated for 24 to 48 hours at 37° C. For fastidious organisms, such as *Streptococcus* species, approximately 5 drops of sterile serum should be added to the peptone water medium or growth may not occur.

ANTIBIOTIC SENSITIVITY TESTING

When bacteria are isolated from a patient, an antimicrobial sensitivity test may be performed to determine the susceptibility or resistance to specific antimicrobial drugs. The results of this test indicate which antimicrobial to use in treatment. Ideally, the specimen used for antimicrobial susceptibility testing is taken from the animal before treatment begins. The veterinarian may begin treatment before obtaining susceptibility results but then may change to a more appropriate drug when the results are available.

Agar Diffusion Method

The agar diffusion test is the most commonly performed method for antimicrobial susceptibility testing and uses paper disks impregnated with antimicrobials. It is quantitative and requires measurement of inhibitory zone sizes to give an estimate of antimicrobial susceptibility. The concentration of drug in the disk is chosen to correlate with therapeutic levels of the drug in the treated animal. Diffusion methods in common use include the U.S. Food and Drug Administration (FDA) method; standardized disk susceptibility method, which is a modified Bauer-Kirby technique; and the International Collaborative Study standardized disk technique. The most commonly used method of antibiotic susceptibility testing is the Kirby-Bauer.

A similar method can be used to determine the minimum inhibitory concentration (MIC) of an antimicrobial. This is the smallest concentration of the specific antimicrobial that can inhibit the growth of a given bacteria. Paper disks with varying concentrations of the chosen antimicrobial are placed on a freshly inoculated culture plate and incubated. Measuring the zones of inhibition around each of these disks will aid in choosing an appropriate concentration of medication to be given to the patient.

Although cultures can be performed in the classic manner by using individual Mueller-Hinton agar plates, modular culture systems or specialized media are more commonly used in the veterinary practice. Some organisms, such as streptococci, do not grow sufficiently well on plain Mueller-Hinton agar for a test to be read. In these cases, Mueller-Hinton agar plus 5% blood must be used. However, having departed from the standardized method, the inhibitory zone sizes must be interpreted with caution. For example, the zone sizes for novobiocin are smaller if the medium contains blood. Most streptococci are still susceptible to penicillin.

A supply of antibiotic disks is needed corresponding to the antibiotics commonly used in the clinic and the dosages most often needed. The antimicrobial content in a disk is indicated in Table 4-4. Only one disk representative each of the tetracyclines and one for the sulfonamides is necessary because of the phenomenon of cross-resistance. For example, if the bacterial species is resistant to one of the tetracyclines, it is usually resistant to all members of the group.

Antimicrobial disks always should be kept in the refrigerator (4° C) when not being used and replaced as soon as possible after use. Outdated disks should never be used. The potency of the antimicrobial disks can be monitored with control organisms of known sensitivity patterns. A disk dispenser and a caliper or clear overlays for measuring inhibitory zones is also required. Disk dispensers should be obtained from the same manufacturer as the disks. Not all products are interchangeable. Inoculation of a thioglycollate or trypticase soy broth tube is recommended at the same time that plates are streaked. If the in-house culture results prove inconclusive, the broth culture can then be sent to an outside laboratory for confirmation.

Indirect sensitivity testing requires that colony samples be taken from the culture plate, subcultured in broth media, and incubated to achieve a turbidity that matches a standardized 0.5 McFarland suspension. The broth suspension is then applied to Mueller-Hinton media with a swab or loop to cover the plate evenly. To obtain the broth solution, just the surfaces of three or four colonies should

TABLE 4-4

Chart of Inhibitory Zones to Determine the Relative Resistance of the Bacterium to the Antibiotics Being Tested

Antimicrobial Agent	Disk Content	Susceptible	Intermediate	Resistant
Amikacin	30 µg	≥17	15-16	≤14
Amoxicillin/clavulanic acid (staphylococci)	20/10 µg	≥20		≤19
Amoxicillin/clavulanic acid (other organisms)	20/10 µg	≥18	14-17	≤13
Ampicillin* (gram-negative enteric organisms)	10 µg	≥17	14-16	≤13
Ampicillin* (staphylococci)	10 µg	≥29		≤28
Ampicillin* (enterococci)	10 µg	≥17		≤16
Ampicillin* (streptococci)	10 µg	≥26	19-25	≤18
Cefazolin	30 µg	≥18	15-17	≤14
Ceftiofur (respiratory pathogens only)	30 µg	≥21	18-20	≤17
Cephalothin†	30 µg	≥18	15-17	≤14
Chloramphenicol	30 µg	≥18	13-17	≤12
Clindamycin‡	≥2 µg	≥21	15-20	≤14
Enrofloxacin	5 µg	≥23	17-22	≤16
Erythromycin	15 µg	≥23	14-22	≤13
Florfenicol	30 µg	≥19	15-18	≤14
Gentamicin	10 µg	≥15	13-14	≤12
Kanamycin	30 µg	≥18	14-17	≤13
Oxacillin§ (staphylococci)	1 µg	≥13	11-12	≤10
Penicillin G (staphylococci)	10 U	≥29		≤28
Penicillin G (enterococci)	10 U	≥15		≤14
Penicillin G (streptococci)	10 U	≥28	20-27	≤19
Penicillin/novobiocin‖	10 U/30 µg	≥18	15-17	≤14
Pirlimycin‖	2 µg	≥13		≤12
Rifampin	5 µg	≥20	17-19	≤16
Sulfonamides	250 or 300 µg	≥17	13-16	≤12
Tetracycline¶	30 µg	≥19	15-18	≤14
Ticarcillin (Pseudomonas aeruginosa)	75 µg	≥15		≤14
Ticarcillin (gram-negative enteric organisms)	75 µg	≥20	15-19	≤14
Tilmicosin	15 µg	≥14	11-13	≤10
Trimethoprim/sulfamethoxazole**	1.25/23.75 µg	≥16	11-15	≤10

Modified from National Committee for Clinical Laboratory Standards document M31-A2, Table 2, pp. 55-59, 2002.

* Ampicillin is used to test for susceptibility to amoxicillin and hetacillin.

†Cephalothin is used to test all first-generation cephalosporins, such as cephapirin and cefadroxil. Cefazolin should be tested separately with the gram-negative enteric organisms.

‡Clindamycin is used to test for susceptibility to clindamycin and lincomycin.

§Oxacillin is used to test for susceptibility to methicillin, nafcillin, and cloxacillin.

‖Available as an infusion product for treatment of bovine mastitis during lactation.

¶ Tetracycline is used to test for susceptibility to chlortetracycline, oxytetracycline, minocycline, and doxycycline.

** Trimethoprim/sulfamethoxazole is used to test for susceptibility to trimethoprim/sulfadiazine and ormetoprim/sulfadimethoxine.

Reprinted from McCurnin DM, Bassert JM: *Clinical textbook for veterinary technicians,* ed 6, St Louis, 2006, Saunders.

be touched with a sterile loop. The loop should be placed in saline or broth to make a suspension. If bacteria are taken from just the surface of the colony, less likelihood exists of picking up an unseen contaminant growing at the base of the colony. More than one colony of a bacterial species always should be taken because a single colony may represent a variant that has a susceptibility pattern different from that of the parent strain. A correct density is an important aspect of getting reproducible results. The "lawn" of cells that grows after inoculation should be evenly distributed. Extremes in concentration must be avoided.

Application of undiluted samples, such as urine, directly to the Mueller-Hinton plate is referred to as direct sensitivity testing. Although not as precise as indirect testing, reasonable results can be expected when only one organism is present. Antibiotic susceptibility should be interpreted with caution when the culture shows multiple organisms.

The antimicrobial disks are placed on the inoculated agar surface with a disk dispenser or sterile forceps that have been flamed and cooled between each use. The disks should be no closer than 10 to 15 mm to the edge of the plate and sufficiently separated from each other to avoid overlapping of the zones of inhibition. Unless the disks were placed with a self-tamping dispenser, use a second sterile swab to gently press the antibiotic disks into the agar. The plates are incubated aerobically at 37° C and should be placed in the incubator within 15 minutes after placing the disks on the inoculated agar. Inoculated plates should be inverted before placing in the incubator to avoid condensation collecting on the surface of the agar. The plates should be kept in stacks of four or fewer because plates in the center of a tall stack take longer to reach incubation temperature.

Whether performed by the direct or indirect method, antibiotic susceptibility must be determined by physical measurement of the inhibitory zones (Fig. 4-23). That measurement is then compared with a chart of inhibitory zones to determine the relative resistance of the bacterium to the antibiotics being tested (see Table 4-4).

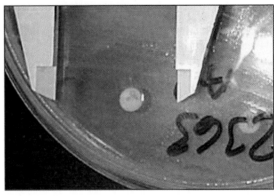

Figure 4-23. The use of a caliper to measure zone of inhibition. (Courtesy of B. Mitzner, DVM.)

Reading the Zones of Inhibition

The plates should be read after a constant period, most satisfactorily after overnight incubation (18 to 24 hours). Prolonged incubation may alter the size of the zone of inhibition with antimicrobials that are not stable at 37° C or at best make the zones hard to read. If rapid results are imperative, the diameters of the zones of inhibition may be read after 6 to 8 hours' incubation. These results should be confirmed by reading them again after overnight incubation. The diameter of each inhibition zone (including the diameter of the disk) is measured from the underside of the plate using calipers, a transparent ruler, or a template. The zones are measured and recorded to the nearest millimeter. If Mueller-Hinton agar with blood has been used, the zone size must be read from the top surface, with the lid of the plate removed.

Interpretation of Zone Sizes

Table 4-4 lists some of the commonly used antimicrobials and gives the suggested interpretation of zone sizes with the FDA standardized disk method. The zone sizes are divided into two major categories: resistant and susceptible to the particular antimicrobial agent. The latter category is subdivided into intermediate susceptibility and susceptible. For predictive purposes, a resistant organism is not likely to respond to therapy with the drug.

A susceptible organism is susceptible to ordinary doses of the antimicrobial. Intermediate susceptibility implies that the organism is susceptible to ordinary doses when the drug is concentrated in the urine or tissues, or the antimicrobial may be used for treatment of systemic infections if a high dosage is safe.

The zone size alone is not indicative of the efficacy of an antimicrobial. Some drugs, such as vancomycin and colistin, do not readily diffuse through agar and give small inhibition zones, even when the test organism is fully susceptible. Therefore direct comparisons of zone diameter, produced by unrelated antimicrobials, are misleading and should not be made.

Control Organisms

Susceptible reference organisms, such as *S. aureus,* American Type Culture Collection (ATCC) 25923, and *E. coli,* ATCC 25922, should be tested regularly, preferably in parallel with each batch of antimicrobial susceptibility tests. These control organisms are used to check such factors as the growth-supporting capability of the medium, potency of antimicrobial disks, and other variable conditions that can affect results.

Limitations of the Test

The FDA method is designed for rapidly growing bacteria. Caution is needed for tests of anaerobes or slow-growing organisms for which the criteria for interpretation of zone diameters have not yet been established with certainty. In general, the zone diameters are somewhat larger for an equivalent minimal inhibitory concentration with slow-growing organisms than with rapid growers.

Some rare strains of staphylococci are resistant to methicillin and other penicillinase-stable penicillins. The routine test cannot be relied on to detect these strains, but they may be detected by incubation of an additional susceptibility test plate, containing a methicillin disk, at 30° C. A reduced zone diameter or no zone surrounding the methicillin disk on the plate incubated at 30° C is presumptive evidence of methicillin resistance.

COLONY COUNT

The presence of pathogenic bacteria does not necessarily indicate infection. For example, although normal urine is considered sterile, small numbers of organisms may occasionally be found even when collecting by cystocentesis. A colony count on cultured urine samples can help support a diagnosis of urinary tract infection. Colony counts can be performed by streaking a blood agar or other nonselective agar plate using a calibrated loop containing 10 µl of urine (Fig. 4-24). After incubation, all colonies are counted and multiplied by 100 to determine the number of colony-forming units (CFUs) per milliliter of urine. Although only a guideline, significant numbers of CFUs are more than 1000 for samples collected by cystocentesis and more than 10,000 for those collected by catheter. Voided samples, although not recommended for culture, should have more than 100,000 CFUs in dogs and 10,000 in cats to be deemed significant.

CALIFORNIA MASTITIS TEST

Mastitis may be caused by bacterial or mycotic organisms. Several laboratory tests are available to diagnose mastitis, including the California mastitis test (CMT), somatic cell count, and milk

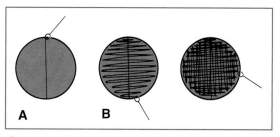

Figure 4-24. Procedure for inoculating media for semiquantitative bacterial colony counts when culturing urine. **A,** Primary inoculation with calibrated loop. **B,** Streak at right angles to previous streak. (Reprinted from McCurnin DM, Bassert JM: *Clinical textbook for veterinary technicians,* ed 6, St Louis, 2006, Saunders.)

culture. A quick check to detect bacteria can be performed by preparing a thin smear of mastotic milk. The smear is heat fixed and stained with Gram stain or methylene blue. The most common microorganisms involved with mastitis are *S. aureus, Streptococcus agalactiae, Streptococcus uberis, E. coli, Corynebacterium* species, and *P. aeruginosa.*

The CMT is a qualitative screening test that can be used as a "cowside" test. The test is based on gel formation when the test reagent reacts with DNA in somatic cells. As the cell count of the milk increases, the gelling action increases. Therefore the test provides an indirect measure of the cell count. The degree of gel formation is scored as negative, trace, 1, 2, or 3, and γ and +.

To perform the CMT, approximately 2 ml of milk is placed in each of the four cups on the CMT paddle and an equal amount of reagent is added. The paddle is gently rotated for approximately 10 seconds in a circular pattern to mix the milk and reagent. A score is then assigned for each quarter according to the chart of grading and interpretation (Table 4-5).

Precautions to be considered in this test are as follows:

1. DNA in somatic cells deteriorates upon standing. If the test is to be used as a laboratory test, the milk samples should be kept refrigerated, but not for more than 48 hours. Unrefrigerated milk cannot be tested accurately after about 12 hours.
2. White blood cells tend to migrate with milk fat. Therefore thorough mixing of samples just before testing is essential.
3. CMT reaction must be scored 10 to 15 seconds after mixing starts. Weaker reactions fade thereafter.

MILK CULTURE

Only positive milk samples identified by CMT or direct somatic cell count should be cultured. The milk sample is inoculated on blood agar and MacConkey agar and incubated at 37° C for 24

hours. Milk samples also are incubated simultaneously. If the cultures show minimal or no growth after 24 hours of incubation, a subculture is made on the blood and MacConkey agar plates from the incubated milk samples. The subcultured plates and the original culture plates are incubated for 24 hours at 37° C. A rapid but presumptive identification of the organism may be made on colonial morphologic characteristics, followed by confirmatory tests (e.g., triple sugar iron, lysine, SIM, methyl red, citrate, coagulase, and/or catalase).

IMMUNOLOGIC EXAMINATION

Numerous immunologic tests are available for identification of bacterial pathogens, particularly obligate intracellular bacteria. See Chapter 8 for more information on immunologic testing.

MYCOLOGY

Fungal Characteristics

Fungi are heterotrophs and may be parasitic or saprophytic. Most are multicellular, except yeasts. They contain eukaryotic cells with cell walls composed of chitin. Fungal organisms consist largely of webs of slender tubes, called hyphae, which grow toward food sources. Fungi digest their food externally, through release of digestive enzymes, then bring the resulting small molecules into the hyphae. Hyphae make up a branching web called a mycelium. Fungal organisms may also have a reproductive structure called a fruiting body that produces and releases reproductive cells called spores. Different groups of fungi produce different types of spores. Yeasts reproduce by budding rather than spore formation.

Most fungi rely on both sexual and asexual reproductive systems. Asexual spores produced by some fungi are either sporangiospores or conidia (Fig. 4-25). Sexual spores include ascospores, basidiospores, and zygospores (Fig. 4-26). Fungi can be differentiated on the basis of structure of the hyphae and on the presence of spores.

TABLE 4-5

Grading of California Mastitis Test Results

Symbol	Meaning	Visible Reaction	Interpretation
—	Negative	Mixture remains liquid with no evidence of a precipitate.	0-200,000 cells/mL 0%-25% PMNs
T	Trace	Slight precipitate forms and is seen to best advantage by tipping the paddle back and forth and observing the mixture as it flows over the bottom of the cup. Trace reactions tend to disappear with continued movement of the fluid.	150,000-500,000 cells/mL 30%-40% PMNs
1	Weak positive	A distinct precipitate but no tendency toward gel formation. With some samples the reaction is reversible. With continued movement of the paddle, the precipitate may disappear.	400,000-1,500,000 cells/mL 40%-60% PMNs
2	Distinct positive	Mixture thickens immediately, with some suggestion of gel formation. As the mixture is swirled, it tends to move toward the center, leaving the bottom of the outer edge of the cup exposed. When the motion is stopped, the mixture levels out again and covers the bottom of the cup.	800,000-5,000,000 cells/mL 60%-70% PMNs
3	Strong positive	Gel formation causes the surface of the mixture to become convex. Usually a central peak remains projecting above the main mass after the motion of the paddle has been stopped. Viscosity is greatly increased, so there is a tendency for the mass to adhere to the bottom of the cup.	Cell number generally 5,000,000/mL, 70%-80% PMNs
+	Alkaline milk pH ≥7.0	This notation should be added to the score when the reaction is distinctly alkaline, as indicated by a contrasting deeper purple color.	An alkaline reaction reflects depressed secretory activity as a result of inflammation or in drying off of the gland.
γ	Acidic milk	Bromcresol purple is distinctly yellow at pH 5.2. This notation should be added to the score when the mixture is yellow.	Distinctly acidic milk in the udder is rare. When encountered, it indicates fermentation of lactose by bacterial action within the gland.

PMN, Polymorphonuclear leukocyte.

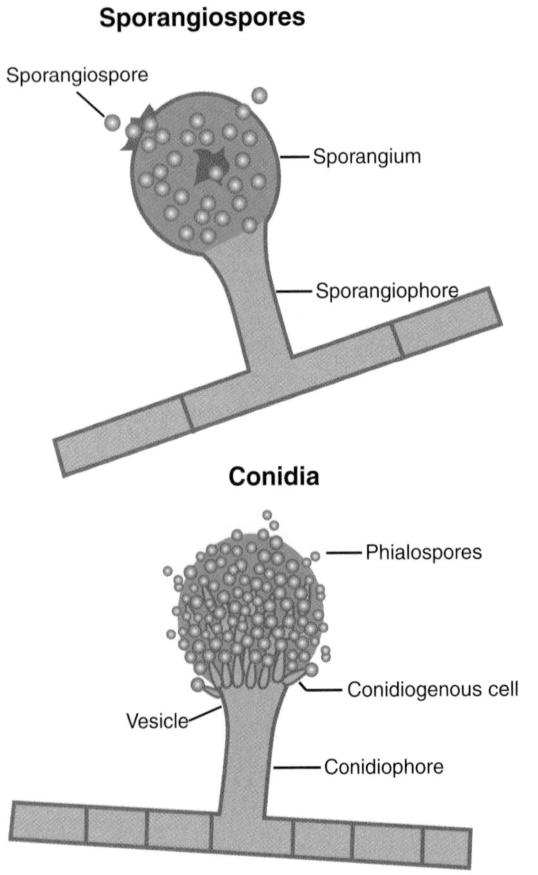

Sporangiospores

Sporangiospore

Sporangium

Sporangiophore

Conidia

Phialospores

Conidiogenous cell

Vesicle

Conidiophore

Figure 4-25. Sporangiospores and conidia, the two main types of asexual spores. (Courtesy Ashley E. Harmon. From Songer JG, Post KW: *Veterinary microbiology: bacterial and fungal agents of animal disease,* St Louis, 2005, Saunders.)

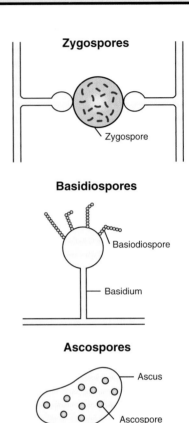

Zygospores

Zygospore

Basidiospores

Basiodiospore

Basidium

Ascospores

Ascus

Ascospore

Figure 4-26. Sexual spores (zygospores, basidiospores, and ascospores) are produced through fusion of the protoplasm and nuclei of two cells by meiosis. (Courtesy Ashley E. Harmon. From Songer JG, Post KW: *Veterinary microbiology: bacterial and fungal agents of animal disease,* St Louis, 2005, Saunders.)

Pathogenic fungal organisms can be categorized into one of the following four groups on the basis of the type of reproductive structures present:

1. Basidiomycetes: the mushrooms or club fungi
2. Ascomycetes: cup fungi
3. Zygomycetes: molds
4. Deuteromycetes: also known as fungi imperfecti because no known sexual stage occurs

Supplies and Equipment

Supplies needed for collection and examination of fungal samples are much the same as those used for bacterial samples. Specifically, forceps, swabs, lactophenol cotton blue stain, potassium hydroxide solution, and culture media (DTM and/or Sabouraud agar). A Woods lamp may prove helpful, and cellophane tape may also be used to collect certain types of samples for fungal analysis.

Ideally a separate room and incubator should be used for fungal culture because fungal spores may contaminate plates used for bacteriologic culture.

If an incubator is inadvertently contaminated with fungal spores, the interior should be swabbed thoroughly with 70% ethyl or isopropyl alcohol, or one bowl of water and one of alcohol should be placed at the bottom of the incubator and the incubator left empty of plates for 24 hours, with the door shut, at 37° C. Table 4-6 summarizes sample collection for mycology samples.

Most fungal agents of clinical importance in the veterinary practice are the cutaneous mycotic organisms, the dermatophytes. These organisms are often referred to as the ringworm fungi because of the characteristic circular lesions on the skin of infected animals. The dermatophytes are saprophytic mycelial-forming fungi that possess keratolytic properties that allow them to invade skin, nails, and hair. Some of these agents can infect human beings.

The dermatophytes comprise more than three dozen different organisms in the taxonomic genera *Microsporum* and *Trichophyton*. The most commonly seen species are *Microsporum canis, M. gypseum,* and *Trichophyton mentagrophytes*. Dermatophytes can be classified by the habitat in which they are most likely to be found: anthropophilic, confined to human beings; zoophilic, parasites of animals; and geophilic, normally existing as free-living saprophytes in the soil. Of the 15 known geophilic species, five may occasionally be opportunist pathogens, and only one, *M. gypseum*, commonly causes lesions in animals. These geophilic species pose a certain difficulty in diagnosis because they must be differentiated from zoophilic species.

Dermatophyte Testing

Most dermatophytes will grow on the outside of the hair shaft and in some cases can be visualized microscopically by mounting in 10% KOH or a combination of KOH and DMSO (DermatoPlate, Vetlab Supply, Palmetto Bay, FL.). The DMSO eliminates the need to warm the slide and provides more rapid clearing of the sample. To examine for dermatophytes, a few hairs plucked from the periphery of the suspect lesion are placed on a slide with 1 or 2 drops of the clearing solution. A cover glass is applied and the slide warmed gently

if using just 10% KOH. After 2 to 10 minutes small globular arthrospores attached to the hair shafts are visible, indicating a positive test result.

A Woods lamp is an ultraviolet light source that may be used to screen suspect lesions for dermatophytes infection, but results may be ambiguous. Hair samples from dogs and cats, or the animals themselves, can be examined under the Woods lamp. Hairs infected with some species of *Microsporum* may fluoresce a clear apple-green under the Woods lamp in a darkened room. Approximately 60% of positive cases involving *Microsporum canis* fluoresce, apparently depending on whether the fungus has reached the right growth stage to produce fluorescence. No fluorescence on Woods lamp examination does not rule out the possibility of ringworm infection.

Several products are available for culturing dermatophytes. The most common is standard dermatophyte test medium (DTM), which contains an indicator that turns red in the presence of most dermatophytes. Rapid sporulation medium (RSM) or enhanced sporulation media (ESM) with color indicators can be used in conjunction with standard DTM to accelerate the formation of macroconidia used for identification and confirmation. Standard Sabouraud dextrose agar will also promote earlier formation of macroconidia but contains no color indicator.

When collecting specimens for dermatophyte culture, clean the skin lesion to remove some of the surface contamination and collect specimens from the lesion periphery. Broken hair shafts and dry scale are most likely to contain viable organisms. Push the specimens into and partially below the surface of the media. Incubate the culture at room temperature with the cap or plate cover loosened and observe daily for growth. At the first sign of color change, perform a wet prep using Fungi-Tape (Scientific Device Laboratory, Des Plaines, IL.) or clear cellophane tape and lactophenol cotton blue stain to confirm the presence of pathogenic forms. Remember, the presence of red coloration (DTM) or teal (ESM and other media) alone is not diagnostic of dermatophyte infection. Both bacterial contaminants and nonpathogenic fungi can, under certain conditions, cause positive color reactions.

TABLE 4-6

Sample Collection for Fungal Testing

Specimen	Container	Comments
Hairs	Paper envelope (dry conditions inhibit overgrowth of bacterial or saprophytic fungal contaminants)	Wash and dry affected area with soap and water. With forceps, epilate hairs from the periphery of an active lesion. Pull hairs in the direction of growth to include the root. Look for broken, stubby hairs, which are often infected. Useful for diagnosis of dermatophytosis.
Skin	Paper envelope	Clean skin with alcohol gauze sponge (cotton leaves too many fibers). Scrape the periphery of an active lesion with a sterile scalpel blade. Also obtain crusts and scabs. Useful for diagnosis of dermatophytosis.
Nails	Paper envelope	Proven nail infections in animals are rare. Cleanse affected nail with alcohol gauze. Scrape with a scalpel blade so that fine pieces are collected. Also collect debris under the nail. Useful for diagnosis of onchyomycosis.
Biopsy	Sterile tube in sterile saline or water	Normal and affected tissue should be included. Important to prevent specimen desiccation.
Urine	Sterile tube	Centrifuge and use sediment for direct examination and culture. Useful for diagnosis of histoplasmosis.
Cerebrospinal fluid	Sterile tube	Useful for diagnosis of cryptococcosis. Make India ink preparation to observe encapsulated yeasts.
Pleural/abdominal fluid	Sterile tube	If fluid contains flakes or granules, they should be included because these are actual colonies or organisms.
Transtracheal/bronchial washings	Sterile tube	Centrifuge and use sediment for direct examination and culture. Useful for diagnosis of systemic mycoses.
Nasal flush	Sterile tube	Centrifuge and use sediment for direct examination and culture. Useful for diagnosis of nasal aspergillosis and guttural pouch mycosis.
Ocular fluid	Sterile tube or syringe	Examine directly. Inoculate onto plated fungal media immediately after collection. Useful for diagnosis of ocular blastomycosis.

From Songer JG, Post KW: *Veterinary microbiology: bacterial and fungal agents of animal disease,* St Louis, 2005, Saunders.

Therefore a diagnosis must be supported by microscopic examination.

Fungal Cultures

Cultures of nondermatophytes are usually streaked out on blood agar or Sabouraud dextrose agar, as for bacteria. For fungal organisms that do not produce spores, cultures may be prepared by cutting 1 cm² agar from the center of a Sabouraud dextrose agar plate with a sterile scalpel. A square of the same size is taken from the edge of the colony to be subcultured. This square is made to fit snugly into the hole in the agar. Taking material for subculture from the edge of a fungal colony is always advisable because the old mycelia at the center of the colony may not be viable.

Fungi that can invade tissue grow at body temperature (37° C). This temperature for incubation of primary cultures of nondermatophytes inhibits many contaminant saprophytic species. The exception to this is examination of specimens for dimorphic fungi, such as *Blastomyces* and *Histoplasma* species. These organisms grow as yeasts when at body temperature and as molds at 25° C. Cultures should be incubated, in parallel, at both temperatures. Characteristics of the systemic dimorphic fungi of veterinary importance are located in Table 4-7.

Because many pathogenic fungi, such as *Candida albicans* and *Aspergillus fumigatus,* are ubiquitous, tissue sections showing invasion may be needed for definitive diagnosis of a mycotic infection. Occasionally, myceliate fungi or yeasts may appear on blood agar plates put up for bacteriology. These fungi or yeasts, of course, may be contaminants, but some of the original specimen, in 10% formalin, should be submitted for histopathologic examination. Examination of a KOH wet preparation for fungal elements is also useful. Table 4-8 summarizes the characteristics of common yeasts of veterinary importance.

After incubation, cultures can be examined to identify the types of spores present. This is done by taking about 2.5 inches of clear cellophane tape and pressing the center of the tape, sticky side down, onto the center of the colony. The tape, with hyphae and fruiting heads adhering to it, is placed with the sticky side down on a microscope slide that has a drop of lactophenol cotton blue on it. The tape acts as its own cover slip. The slide preparation is examined under low power or high dry if necessary. Additional information on microscopic appearance of fungi is located in Table 4-9.

VIROLOGY

Virologic techniques are performed in specialized laboratories. They include histopathologic and serologic examination, electron microscopy, and attempted isolation and identification of the virus. The veterinary technician should contact the diagnostic laboratory to check which facilities

TABLE 4-7

Characteristics of the Systemic Dimorphic Fungi

Agent	Ecology	Saprobic Form	Parasitic Form
Blastomyces dermatitidis	Slightly acidic soils and wood; possible association with animal excreta, water sources, beaver dams	Hyphae, oval to pyriform terminal and lateral conidia, 2-10 μm in diameter	Unencapsulated yeasts with thick, refractile double walls; 5-20 μm in diameter
Coccidioides immitis	Alkaline desert soils with high levels of salt and carbonized organic materials	Hyphae with thick-walled or barrel-shaped arthroconidia alternating with thin-walled empty (disjunctor cells)	Spherules, 10-100 μm in diameter, with doubly refractile cell walls and containing endospores, 2-5 μm in diameter
Histoplasma capsulatum	Humid environments with highly nitrogenous soils, especially those contaminated with bird or bat droppings	Hyphae, globose microconidia, and tuberculate and nontuberculate macroconidia, 8-16 μm in diameter	Tiny, ovoid, budding yeasts with narrow bases, 2-4 μm in diameter

Reprinted from Songer JG, Post KW: *Veterinary microbiology: bacterial and fungal agents of animal disease,* St Louis, 2005, Saunders.

TABLE 4-8

Characteristics of Yeasts of Veterinary Importance

Genus	Pseudohyphae	True Hyphae	Blastoconidia	Arthroconidia	Urease	Growth at 25°C with Cycloheximide	Growth at 37°C on Potato Dextrose Agar
Candida	+	+	+	−	−	Var	+
Geotrichum	−	+	−	+	−	−	−
Malassezia	−	−	−	−	+	+	+
Trichosporon	+	−	+	+	+	+	+

Var, Variable.
From Songer JG, Post KW: *Veterinary microbiology: bacterial and fungal agents of animal disease,* St Louis, 2005, Saunders.

TABLE 4-9

Microscopic Appearance of Fungi in Clinical Specimens

Disease	Microscopic Examination Method	Appearance
Aspergillosis	Wet mount (lactophenol cotton blue or KOH)	Septate hyphae with dichotomous branching; may see fruiting heads
Blastomycosis	Wet mount	Thick, double-walled budding yeasts with broad bases of attachment to mother cells
Candidiasis and other yeast infections	Wet mount	Budding and nonbudding yeasts; pseudohyphae may be present
Coccidioidomycosis	Wet mount	Spherules with and without endospores
Cryptococcosis	India ink	Encapsulated yeasts
Dermatophytosis	Wet mount	Hairs with arthrospores (endothrix or ectothrix), hyphae or sheath of spores around skin and nails
Histoplasmosis	Hematologic stain	Small yeasts with narrow necks of attachment to mother cells, often within macrophages
Mycetoma	Wet mount	Dark brown chlamydospores and hyaline hyphae in crushed granules
Phaeohyphomycosis	Wet mount	Dark hyphae
Pneumocystosis	Hematologic stain	Cysts and trophozoites
Protothecosis	Wet mount	Spherical to oval nonbudding, small and large cells containing two or more autospores
Rhinosporidiosis	Wet mount	Spherules (some large) with and without endospores
Sporotrichosis	Hematologic stain	Small oval to round to cigar-shaped yeasts
Zygomycosis	Wet count	Broad, relatively nonseptate hyphae

KOH, Potassium hydroxide.
From Songer JG, Post KW: *Veterinary microbiology: bacterial and fungal agents of animal disease,* St Louis, 2005, Saunders.

are available, which samples are preferred, and whether a transport medium is necessary. If an exotic (reportable) disease is suspected, the proper authorities should be notified and no clinical material removed from the farm.

Many of the viral diseases encountered may be diagnosed on clinical and pathologic grounds. Serologic tests are available for most viral diseases. These usually require paired serum samples collected 2 to 3 weeks apart, early in the disease and on recovery. A rising antibody titer indicates recent infection by the virus. Collection of serum samples from contact animals is worth considering because these animals are more likely to have low initial titers to the virus.

Virus isolation is expensive and time-consuming and may provide only a diagnosis after the animals have recovered or died. However, in some instances isolation and identification of a virus should be attempted, such as to establish the identity of a viral disease not previously seen in a practice, discover the exact agent when serologic and other tests have given equivocal results, find the immunologic type of a virus in an epizootic, and verify the etiologic agent if a public health problem is involved.

Isolation of a virus from a diseased animal does not necessarily mean the virus caused the disease because many viruses can persist in animals without clinical signs of illness. Some other pathogen or condition could have been responsible for the disease. Virus isolation is most successful when specimens are collected early in the active infectious phase of the disease.

Viruses vary greatly in their ability to remain viable in tissues and exudates. Contamination with bacteria greatly decreases the success of attempted virus isolation. Specimens should be selected on the basis of their likelihood to contain large numbers of virus particles. They should be collected from live or very recently dead animals, even if this means sacrificing an affected animal. Samples for virology testing must be collected aseptically, kept at 4°C, and taken to a laboratory in the shortest time possible.

Collection of Specimens

Viruses are often present in the nasal or pharyngeal secretions early in the acute stage of respiratory diseases. Mucosal scrapings rather than swabs of the secretions should be taken. Sterile wooden tongue depressors are useful for mucosal scrapings. Attempted isolation from blood samples may be considered in generalized catarrhal diseases that tend to have a viremic stage. Poxviruses often may be demonstrated by electron microscopy in fluid from early vesicular lesions and sometimes in scabs from early lesions.

Specimens should also be selected for indirect studies, such as serologic, hematologic, histologic, and bacteriologic examinations. Viral diseases often are complicated by pathogenic bacteria acting as secondary invaders, which often can turn a mild viral infection into a serious disease. Specimens for histopathologic examination should consist of thin sections of tissue placed immediately in 10% formalin. Sections for histologic examination must never be frozen because this causes tissue artifacts that may be difficult to differentiate from a pathologic process.

Tissue samples for attempted virus isolation should be 2-inch cubes that contain both diseased and normal tissue, if possible. Mucosal scrapings should be obtained instead of swabs. Sterile screw-capped containers should be used for collection, with a separate container for each sample. Veterinary technicians must use strict aseptic technique and label the containers carefully.

Submission of Samples

Specimens should be refrigerated (4° C) when possible because virus titers decrease as temperature increases. If the specimens are to be delivered to the virology laboratory within 24 hours, they may be stored at 4° C and packed with coolant packs or ice in a polystyrene-insulated carton for shipment. If the time delay will be longer than 24 hours, snap freezing at −70° C and shipping on dry ice is desirable, except for specimens of suspected parainfluenza and influenza virus, in which case the integrity of these viruses is best preserved at −20° C. Specimens must be shipped in airtight containers to prevent entry of carbon dioxide into the container. Carbon dioxide gas from the dry ice can lower the pH of fluid, killing any pH-labile viruses.

Small pieces of tissue, fecal material, or mucus can be preserved in vials filled with 50% glycol and stored at 4° C. A virus transport medium is available commercially (NCS Diagnostics, Mississauga, ON, Canada). Because viruses vary in their longevity, a reference laboratory should be contacted for recommendations on the appropriate transport medium and sampling procedure.

Fecal materials and fluids often are submitted for electron microscopic examination. A fixative, such as universal or 10% buffered neutral formalin, should be added to the sample at a maximum of 1:1 fixative to sample to prevent overdilution of virus particles.

For urine samples, approximately 5 ml is sent in a sterile container. Virus transport medium should not be used. The specimen must be kept chilled if it is to arrive at the laboratory within 24 hours of collection; otherwise, it should be frozen at −270° C and shipped frozen.

If blood samples have been collected for serologic examination, they should be left at room temperature and the clot allowed to retract. Then they are refrigerated. Blood samples should not be frozen because freezing causes hemolysis and may render serum samples useless for serologic examination.

Cell Culture

To demonstrate the presence of a virus in a specimen, the virus is grown (isolated) in the laboratory, or the virus antigens or antibodies are assayed. Unlike bacteria, which can be grown on nutrient agar, viruses need living cells in which to grow and replicate. The tissue cells are placed into a suitable glass bottle or chamber containing a medium rich in nutrients. The cells settle and begin to grow in a confluent monolayer across the surface of the container. Various types of cells have been used for tissue culture of viruses. Most animal cells can be grown in vitro for some generations, but some cells divide indefinitely and are used for virus isolation. These cells are called continuous cell lines and are of a single type of cell. Continuous cell lines, such as those from fetal kidney, embryonic trachea, skin, and other cells, are derived from monkeys, dogs, cattle, pigs, cats, mice, hamsters, rabbits, and other animals. The virus specimen is commonly inoculated into a primary culture of cells derived from the same species of animal from which the specimen was taken.

After the cell culture has been inoculated with the virus specimen and incubated, it is examined. If the virus is present, cell damage may be visible as the virus particles invade the tissue cells. This damage is referred to as a cytopathic effect. Different types of cytopathic effects are used to identify viruses. Some viruses cause cell lysis, and others cause the cells to fuse and form syncytiae (sheets) and giant cells. An inclusion body is another type of cytopathic effect that may be seen.

Immunologic Examination

Clinical signs and cell culture examination may identify the virus to a family level and perhaps to the genus and species level, but definitive identification requires serologic procedures based on immunologic principles. Sometimes these serologic procedures may be used on the specimens directly, which saves the time and expense of cell culture. Chapter 8 contains more details on the immunologic tests used for detection of viral antigens and antibodies.

Recommended Reading

Anthony A, Sirois M: Microbiology, cytology, and urinalysis. In Sirois M: *Principles and practice of veterinary technology,* ed 2, St Louis, 2004, Mosby.

Hirsh DC, Walker RL, Maclachlan NJ, editors: *Veterinary microbiology,* ed 2, Ames, IA, 2004, Iowa State Press.

Latimer KS, Prasse KW, Mahaffey EA: *Duncan and Prasse's veterinary laboratory medicine: clinical pathology,* Ames, IA, 2003, Blackwell.

Songer J, Post K: *Veterinary microbiology: bacterial and fungal agents of animal disease,* St Louis, 2005, Saunders.

CHAPTER 5

Urinalysis

Lisa Martini-Johnson

KEY POINTS

- Consistency in laboratory methods is the key to obtaining accurate urinalysis results.
- The best samples for urinalysis are morning samples or samples collected after several hours of water deprivation.
- Preferred methods of urine collection are cystocentesis and catheterization.
- All samples should be labeled immediately after collection.
- Urine samples should be analyzed within 30 minutes to 1 hour of collection.
- Always note the method of urine sample collection on the urinalysis report.
- If the sample cannot be examined within 1 hour of collection, it should be refrigerated or preserved.
- A refrigerated sample should be allowed to warm to room temperature before evaluation.
- Physical properties of urine include volume, color, odor, transparency, and specific gravity.
- Normal urine of most animals is yellow to amber in color and clear.
- Specific gravity is most commonly determined by a refractometer.
- Isosthenuria occurs when the urine specific gravity approaches that of glomerular filtrate (1.008 to 1.012).
- Testing of chemical properties of urine uses dry reagent strips.
- The manufacturer's directions must be precisely followed regarding the timed intervals and color analysis when using the reagent strips.
- Subdued light must be used when examining sediment under the microscope.
- The fine adjustment knob on the microscope should be continuously adjusted to see structures.
- To identify different cell types and bacteria accurately, the high power objective (40×) is used.
- Red blood cells in urine sediment have several different appearances depending on the concentration, pH, and time elapsed between collection and examination.
- White blood cells are larger than red blood cells and are identified by the characteristic granules or the lobulations of the nucleus.
- Casts are formed in the lumen of the distal and collecting tubules of the kidney.
- Casts are cylindrical structures with parallel sides present in acid urine.
- Crystal formation depends on the urine pH, concentration, and temperature and the solubility of the elements.

Urinalysis is a relatively simple, rapid, and inexpensive laboratory procedure. It evaluates the physical and chemical properties of urine, as well as the sediment. A urinalysis provides information to the veterinarian on the status of the urinary system, metabolic and endocrine systems, and electrolyte and hydration status. Therefore the veterinarian may request that the owner bring a urine sample for initial testing.

SPECIMEN COLLECTION

The first step in performing a urinalysis is proper collection of a urine sample, which must be carefully obtained to ensure accurate results. Analysis of urine samples should be performed only on samples taken before administration of therapeutic agents. Urine specimens may be obtained by natural voiding of urine, bladder expression, catheterization, or cystocentesis. The two preferred methods are cystocentesis and catheterization; these methods provide optimal samples for all aspects of urinalysis by avoiding contamination from the distal genital tract and external areas. Collecting samples by voiding or expression of the bladder may be easier, but urine collected in these ways may be of limited diagnostic value. Except for cytologic examination, performing a urinalysis on preprandial morning samples is best. Morning samples tend to be the most concentrated and least affected by dietary factors, which increases the chances of finding formed elements.

Voided or "Free Catch" Sample

The easiest sample to obtain is the voided sample, which is collected as the animal urinates. A sample collected in this manner is not satisfactory for bacteriologic examination because it is often contaminated during urination. Occasionally voided samples contain increased white blood cell (WBC) counts because of contamination from inflammatory lesions of the distal genital tract. Results of other evaluations are usually unaffected.

A voided sample is collected in a clean, although not necessarily sterile, container. If possible, the vulva or prepuce should be washed to decrease contamination of the sample before collection. Animals' owners may not be able to do this because they may be asked to collect a sample when the animal spontaneously urinates. Furthermore, the cleansed tissue in the external orifice area does not remain clean for long. A midurination (midstream) sample is best because it is less likely to be contaminated. However, the initially voided urine is sometimes collected as a precaution against not being able to collect a midurination sample.

Dogs may begin to urinate and then stop when collection is attempted. Chances of successfully obtaining urine may be increased by attaching a paper cup to a long pole and collecting the sample without disturbing the animal. A voided sample from a cat is difficult to obtain. Occasionally cats urinate in an empty litter box. Veterinarians prefer to give cat owners nonabsorbent granules to use in the litter box. Cows may be stimulated to urinate by rubbing a hand or dry hay ventral to the vulva in a circular fashion. Sheep may be stimulated to urinate by occluding their nostrils. Horses may be stimulated to urinate by rubbing a warm, wet cloth on their ventral abdomen or by placing them in a clean stall with fresh hay.

Bladder Expression

Urine may be collected in small animals by manual compression of the bladder. Samples obtained in this manner are also unsatisfactory for bacteriologic culturing. As with collection of a voided sample, the external genitalia should be cleansed before bladder expression. With the animal standing or in lateral recumbency, the bladder is palpated in the caudal abdomen and gentle, steady pressure is applied. Care must be taken not to exert too much pressure and injure or rupture the bladder. Relaxation of the bladder sphincters often takes a few minutes. Occasionally an increase in red blood cells (RBCs) will be found because of pressure applied to the bladder and an increase in WBCs resulting from contamination originating in the distal genital tract. If bacteria are in the urine, the kidneys may become infected from these bacteria. This method should never be used on animals whose urethra may be obstructed or whose bladder wall may be fragile because excessive pressure can cause the bladder to rupture. In large animals, urination may be stimulated by maintaining pressure on the bladder through the rectal wall while performing rectal palpation.

Catheterization

Catheterization is the insertion of a polypropylene or rubber catheter into the bladder by way of the urethra. A variety of catheters exist for different species and sexes. As with the previous two methods of collection, the external genitalia should be cleansed before the procedure. Sterile catheters should always be used and sterile gloves worn. Care must be taken to maintain sterility and prevent trauma to the urinary tract. This method may be used for culture and sensitivity if a cystocentesis cannot be performed. For female animals a speculum improves visualization of the urethral orifice and thus facilitates the catheterization. The catheter should pass easily through the urethra. A small amount of sterile, water-soluble lubricating jelly, such as K-Y Jelly (Johnson & Johnson, Arlington, TX), should be placed on the tip of the catheter. Care must be taken to avoid trauma to the sensitive urethral mucosa. The distal end of many catheters is designed for attachment to a syringe so that urine can be collected with gentle aspiration. Collection into a sterile syringe is especially advantageous if bacteriologic culture is anticipated. Often the first portion of the sample obtained is discarded because of possible contamination as the catheter was advanced through the distal urethra. Occasionally an increase in RBCs and epithelial cells may be seen in the sample because of urethral mucosa damage from the catheter.

Cystocentesis

Cystocentesis is used often to collect sterile urine samples from dogs and cats only when the bladder is sufficiently distended so that it can be easily isolated. This procedure should be performed only on calm, easily restrained patients (Fig. 5-1). An ultrasound-guided cystocentesis may also be performed. The bladder must be palpated before the

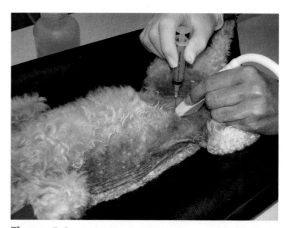

Figure 5-1. Collection of a urine sample through ultrasound-guided cystocentesis.

procedure to avoid damage to other internal organs. When performing a cystocentesis, a 22- or 20-gauge needle by 1 inch or $1\frac{1}{2}$ inches and a 10-ml syringe should be used. Once the needle is through the skin, it should never be redirected because of the potential for damage to other internal organs. With the animal in lateral recumbency or ventral recumbency or standing, the bladder is gently palpated and immobilized and the needle is inserted into the caudal abdomen. For male dogs, insert the needle caudal to the umbilicus and to the side of the sheath. For female dogs and for cats, insert the needle on the ventral midline caudal to the umbilicus. Gently aspirate urine into the syringe and properly label it with the patient information. This sample can also be used for culture and sensitivity testing. Occasionally samples contain an increase in RBCs caused by bladder trauma. The urine S-Monovette system (Sarstedt AG & Co., Nümbrecht, Germany) is a commercially available urine collection device that consists of a sterile, individually wrapped syringe with a disposable tube (Fig. 5-2). This system can simplify cystocentesis collection and minimizes the potential for contamination when samples are transferred between a syringe and collection tube. The sample is drawn directly into the tube. The tube can also be centrifuged for urine sediment examination. A special tip is also included to collect catheter specimens.

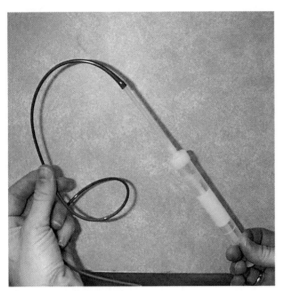

Figure 5-2. Urine S-Monovette system. (Courtesy of B. Mitzner, DVM.)

All the aforementioned methods of collection are satisfactory for qualitative analysis. However, for quantitative analysis, a 24-hour sample must be collected. Ratios of certain urine constituents, such as protein/ creatinine, have recently been used to obtain data that may be interpreted in a similar manner to 24-hour urinary excretions.

QUALITY ASSURANCE

Quality assurance begins with proper specimen identification and handling. All samples should be labeled immediately after collection, and urinalysis should be performed as soon as possible. Reagent strips and tablets must be kept in tightly sealed bottles, and outdated reagents must be replaced with fresh reagents. Reactions for most constituents in urine may be checked against available controls (e.g., Chek-Stix, Bayer Corporation, Leverkusen, Germany; Uritrol, YD Diagnostics, Seoul, Korea; Liquid Urine Control, Kenlor Industries, Inc., Santa Ana, CA). In addition, urine samples with distinct reactions for certain constituents sometimes may be preserved and used as positive controls. The results obtained from control samples and made-up

controls should be plotted to determine whether observer drift or reagent decomposition is occurring. The urinalysis laboratory report should include patient information, collection technique, date and time collected, method of preservation (if used), complete urinalysis results, including the results of microscopic examination results. Precision and accuracy need to be maintained by the veterinary technician for proper interpretation of results.

SPECIMEN STORAGE AND HANDLING

Ideally, samples should be analyzed within 30 minutes to 1 hour of collection to avoid post-collection artifacts and degenerative changes. If immediate analysis is not possible, refrigeration preserves most urine constituents for an additional 6 to 12 hours. Refrigeration may have an impact on urine specific gravity, so this test should be done before refrigeration. If a urine sample is going to be refrigerated, it should have a tight-fitting lid to prevent evaporation and contamination. Crystals may form when the urine cools. Decreased glucose and bilirubin concentrations, increased pH resulting from bacterial breakdown of urea to ammonia, crystal formation with increased sample turbidity, breakdown of casts and RBCs (especially in dilute or alkaline urine), and bacterial proliferation may occur in samples allowed to stand for long periods at room temperature. Many crystals may form in refrigerated samples. Refrigerated urine should be warmed to room temperature before evaluation, and crystals that formed during cooling may not dissolve when the sample is brought to room temperature. The urine sample should be mixed by gentle inversion before evaluation so that formed elements are evenly distributed. Cells tend to break down rapidly in urine, so if cytologic evaluation is to be performed, the urine should be centrifuged soon after collection and 1 to 2 drops of the patient's serum or bovine albumin added to the sediment to preserve cell morphologic characteristics.

Samples to be transported to an outside laboratory or held for longer than 6 to 12 hours may be preserved by adding one of the following: 1 drop of 40% formalin in 1 oz of urine; toluene sufficient to form a layer on top of the sample; a single thymol crystal; or one part 5% phenol to nine parts urine. If formalin is used as a preservative, chemical tests should be performed before the addition of formalin because it interferes with some chemical analyses, especially that for glucose. Formalin, however, is the best preservative for formed elements in urine.

PHYSICAL PROPERTIES

Physical properties of urine include all the observations that may be made without the aid of a microscope or chemical reagents. Volume, color, odor, transparency, and specific gravity of urine are evaluated. (Procedure 5-1 describes the procedure for a routine urinalysis.)

Urine Volume

The animal's owner often provides information concerning the amount of urine passed. However, owners may mistake frequent urination, or pollakiuria, for increased urine production, or polyuria. Therefore obtaining an estimate of the amount of urine an animal is producing is important. Many factors unrelated to disease influence the amount of urine produced. Some of these factors include fluid intake, external losses (especially through the respiratory system and the intestinal tract), environmental temperature and humidity, amount and type of food, level of physical activity, size of the animal, and species. Observing a single urination is not reliable for estimating urine output of an animal. Ideally, 24-hour urine volume should be determined,

PROCEDURE 5-1

Routine Urinalysis

1. Prepare a laboratory sheet with patient information, date, time, and method of urine collection.
2. If sample was refrigerated, make note on the record and allow the sample to warm to room temperature.
3. Properly mix the sample.
4. Record the physical characteristics: color, clarity, volume, and odor of sample by gentle inversion.
5. Calibrate the refractometer with distilled water to 1.000.
6. Determine and record the specific gravity of the sample.
7. Dip a reagent test strip into the urine sample and remove promptly, making sure to lightly tap the edge of the strip onto a paper towel to remove excess urine.
8. Read the pad's color at the appropriate time intervals as stated by the manufacturer's directions and record the results.
9. Properly label a 15-ml conical centrifuge tube.
10. Pour approximately 5-10 ml of the urine sample into the centrifuge tube.
11. Centrifuge the sample for 5 to 6 minutes at 1000-2000 rpm.
12. Make note of the amount of sediment.
13. Pour off the supernatant, leaving approximately 0.5 to 1 ml in the tube.
14. Resuspend the sediment by gently mixing with a pipette or flicking the tube with the fingers.
15. Transfer a drop of reconstituted sediment to a microscope slide with a transfer pipette and place a cover slip over it.
16. Alternatively, place 1 drop of Sedi-Stain to 1 drop of urine on a microscope slide and place a cover slip over it.
17. Subdue the light of the microscope by partially closing the iris diaphragm.
18. Examine the entire specimen under the cover slip with the high power (40×) objective to identify cells, casts, crystals, and bacteria.
19. To aid in the detection of these elements, the fine adjustment knob should be continuously focused.
20. Record results.

TABLE 5-1

Normal Daily Urine Production for Domestic Species

Species	Daily Urine Output (ml/kg)
Dogs	20-40
Cats	20-40
Cattle	17-45
Horses	3-18
Sheep and goats	10-40

TABLE 5-2

Significance of Urine Colors

Color	Significance
Pale Yellow	low SG; decrease concentration of urine
Very Yellow	high SG; oliguria (yellow-brown)
Brown/Green	bile pigment (plus green foam)
Red/Brown	hematuria; hemoglobin
Brown	myoglobin
Orange	drugs (e.g., tetracycline)

although this is often impractical. Observing an animal in its cage or outdoors may provide a rough estimate of the volume of urine being produced. Table 5-1 lists the approximate daily urine production for common domestic species. The amount of urine produced per day is variable. Normal urine output for adult dogs and cats is approximately 20 to 40 ml/kg body weight per day.

An increase in daily urine output or production is termed polyuria and is usually accompanied by polydipsia. Polydipsia is defined as an increase in water consumption. With polyuria the urine is usually pale or light yellow in color and has a low specific gravity. Polyuria occurs in many diseases, including nephritis, diabetes mellitus, diabetes insipidus, pyometra in dogs and cats, and liver disease. It also is seen after administration of diuretics, corticosteroids, or fluids.

Oliguria, a decrease in daily urine output, may occur when an animal has restricted access to water. It can be severe when the environmental temperature increases and causes excess water loss through the respiratory system. With oliguria the urine is usually concentrated and has a high specific gravity. Oliguria also occurs with acute nephritis, fever, shock, heart disease, and dehydration. Anuria, the absence of urine production, may be seen in complete urethral obstruction, urinary bladder rupture, and renal shut down.

Color

Normal urine color is light yellow to amber as a result of the presence of pigments called urochromes. The magnitude of yellow color in urine varies with the degree of urine concentration or dilution (Table 5-2). Colorless urine usually has a low specific gravity and is often associated with polyuria. Dark yellow to yellow-brown urine generally has a high specific gravity and may be associated with oliguria. Yellow-brown or green urine that produces a greenish-yellow foam when shaken is likely to contain bile pigments. Red or red-brown urine indicates the presence of RBCs (referred to as hematuria) or hemoglobin (referred to as hemoglobinuria). Urine that is brown when voided may contain myoglobin (referred to as myoglobinuria) excreted during conditions that cause muscle cell lysis, such as rhabdomyolysis in horses. Some drugs may alter the color of urine; red, green, or blue urine may be observed. When observing urine it should be in a clear plastic or glass container against a white background to be properly evaluated for color.

Clarity/Transparency

In most species freshly voided urine is transparent or clear. Normal equine urine is cloudy because of a high concentration of calcium carbonate crystals and mucus secreted by glands in the renal pelvis. Normal rabbit urine also has high concentrations of calcium carbonate crystals and appears milky. When observing urine for the degree of transparency, it should be placed against a letter-print background. Transparency is noted as clear, slightly cloudy, cloudy, or turbid (flocculent) depending on how well the letters can be read through the sample. Clear samples usually do not have much sediment on centrifugation. Cloudy samples usually contain large particles and often yield a significant amount of sediment on centrifugation. Urine may become cloudy while standing because of bacterial multiplication or crystal formation. Substances that cause urine to be cloudy include RBCs, WBCs, epithelial cells, casts, crystals, mucus, fat, and bacteria. Other causes of turbidity can include contaminants from the collection container or surface and contamination with feces. Flocculent samples contain suspended particles that are sometimes large enough to be seen with the naked eye.

Odor

The odor of urine is not highly diagnostic but sometimes may be helpful. Normal urine has a distinctive odor that varies among species. The urine of male cats, goats, and pigs has a strong odor. An ammonia odor may occur with cystitis caused by bacteria that produce urease (*Proteus* spp. or *Staphylococcus* spp.) that has metabolized urea to ammonia. Samples left standing at room temperature may occasionally develop an ammonia odor as a result of bacterial growth. A characteristic sweet or fruity odor to urine indicates ketones and is most commonly found with diabetes mellitus, ketosis in cows, and pregnancy disease in ewes.

Specific Gravity

Specific gravity is defined as the weight (density) of a quantity of liquid compared with that of an equal amount of distilled water. The number and molecular weight of dissolved solutes determine the specific gravity of urine. Specific gravity may be determined before or after centrifugation because the particles that settle during centrifugation have little or no effect on specific gravity. Whichever method is used to perform the specific gravity in a specific clinic, whether before or after centrifugation, the same method must be consistently performed by all clinic personnel. If the urine is turbid, the sample should be centrifuged and the supernatant used to determine the specific gravity. The specific gravity of urine from polyuric patients tends to be low, and urine from oliguric patients tends to be high. The specific gravity of normal urine depends on eating and drinking habits, envi-

ronmental temperature, and when the sample was collected. An early morning, midurination sample tends to be the most concentrated. Interpretation of urine specific gravity yields information on the hydration status and the ability of the kidneys to concentrate or dilute urine. Specific gravity of normal animals is extremely variable and fluctuates throughout the day. Table 5-3 lists the urine specific gravity ranges for normal domestic animals. In normal dogs the urine specific gravity may range from 1.001 to 1.060 and in normal cats from 1.001 to 1.080.

To determine specific gravity of urine, the refractometer, urinometer, or reagent strips can be used. Urine specific gravity is less frequently determined by use of a urinometer. This instrument requires a large amount of urine (approximately 10 ml) and generally provides less-reproducible results than a refractometer.

Refractometer
Specific gravity is most commonly determined by a refractometer. More information on the principle of the refractometer is presented in Chapter 1. Urine contains substances that absorb various wavelengths of light. The light waves bend as they pass through the medium, and this bend is measured by the refractometer. The refractive index of a fluid is influenced by the same factors that determine specific gravity and therefore provides an estimate of urine specific gravity.

Reagent Strips
Several reagent strips have been developed to determine urine specific gravity. Reagent strip specific gravity is the least reliable method for determining urine specific gravity in animals.

Causes of Altered Urine Specific Gravity
Increased urine specific gravity is seen with decreased water intake, increased fluid loss through sources other than urination (e.g., sweating, panting, diarrhea), and increased excretion of urine solutes. Decreased water intake in animals with normal renal function rapidly causes increased urine specific gravity. Increased urine specific gravity may occur in acute renal failure, dehydration, and shock.

TABLE 5-3

Urine Values for Common Domestic Species

Dog	Cat	Horse	Cattle	Sheep
Specific Gravity				
1.025	1.030	1.035	1.015	1.030
(1.001-1.060)	(1.001-1.080)	(1.020-1.050)	(1.005-1.040)	(1.020-1.040)
pH				
6-7	6-7	7-8.5	7-8.5	6-8.5
Glucose				
None	None	None	None	None
Protein				
None/trace	None/trace	None	None/trace	None/trace
Bilirubin				
None/trace	None/trace	None/trace	None	None/trace
Ketones				
None	None	None	None	None
Occult Blood				
None	None	None	None	None

Decreased urine specific gravity is seen in diseases in which the kidneys cannot resorb water and with increased fluid intake, such as with polydipsia or excessive fluid administration. Pyometra, diabetes insipidus, psychogenic polydipsia, some liver diseases, certain types of renal disease, and diuretic therapy may also cause decreased urine specific gravity.

Isosthenuria occurs when the urine specific gravity approaches that of glomerular filtrate (1.008 to 1.012). In other words, urine with this specific gravity range has not been concentrated or diluted by the kidneys. Animals with chronic renal disease frequently produce isosthenuric urine. In animals with kidney disease, the closer the specific gravity is to isosthenuric, the greater the amount of kidney function that has been lost. When these animals are deprived of water, their urine specific gravity usually remains in the isosthenuric range. Animals with decreased renal function are often slightly to moderately dehydrated and have urine specific gravity slightly greater than isosthenuric (1.015 to 1.020).

CHEMICAL PROPERTIES

Testing for various chemical constituents of urine is usually performed with reagent strips that are impregnated with appropriate chemicals or reagent tablets. The container of reagent strips must be stored at room temperature with the lid tightly closed. The expiration date should also be noted. Some reagent strips simultaneously test for numerous constituents, and other strips exist for individual tests. Urine is added to the reagent strip from a pipette, or the strips are dipped in the urine sample and the color changes are noted at specific time intervals. The concentration of various constituents is determined by comparing the colors on the strip with the color chart on the label of the strip container (Fig. 5-3). The manufacturer's directions must be carefully followed.

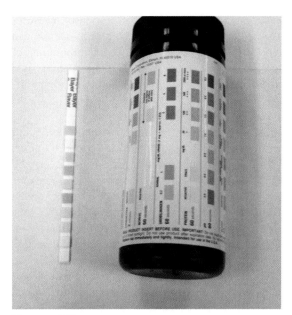

Figure 5-3. Reagent strip test container and combination dipstick strip.

pH

The pH expresses the hydrogen ion (H^+) concentration. Essentially, pH is a measure of the degree of acidity or alkalinity of urine. A pH above 7.0 is alkaline, whereas a pH below 7.0 is acidic. Proper technique must be used to obtain accurate results. The urine sample must be fresh to obtain accurate results. The pH of samples left standing open at room temperature tends to increase resulting from a loss of carbon dioxide, whereas delays in reading the reaction may lead to color changes and false readings. If samples containing urease-producing bacteria (*Proteus* spp. or *Staphylococcus* spp.) are left standing, the pH is usually increased.

The kidneys play a role in acid-base regulation of the body. Kidneys must vary the pH of urine to compensate for diet and products of metabolism. The pH of a healthy animal's urine depends largely on its diet. Alkaline urine usually is found in animals on plant diets, whereas high-protein cereal diets or diets of animal origin cause acidic urine. Therefore herbivores normally have alkaline urine, carnivores have acidic urine, and omnivores have either acidic or alkaline urine depending on what was ingested. Many dog foods contain substantial amounts of plant material that may cause the urine to be slightly alkaline. Nursing herbivores have acidic urine from the consumption of milk. Other factors such as stress and excitement, especially in cats, increase the urine pH and may create a transient glucosuria. Table 5-3 lists the normal urine constituents and characteristics, including pH, for common domestic species.

Urine pH is usually measured with reagent strips or a pH meter. Factors that may decrease the pH (acidity) include fever, starvation, high-protein diet, acidosis, excessive muscular activity, or administration of certain drugs. Increased pH (alkalinity) may be caused by alkalosis, high-fiber diets (plants), infection of the urinary tract with urease bacteria, use of certain drugs, or urine retention such as occurs with urethral obstruction or bladder paralysis. If the pH of the urine is too acidic or too alkaline specific crystals or uroliths can form. The pH can be manipulated with diet to help dissolve the solids or prevent them from forming.

Protein

Protein is usually absent or present in only trace amounts in normal urine obtained by catheterization or cystocentesis. In healthy animals, plasma proteins that pass into the glomerular filtrate are resorbed in the renal tubules before the filtrate reaches the renal pelvis. However, voided samples or those obtained by expressing the bladder may contain a small amount of protein from secretions that may contaminate urine during its passage along the urinary tract. Trauma to the urinary tract that results from cystocentesis, catheterization, or bladder expression may occasionally cause sufficient bleeding that results in a trace of protein in the urine. Urine protein measurements are interpreted in light of the collection method, urine specific gravity, rate of urine formation, and contributions from any hemorrhage or inflammation noted by sample analysis. Protein levels in the urine may be measured by several methods, including reagent test strips, sulfosalicylic acid turbidity test, and urine protein/creatinine ratio.

Protein Determination by Reagent Test Strips

Urine dipsticks allow semiquantitative measurement of protein in urine by progressive color changes on the reaction pad. Reagent strip analysis is a rapid, convenient, and reasonably accurate method of determining urinary protein levels. The accuracy of these methods is variable. Reagent strips primarily detect albumin (protein soluble in water) and are much less sensitive to globulins (proteins insoluble in water). False-positive results may occur in alkaline urine depending on factors such as diet, urinary tract infection, or urine retention (urethral obstruction). Protein measurements considered excessive or pathologic should be confirmed by sulfosalicylic acid turbidity test or specific biochemical analysis. Microalbuminuria is the presence of an abnormal amount of albumin (1 to 30 mg/dl) in urine that is not detected by the reagent strip method. The reagent strip method detects urine protein concentrations that are greater than 30 mg/dl. The albumin-capture enzyme linked immunosorbent assay (ELISA) method is used to measure albumin levels 1 to 30 mg/dl in the urine (Fig. 5-4). See Chapter 8 for more information on the principles of ELISA tests.

Protein Determination by Sulfosalicylic Acid Turbidity Test

Sulfosalicylic acid turbidity determines urine protein levels by acid precipitation. The resultant turbidity is proportional to the concentration of protein. Results are compared with levels in prepared standards and thus may be reported in semiquantitative units. The advantage of this method is that it is equally sensitive to albumin and globulins and is quite useful to confirm strip methods, especially in alkaline urine. This test also measures Bence Jones proteins (light chain proteins that can pass through the glomerulus). Components of extremely alkaline urine may interact with the acid and decrease the amount of protein precipitated.

Urine Protein/Creatinine Ratio

This test is used to help confirm significant amounts of protein in the urine. To determine its significance, urine protein concentration can be compared with that of creatinine. The sample is centrifuged to separate particulate matter (cells) from dissolved substances (protein) and the creatinine and protein concentration of the supernatant is used. The ratio is obtained by dividing the protein concentration by the creatinine concentration. The ratio is not affected by urine concentration and volume and therefore aids in the accurate assessment of urine protein loss in patients with low specific gravity.

Interpretation of Protein in Urine

Very dilute urine may yield a false-negative result because the protein concentration may be below the sensitivity of the testing method. A trace amount of protein in a very dilute sample may be clinically significant because dilute urine often occurs when a large volume of urine is being produced, such as in a patient with chronic renal failure.

Occasionally a small amount of protein is found in the urine of normal animals. Transient proteinuria may result from a temporary increase in glomerular permeability, allowing excessive protein to enter the filtrate. This condition is caused by increased pressure in the glomerular capillaries and may be found with muscle exertion, emotional stress, or convulsions. Occasionally a small amount of urine protein is found after parturition, during the first few days of life, and during estrus. The presence of protein in the urine is usually abnormal and is primarily attributable to disease of the urinary tract (or possibly the genital system).

In most cases proteinuria indicates disease of the urinary tract, especially of the kidneys. Both acute and chronic renal diseases lead to proteinuria. Acute nephritis is characterized by marked

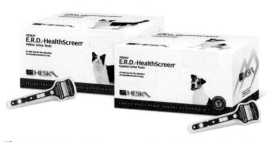

Figure 5-4. An in-house test for microalbuminuria.

proteinuria with WBCs and casts in the urine, whereas in chronic renal disease the degree of proteinuria is qualitatively less. However, in chronic renal disease urine output is usually excessive with low specific gravity; therefore the total protein excreted is actually quite significant. The ratio of urine protein to creatinine is used to determine the degree of protein loss in chronic renal disease.

Multiple myeloma, a cancer of plasma cells, may produce large quantities of light chain proteins (Bence Jones protein) that may leak through the glomerulus. In patients with myeloma, proteins may be passed in the urine because they have damaged the glomerulus or because they are the "light chains" that freely pass through the glomerulus. Because these proteins do not react with the protein pads on the reagent strips, the sulfosalicylic acid method is necessary to detect and quantify them.

Mild proteinuria is seen with passive congestion of the kidneys, as in congestive heart failure or any other impediment of blood flow from the kidneys. Proteinuria of renal origin may also be caused by trauma; tumors; renal infarcts; or necrosis resulting from drugs and chemicals such as sulfonamides, lead, mercury, arsenic, and ether.

Inflammation of the urinary or genital tract may cause proteinuria of postrenal origin. Proteinuria also may be seen with traumatic catheterization or bladder expression.

Glucose

The presence of glucose in urine is known as glucosuria or glycosuria. Glucose is filtered through the glomerulus and resorbed by the kidney tubules. The amount of glucose in the urine depends on blood glucose levels and the rates of glomerular filtration and tubular resorption. Glucosuria usually does not occur in normal animals unless the blood glucose level exceeds the renal threshold (approximately 170 to 180 mg/dl for dogs). At this concentration tubular resorption cannot keep up with the glomerular filtration of glucose, and glucose passes into the urine.

Glucosuria occurs in diabetes mellitus as a result of a deficiency of insulin or an inability of insulin to function. Insulin is necessary to transport glucose into body cells, and a deficiency causes hyperglycemia and spilling of glucose into the urine. A high-carbohydrate meal may lead to blood glucose levels exceeding the renal threshold and thus glucosuria. Because of this, a period of fasting is recommended before urine glucose concentration is determined. Fear, excitement, or restraint, especially in cats, often causes hyperglycemia and glucosuria as a result of epinephrine release. Glucosuria often occurs after intravenous administration of fluids containing glucose and occasionally after general anesthesia. Rarely glucosuria is found in hyperthyroidism, Cushing's disease, and chronic liver disease. A rare condition called renal glucosuria may occur when the blood glucose concentration is in the normal range. Renal glucosuria is caused by reduced resorption of glucose in the renal tubules. Glucosuria may occur in some cats with chronic disease, possibly as a result of altered proximal renal tubular function.

False-positive results for glucose may be seen after the use of various drugs, including ascorbic acid (vitamin C), morphine, salicylates (e.g., aspirin), cephalosporins, and penicillin.

Various reagent test strips are available to detect glucose in urine. Clinitest Reagent Tablets (Bayer Corporation) are also available. These tablets detect any sugar in the urine, whereas most reagent test strips detect only glucose.

Ketones

Ketones include acetone, acetoacetic acid, and β-hydroxybutyric acid. Ketone bodies are formed during incomplete catabolism of fatty acids. Normal animals may have small amounts of ketones in the blood. Conditions characterized by altered carbohydrate metabolism may result in excessive amounts of fat catabolism to provide energy. When fatty acid metabolism is not accompanied by sufficient carbohydrate metabolism, excess ketones are present in the urine, a condition called ketonuria.

A common cause of ketonuria is ketonemia, or ketosis, in lactating cows and pregnant ewes and cows. Ketosis usually occurs early in lactation (3 to 6 weeks after freshing), when the energy for milk production exceeds the capacity of the cow to ingest sufficient feed to meet its energy requirements. In ewes, this condition is called pregnancy toxemia and is seen when the ewe is carrying twins or triplets. Ketosis is associated with hypoglycemia and is caused by carbohydrate intake insufficient to meet energy requirements. Body fat is then rapidly metabolized, resulting in ketonemia and ketonuria.

Ketonuria frequently occurs in animals with diabetes mellitus. Because the animal lacks the insulin necessary for carbohydrate metabolism, fat is broken down to meet the animal's energy needs and excess ketones are excreted in the urine. Ketones are important sources of energy and are normally produced during fat metabolism. Problems develop, however, when excessive ketones are produced. Ketones are toxic, causing central nervous system depression and acidosis. Acidosis resulting from ketonemia is termed ketoacidosis.

Ketonemia with ketonuria also occurs with high-fat diets, starvation, fasting, long-term anorexia, and impaired liver function. With a high-fat diet, carbohydrates meet a relatively low percentage of energy needs, so a great amount of fat is used to meet energy needs. In the fasting, starved, or anorexic animal, body fat is used to meet energy needs, producing a greater than normal amount of ketones. With liver damage, impaired carbohydrate metabolism leads to fat serving as the main energy source, especially when the damaged liver cannot store adequate amounts of glycogen.

Measurement of Urine Ketone Content

Urinary ketones are detected by using urinary reagent strips with a ketone reagent pad. The color intensity is roughly proportional to the concentration of urine ketones. These methods are most sensitive to acetoacetic acid and less sensitive to acetone and do not detect β-hydroxybutyric acid. β-Hydroxybutyric acid is the first ketone produced by the body in any condition that causes ketosis. Urine reagent test strips may not adequately identify these patients until the ketosis has been present for some time.

Bile Pigments

Bile pigments commonly detected in urine are bilirubin and urobilinogen. Only conjugated bilirubin (water soluble) is found in urine because unconjugated bilirubin does not pass through the glomerulus into the renal filtrate; it is bound to albumin and is not water soluble. Normal dogs, especially males, occasionally have bilirubin in their urine because of a low renal threshold for conjugated bilirubin and the ability of their kidneys to conjugate bilirubin. Many normal cattle also have small amounts of bilirubin in their urine. Bilirubin is usually not found in the urine of cats, pigs, sheep, or horses. In cats the renal threshold is many times that of dogs, and any amount of bilirubin in the urine is considered abnormal and suggests disease.

Bilirubinuria is seen in a number of diseases, including obstruction of bile flow from the liver to the small intestine and in liver disease. Bilirubinuria results from accumulation in hepatic cells of conjugated bilirubin that is released into the blood and excreted in the urine. Conditions causing biliary obstruction include calculi in the bile duct, tumors in the area of the bile duct, acute enteritis, pancreatitis, and obstruction of the upper intestinal tract. When conjugated, bilirubin enters the bloodstream after being released from damaged liver cells and passes into the urine.

Hemolytic anemia (RBC destruction) may also cause bilirubinuria, especially in dogs. In hemolytic anemia, the liver's ability to metabolize the excess bilirubin may be exceeded, resulting in release of conjugated bilirubin into the blood and ultimately bilirubinuria. In dogs, unconjugated bilirubin from hemoglobin catabolism in the mononuclear phagocytic system can be conjugated in the kidney and passed in the urine.

Bilirubinuria is detected with the Ictotest (Bayer Corporation). A diazo compound in reagent the tablet reacts with bilirubin to produce a blue or purple color. The speed with which the color change occurs and the degree of color change indicates the amount of bilirubin present. Reagent strips are less sensitive than Ictotest tablets. Urine to be tested for bilirubin must not be exposed to light because bilirubin is broken down by short-wave light. False-negative results for bilirubin occur in urine that is exposed to sunlight or artificial light.

In the intestines, bacteria convert bilirubin to stercobilinogen and urobilinogen. The bulk of these products are excreted in the feces, but some are resorbed into the bloodstream and excreted by the liver into the intestinal tract. A small amount of resorbed urobilinogen is excreted by the kidneys into the urine. Urobilinogen in a urine sample is considered normal. The reliability of screening tests for detection of urobilinogen is questionable because of the instability of urobilinogen.

Blood (Hemoprotein)

Tests for blood in urine detect hematuria, the presence of intact RBCs in urine; hemoglobinuria, the presence of free hemoglobin in urine; and myoglobinuria, the presence of myoglobin in the urine. Hematuria, hemoglobinuria, and myoglobinuria may occur simultaneously. The presence of one does not rule out the others. The urine sediment should also be examined for intact RBCs.

Hematuria

Hematuria usually is a sign of disease causing bleeding somewhere in the urogenital tract, whereas hemoglobinuria usually indicates intravascular hemolysis. Some systemic conditions may also cause hematuria. In very dilute or highly alkaline urine, RBCs often lyse to yield hemoglobin. Therefore in dilute or highly alkaline urine, hemoglobinuria may not be the result of hemoglobin entering the urine through the glomerulus. Ghost cells (the shells of lysed RBCs) may be seen on microscopic examination of sediment if the source of hemoglobin is lysis of RBCs within the excretory pathway or in vitro.

Moderate to large amounts of blood impart a cloudy red, brown, or wine color to urine. Similar colors, but with a transparent appearance that remains after centrifugation, indicate hemoglobinuria. With minute amounts of blood in the urine, a visible color change usually is not evident. Occult, or hidden, blood occurs when the urine is not obviously discolored by blood but blood is detected by chemical analysis. More information on hematuria is found in the section on microscopic examination of urinary sediment.

Hemoglobinuria

Hemoglobinuria is usually the result of intravascular hemolysis. Hemoglobin from RBCs broken down intravascularly is normally bound to the plasma protein haptoglobin. When hemoglobin is bound to haptoglobin, it does not pass through glomeruli. If intravascular hemolysis overwhelms the binding ability of haptoglobin, hemoglobinemia leads to hemoglobinuria because free hemoglobin filters through glomeruli. Hemoglobinuria is indicated by a positive test for hemoglobin without RBCs in the urine sediment, or the degree of the test reaction is often greater than may be accounted for by the numbers of RBCs in the urine sediment. When hemoglobin concentration is sufficiently high in the urine to impart red discoloration, the urine remains red after centrifugation. If the discoloration is from intact RBCs, the urine is clear above the pellet after centrifugation. Partial clearing after centrifugation indicates both hemoglobinuria and hematuria. The presence of hemoglobin (either as free hemoglobin or in RBCs) must be confirmed by urine dipstick test and further evaluation by microscopic examination.

Hemoglobinuria may be seen with many conditions that cause intravascular hemolysis. Conditions that can cause intravascular hemolysis include immune-mediated hemolytic anemia, isoimmune hemolytic disease of neonates, incompatible blood transfusions, leptospirosis, babesiosis, certain heavy metals (e.g., copper), and ingestion of certain poisonous plants. Other conditions that cause hemoglobinuria include severe hypophosphatemia, postparturient hemoglobinemia in cattle, and hemolysis that occurs when cattle drink large quantities of water after being unable to obtain water (e.g., after a long period of low temperatures has frozen their usual water source).

If the urine is dilute or very alkaline, hemoglobinuria can originate from lysis of RBCs in the urine. This condition must be considered hematuria because intact RBCs were initially present. Often ghost RBCs may be found when hemoglobinuria is caused by release of hemoglobin from RBCs in vitro.

Because the test for blood in the urine detects hemoglobinuria, hematuria, and myoglobinuria, other considerations include sediment examination, history, physical examination findings, and additional laboratory procedures to determine the cause of the positive test for blood in the urine.

Myoglobinuria

Myoglobin is a protein found in muscle. Severe muscle damage causes myoglobin to leak from muscle cells into the blood. Myoglobin passes through the glomeruli and is excreted in the urine. Urine containing myoglobin is usually very dark brown to almost black, but at low concentrations the urine may have a similar color to that seen with hemoglobin. Distinguishing myoglobinuria from hemoglobinuria may be difficult. History and clinical findings that suggest muscle damage help determine whether a positive hemoglobin test is due to the presence of myoglobin. Myoglobinuria is frequently seen in horses with exertional rhabdomyolysis.

Several methods have been used to try to distinguish hemoglobin from myoglobin. None of the methods is completely reliable. They sometimes may be differentiated on the basis of their different molecular weights and different solubility in ammonium sulfate.

Leukocytes

Presumptive evidence of leukocytes (WBCs) in urine may be obtained with the leukocyte reaction of certain reagent strips. However, many false-negative reactions occur with animal species, and microscopic evaluation is necessary to confirm a positive result. The leukocyte reagent strip test is not valid for cats because of false-positive results.

MICROSCOPIC EXAMINATION OF URINE SEDIMENT

Microscopic examination of urine sediment is an important part of a complete urinalysis, especially for recognizing diseases of the urinary tract. Many abnormalities in a urine sample cannot be detected with reagent test strips or tablets, but often more specific information may be obtained by obser-

vation of the urine sediment. In addition, urine sediment examination is occasionally an aid in diagnosing systemic disease. In human medicine, microscopic analysis of urine sediment is usually performed only when patients are symptomatic or abnormalities are evident on the physical and chemical urine examinations. However, many veterinary practitioners routinely request a urine sediment examination on every urine sample.

With the exception of horse and rabbit urine, normal urine of domestic animals does not contain a large amount of sediment. Small numbers of epithelial cells, mucus threads, RBCs, WBCs, hyaline casts, and crystals of various types can be found in the urine of normal animals. The urine of horses and rabbits usually has large amounts of calcium carbonate crystals. Urine must be collected cleanly because bacteria and aberrant substances may be present in a urine sample that has been contaminated during collection.

The best samples for sediment examination are morning samples or samples collected after several hours of water deprivation. Because such samples are more concentrated, the chances of finding formed elements are increased. Sediment should be examined while the urine is fresh because bacteria will multiply if allowed to stand at room temperature for a period of time. Also, as previously discussed, other changes may occur in a sample as it ages. Crystals may form as the sample cools and casts may dissolve in alkaline urine. If a voided sample is collected, a midstream sample is preferred because it is less likely to be contaminated by cells, bacteria, and debris from the external genital surfaces. Urine collected by cystocentesis is the best sample for microscopic examination. If the sample cannot be examined within 1 hour of collection, it should be refrigerated or preserved.

For semiquantitative measurements of the formed elements in urine, the volume of urine used and the volume of sediment obtained should be recorded. If a sufficient volume has been obtained, 5 to 10 ml of a well-mixed sample should be placed in a graduated, conical centrifuge tube and centrifuged for 3 to 5 minutes at approximately 1000 to 2000 rpm depending on the radius of the centrifuge. Excessive force compacts the sediment and may distort or disrupt formed elements. The procedure should be standardized for a particular centrifuge to yield uniform results. After centrifugation, the volume of sediment is recorded, and the supernatant is gently poured off, leaving approximately 0.5 ml of urine in the bottom of the tube. The sediment is resuspended by gently flicking the bottom of the centrifuge tube with the fingers or by mixing gently with a pipette (Procedure 5-2).

The Kova urine sediment system (Hycor Biomedical Inc., Garden Grove, CA) provides a method for standardization of initial sample volume, the volume of sample used to resuspend the packed sediment, and the distribution of elements on the slide. Each specimen is processed in a specially shaped conical plastic tube with a flared opening for easy filling. When the supernatant is poured off after centrifuging, a fixed volume is retained along with the sediment. The specially designed pipette is then used to dispense a fixed volume of the resuspended sediment into a special chambered slide for microscopic examination (Fig. 5-5).

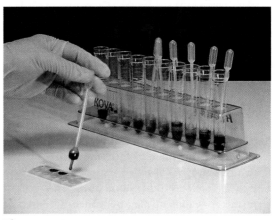

Figure 5-5. The Kova urine sediment system. (Courtesy of B. Mitzner, DVM.)

This unique system provides an even distribution of microscopic elements that improves visualization.

The sediment may be examined stained or unstained. Examining the sediment unstained first allows better evaluation of the specimen. To exam-

PROCEDURE 5-2

Preparing Urine Sediment for Microscopic Examination

1. Pour approximately 10 ml of the urine sample into a labeled conical centrifuge tube.
2. Centrifuge the sample for 3 to 6 minutes at 1000 to 2000 rpm.
3. Pour off the supernatant leaving approximately 0.5 to 1 ml in the tube.
4. Resuspend the sediment by flicking the tube with your fingers or gently mixing the sediment and supernatant with a pipette.
5. Transfer a drop of resuspended sediment near the end of a microscope slide with a transfer pipette and place a coverslip over it.
6. *Optional.* Add 1 drop of Sedi-stain or new methylene blue to 1 drop of urine sediment on the other end of the microscope slide and place a coverslip over it.
7. Subdue the light of the microscope by partially closing the iris diaphragm.
8. Scan the entire unstained slide for the presence of large formed elements such as casts and clusters of cells.
9. Examine the entire specimen under the coverslip with the high power (40 x) objective to identify and quantify formed elements. Use the stained sediment as needed to confirm identification of formed element.
10. Examine a minimum of 10 microscopic fields with the high power lens.
11. Record results. Report cells and bacteria in numbers/HPF and casts in numbers/LPF. The report can list either the average number seen in 10 microscope fields or a range representing the lowest and highest number of each element seen in 10 microscopic fields.

ine unstained sediment, a small drop of the suspended sediment is placed on a clean glass slide, covered with a cover slip, and examined immediately. Subdued light that partially refracts the elements must be used to examine unstained urine sediment. This is achieved by partially closing the diaphragm and adjusting the condenser downward until optimal contrast is achieved. If too much light is present, some structures may be missed. The fine adjustment knob of the microscope should be continuously adjusted to see the depth of the object, as well as other structures. The use of stain in the sediment may help identify different cell types. However, stains often introduce artifacts into the sediment, particularly precipitate material and bacteria. Available urine sediment stains include Sternheimer-Malbin stain (Sedi-Stain, Becton, Dickinson, Franklin Lakes, NJ) (Fig. 5-6) or 0.5% new methylene blue containing a small amount of formalin. One drop of stain is mixed with the suspended sediment before placing a drop of sediment on a microscope slide. A cover slip is placed over the drop of stained sediment. The amount of illumination is less critical when examining a stained specimen than with an unstained one, although reduced illumination also aids visualization of substances by providing contrast. Quantifying elements in the sediment should never be done with a stained slide because the stain dilutes the sample significantly. One method that may simplify the urinalysis procedure is to prepare two drops of urine sediment side by side on the same microscope slide (Fig. 5-7). One drop has stain added and can be used to identify cells while the unstained side is used to quantify elements in the urine.

The specimen must be initially scanned under low power (10× objective) to evaluate the overall quality of the preparation and identify larger elements, such as crystals or aggregates of cells. The entire area under the cover slip should be examined because casts tend to migrate toward the edge of the cover slip. Casts and crystals are identified and reported as the number observed per low power field (lpf). The high power lens (40× objective) is necessary to identify most objects accurately, detect bacteria, and differentiate cell types. A minimum of 10 microscopic fields with a

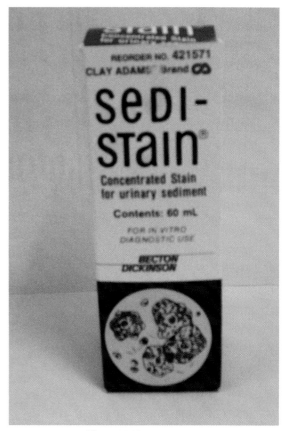

Figure 5-6. Sedi-Stain.

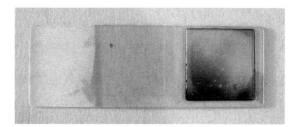

Figure 5-7. Stained and unstained urine sediment prepared for microscopic examination.

high-power lens should be observed. Epithelial cells, RBCs, and WBCs are reported as the average number observed per high power field (hpf). Bacteria are reported as few, moderate, or many, and their morphologic characteristics (cocci, bacilli) are noted. Alternatively, elements can be reported as a range seen. For example, 1 to 4 cells per high power field would indicate that nearly every microscopic field examined had at least one cell and some had as many as four. Bacteria and crystals may also be semi-quantified using a scale of +1 to +4.

CONSTITUENTS OF URINE SEDIMENT

Normal urine sediment in healthy animals may contain a few casts; crystals; epithelial cells; RBCs; WBCs; mucus threads and, in males or recently bred females, spermatozoa. Fat droplets, artifacts, and contaminants may also be seen. If more than a few erythrocytes, leukocytes, hyperplastic and/or neoplastic epithelial cells, casts, crystals, parasite ova, bacteria, and yeast are identified in urine sediment, it is considered abnormal and further diagnostic tests should be performed.

Erythrocytes

Erythrocytes (RBCs) may have several different appearances depending on the urine concentration, pH, and time elapsed between collection and examination. In a fresh sample, RBCs are small, round, usually smooth edged, somewhat refractile, and yellow or orange, but they may be colorless if their hemoglobin has diffused during standing (Figs. 5-8 and 5-9). RBCs are smaller than WBCs and may have a smooth, biconcave disk shape (Fig. 5-10). In concentrated urine, RBCs shrink and

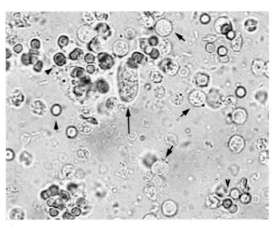

Figure 5-9. Unstained urine sediment with a cast *(long arrow)* and several RBCs *(arrowheads)* and WBCs *(short arrows).* (Reprinted from VanSteenhouse JL: Clinical pathology. In McCurnin DM, Bassert JM, editors: *Clinical textbook for veterinary technicians,* ed. 6, St Louis, 2006, Saunders.)

crenate. Crenated RBCs have ruffled edges, are slightly darker, and may even appear granular as a result of membrane irregularities (see Fig. 5-10). In dilute or alkaline urine, RBCs swell and may lyse. Swollen RBCs have smooth edges and are pale yellow or orange. Lysed RBCs may appear as colorless rings (shadow cells or ghost cells) that vary in size (see Fig. 5-10). However, lysed RBCs, especially when resulting from marked alkalinity, often dissolve and cannot be found on microscopic examination. Normally, urine sediment contains fewer than 2 to 3 RBCs per high power field.

Because mammalian RBCs contain no nucleus, they may be confused with fat globules and yeast. However, their light yellow or orange color usually allows them to be differentiated from these other elements. Furthermore, variation in RBC size is minimal, whereas fat globules vary in size. Erythrocytes in urine usually indicate bleeding somewhere in the urogenital tract or occasionally in the genital system. A voided sample from a female in proestrus or estrus or after parturition may be contaminated with RBCs. Both females and males with inflammatory conditions in the genital system may have RBCs in urine collected by free catch or expression of the bladder. Urine collected by catheterization from females with inflammatory lesions in the

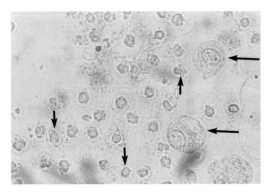

Figure 5-8. Unstained urine showing crenated RBCs *(short arrows)* and two epithelial cells *(long arrows).* (Reprinted from Raskin RE, Meyer DJ: *Atlas of canine and feline cytology,* St Louis, 2001, Saunders.)

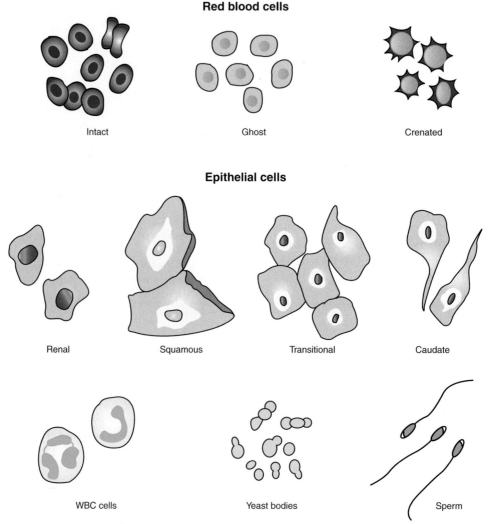

Figure 5-10. Cell types that may be found in urine.

genital tract usually is not contaminated, but urine from males with genital tract inflammation may be contaminated. Even the slight trauma that occurs from catheterization, cystocentesis, and manual expression of the bladder may slightly increase the number of RBCs in the sediment. Generally, cystocentesis does not cause much increase in RBC numbers. The veterinary technician should note the method of urine collection on the laboratory report to help determine the significance of RBCs in urine.

Leukocytes

Leukocytes (WBCs) are larger than erythrocytes and smaller than renal epithelial cells. Leukocytes are spherical and can appear as a dull gray or greenish-yellow color. They are identified in urine sediment by their characteristic granules or by lobulations of the nucleus (Fig. 5-11). Their appearance is attributable to the fact that most WBCs in urine are neutrophils, which contain a large number of granules. Few leukocytes are found

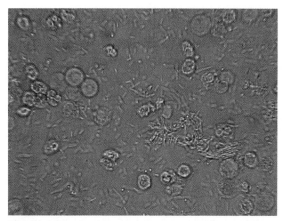

Figure 5-11. WBCs and bacteria in unstained canine urine.

in the urine of animals without urinary or genital tract disease. WBCs shrink in concentrated urine and swell in dilute urine. Leukocytes are usually in low numbers in urine (0 to 1/hpf). Finding more than 2 to 3 per high power field indicates an inflammatory process somewhere in the urinary or genital tracts. The term for excessive WBCs in the urine is pyuria. Pyuria is indicative of an inflammatory or infectious process such as nephritis, pyelonephritis, cystitis, urethritis, or ureteritis. Urine with increased numbers of leukocytes should be cultured for bacteria even if organisms are not observed by microscopic examination.

Epithelial Cells

A few epithelial cells in urine are considered normal and occur as a result of normal sloughing of old cells. A marked increase indicates inflammation. The three types of epithelial cells found in urinary sediment are squamous, transitional, and renal (see Fig. 5-10). Differentiation of transitional from renal epithelial cells is often difficult. In this case, reporting the cells as nonsquamous epithelial cells is acceptable.

Squamous Epithelial Cells

Squamous epithelial cells, derived from the distal urethra, vagina, vulva, or prepuce, are occasionally found in voided samples. Their presence usually is not considered significant. These flat, thin cells with a homogeneous appearance are the largest cells found in urine sediment. They often have straight edges and distinct corners, which sometimes curl or fold (Fig. 5-12, *A*). They may show a small, round nucleus. Squamous epithelial cells are not normally found in samples obtained by cystocentesis or catheterization.

Transitional Epithelial Cells

Transitional epithelial cells come from the bladder, ureters, renal pelvis, and proximal urethra. They are usually round, but they may be pear shaped or caudate. They are granular, have a small nucleus,

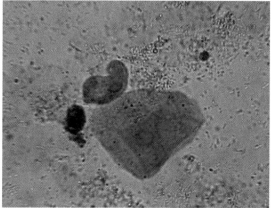

A

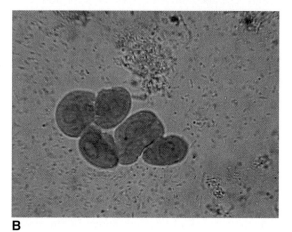

B

Figure 5-12. A, Squamous epithelial cells in stained canine urine. **B,** Transitional epithelial cells in stained canine urine.

and are larger than WBCs (Fig. 5-12, *B*). Low numbers of transitional cells (0 to 1/hpf) may be found in urinary sediment as a result of sloughing of old cells, but an increased number suggests cystitis or pyelonephritis. Increased numbers also may be seen if catheterization was used to obtain the sample.

Renal Epithelial Cells

Renal epithelial cells are the smallest epithelial cells observed in urine. They originate in the renal tubules, are only slightly larger than WBCs, and are often confused with WBCs. Renal epithelial cells are generally round and contain a large nucleus and nongranular or finely granular cytoplasm (see Fig. 5-10). They are rarely found (0 to 1/hpf). Increased numbers of these cells occur in diseases of the kidney parenchyma.

Casts

Casts are formed in the lumen of the distal and collecting tubules of the kidney, where the concentration and acidity of urine are greatest. In the renal tubules, secreted protein precipitates in acidic conditions and forms casts shaped like the tubules in which they form. They are composed of a matrix of protein from plasma and mucoprotein secreted by the tubules. They are commonly classified on the basis of appearance as hyaline, epithelial, cellular (RBCs and/or WBCs), granular, waxy, fatty, and mixed casts. Which cast type is present depends in part on how quickly the filtrate is moving through the tubules and how much tubular damage is present. Faster moving filtrate with minor tubule damage is usually evident as a hyaline cast. Slower moving filtrate allows time for the cells to be incorporated within the cast. If the filtrate is moving very slowly, the cells will degenerate as the cast continues through the tubules; the cast will then appear as a granular cast.

All casts are cylindrical structures, with parallel sides, and their width is determined by the width of the lumen in which they are formed. Their ends may be tapered, irregular, or round. Any cells or structures in the area may also be incorporated into casts, imparting the morphologic features that allow them to be specifically identified (Fig. 5-13). Casts dissolve while in alkaline urine, so cast identification should be performed in fresh samples that have not become alkaline with standing. Because casts dissolve quickly in alkaline urine they are rarely seen in the sediment of herbivores, which characteristically have alkaline urine. Casts may be disrupted with high-speed centrifugation and rough sample handling. A few hyaline casts or granular casts (0 to 1/hpf) may be seen in normal urine, but larger numbers of casts indicate a lesion in the renal tubules. The number of casts observed is not a reliable indicator of the severity of the urinary disease.

Hyaline Casts

Hyaline casts are clear, colorless, and somewhat transparent structures composed only of protein. They are difficult to see and usually are identified only in dim light. Hyaline casts are cylindrical, with parallel sides and usually rounded ends (Fig. 5-14). They are easier to identify in stained sediment than in unstained sediment. Increased numbers of hyaline casts indicate the mildest form of renal irritation. Their numbers also are increased with fever, poor renal perfusion, strenuous exercise, or general anesthesia.

Granular Casts

Granular casts, which are hyaline casts containing granules, are the most common type of cast seen in animals (Fig. 5-15). The granules are from tubular epithelial cells, RBCs, or WBCs that became incorporated in the cast and then degenerated. Cellular degeneration may occur in the tubules producing granular casts, which may be coarse or fine in appearance. Other materials released from cells in the urinary tract may also become embedded in casts. Granular casts are seen in large numbers with acute nephritis and indicate more severe kidney damage than do hyaline casts.

Epithelial Casts

Epithelial casts consist of epithelial cells from the renal tubules imbedded in a hyaline matrix (Fig. 5-16). Epithelial cells in casts are always of

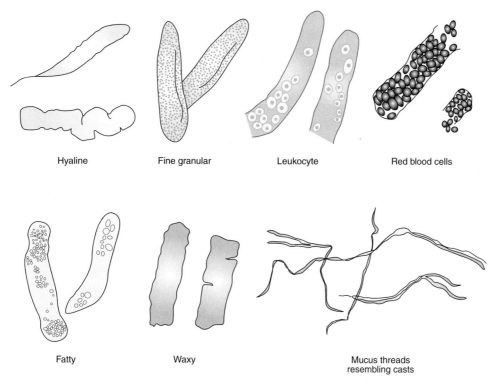

| Hyaline | Fine granular | Leukocyte | Red blood cells |

| Fatty | Waxy | Mucus threads resembling casts |

Figure 5-13. Various types of casts that may be found in urine.

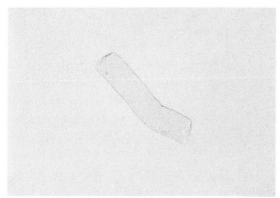

Figure 5-14. Unstained hyaline cast. (Reprinted from Cowell RL, Tyler RD, Meinkoth JH: *Diagnostic cytology and hematology of the dog and cat,* ed 2, St Louis, 1999, Mosby.)

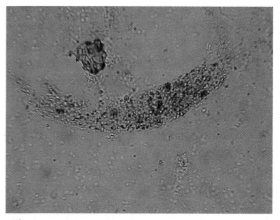

Figure 5-15. Granular cast in stained canine urine.

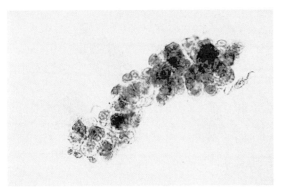

Figure 5-16. Renal epithelial cast, stained. (From Cowell RL, Tyler RD, Meinkoth JH: *Diagnostic cytology and hematology of the dog and cat,* ed 2, St Louis 1999, Mosby.)

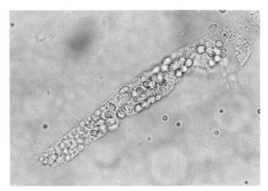

Figure 5-17. RBC cast, unstained. (From Raskin RE, Meyer DJ: *Atlas of canine and feline cytology,* St Louis 2001, Saunders.)

the renal epithelial type because this is the only epithelial cell present at the site of cast formation. These casts are formed by epithelium sloughing in the tubules. These casts are seen in acute nephritis or other conditions that cause degeneration of the renal tubular epithelium.

Leukocyte Casts

Leukocyte casts contain WBCs, predominantly neutrophils (see Fig. 5-13). These casts can be readily identified unless cellular degeneration has occurred. The presence of WBCs and leukocyte casts indicates inflammation in the renal tubules.

Erythrocyte Casts

Erythrocyte casts are deep yellow to orange in color. The RBC membranes may or may not be visible. Erythrocyte casts contain RBCs and form when RBCs aggregate within the lumen of the tubule (Fig. 5-17). Erythrocyte casts indicate renal bleeding. Bleeding may be strictly from hemorrhage resulting from trauma or bleeding disorders, or it may occur as part of an inflammatory lesion.

Waxy Casts

Waxy casts resemble hyaline casts but are usually wider, with square ends rather than round ends and a dull, homogeneous, waxy appearance (Fig. 5-18). They are colorless or gray and highly refractile.

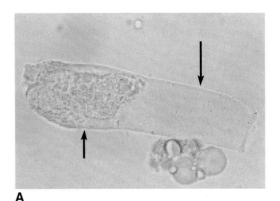

A

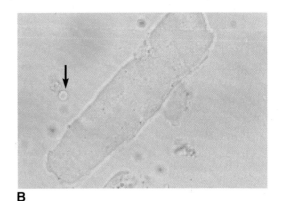

B

Figure 5-18. A, Granular casts unstained develop into waxy cast as illustrated by this cast that has characteristics of both a waxy cast *(long arrow)* and a granular cast *(long arrow).* **B,** Waxy cast, unstained. (From Raskin RE, Meyer DJ: *Atlas of canine and feline cytology,* St Louis, 2001, Saunders.)

They indicate chronic, severe degeneration of the renal tubules.

Fatty Casts

Fatty casts contain many small droplets of fat that appear as refractile bodies (see Fig. 5-13). They are frequently seen in cats with renal disease because cats have lipid in their renal parenchyma. They are occasionally seen in dogs with diabetes mellitus. Large numbers of fatty casts suggest degeneration of the renal tubules.

Crystals

The presence of crystals in the urine is termed crystalluria. Crystalluria may or may not be of clinical significance. Certain crystals form as a consequence of their elements being secreted into the urine by normal renal activity (Fig. 5-19). Some crystals form as a consequence of metabolic diseases. Conditions that lead to crystal formation may also cause formation of urinary calculi. The type of crystals formed depends on the urine pH, concentration and temperature, and the solubility of the elements (see Table 5-4). If a urine sample is allowed to stand and cool before examination, the number of crystals in the sample increases because the materials that make up crystals are less soluble at lower temperatures. Refrigerated samples often have many more crystals than warm, fresh samples. Sometimes crystals dissolve when a refrigerated sample is warmed to room temperature. Crystals are generally reported as occasional, moderate, or many or as +1 to +4. Although crystals (and uroliths) are often identified by their morphologic characteristics, the only definitive methods to identify crystals is with x-ray diffraction or chemical analysis.

Struvite

Struvite crystals are sometimes referred to as triple phosphate crystals or magnesium ammonium phosphate crystals. They are found in alkaline to slightly acidic urine. Generally, struvite crystals are six-to eight-sided prisms, with tapering sides and ends (Figs. 5-20 and 5-21). Struvite crystals typically are described as resembling coffin lids, although they may take on other shapes. Occasionally they may assume a fern-leaf shape, especially when the urine contains a high concentration of ammonia.

Amorphous Phosphate

Amorphous phosphate crystals are common in alkaline urine and appear as a granular precipitate (Fig. 5-22).

Calcium Carbonate

Calcium carbonate crystals are commonly seen in the urine of horses and rabbits. They are round, with many lines radiating from their centers, or appear as large granular masses (Fig. 5-23). They also may have a "dumbbell" shape. They are of no clinical significance.

Amorphous Urates

Amorphous urates appear as a granular precipitate similar to amorphous phosphates (see Fig. 5-15 and Fig. 5-27). Amorphous urates are seen in acidic urine, whereas amorphous phosphates are found in alkaline urine.

Ammonium Biurate

Ammonium biurate crystals are seen in slightly acidic, neutral, or alkaline urine. These crystals are brown in color and round with long, irregular spicules ("thorn apple" shape) (Fig. 5-24; also see Fig. 5-19). Often the spicules fracture and the remaining crystal is brown, with fine radiating lines. They are most common in animals with severe liver disease, such as portacaval shunts.

Calcium Oxalate

Calcium oxalate dihydrate crystals generally appear as small squares, containing an "X" across the crystal resembling the back of an envelope (Fig. 5-25). Calcium oxalate monohydrate crystals may be small and dumbbell shaped or they may be elongated and pointed at each end (resembling a slat from a picket fence) (Fig. 5-26). Calcium dihydrate crystals are found in acidic and neutral urine and are commonly seen in small numbers in dogs and horses. The urine of animals poisoned with

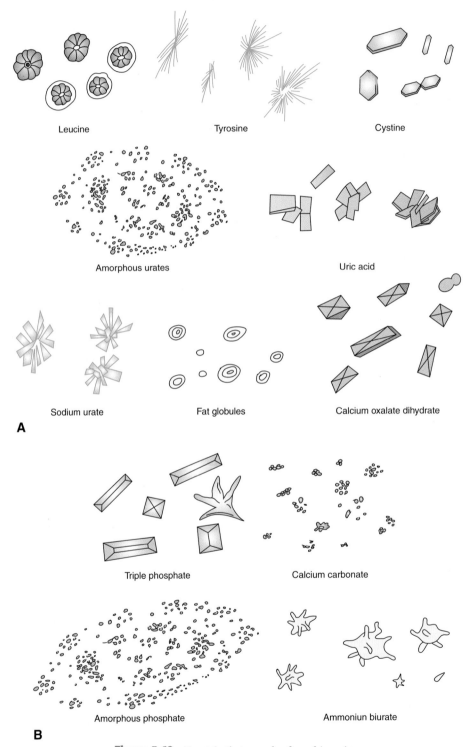

Figure 5-19. Crystals that may be found in urine.

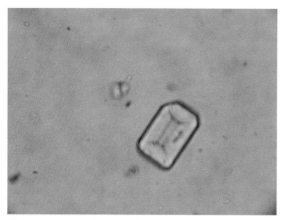

Figure 5-20. Struvite crystal in unstained canine urine, resembling a coffin lid.

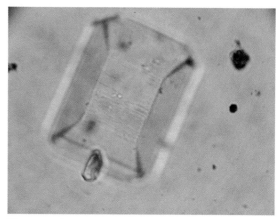

Figure 5-21. Struvite crystal in unstained canine urine.

TABLE 5-4

pH Chart for Urine Crystals

Crystal	pH
Ammonium biurate	Slightly acidic, neutral, alkaline
Amorphous phosphate	Neutral, alkaline
Amorphous urates	Acidic, neutral
Bilirubin	Acidic
Calcium carbonate	Neutral, alkaline
Calcium oxalate	Acidic, neutral, alkaline
Cystine	Acidic
Leucine	Acidic
Triple phosphate	Slightly acidic, neutral, alkaline
Tyrosine	Acidic
Uric acid	Acidic

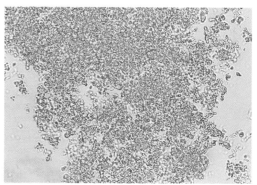

Figure 5-22. Amorphous phosphate crystals, unstained. (Reprinted from Raskin RE, Meyer DJ: *Atlas of canine and feline cytology*, St Louis, 2001, Saunders.)

ethylene glycol (antifreeze) often contains large numbers of calcium oxalate crystals, especially calcium monohydrate crystals. Animals with oxalate urolithiasis may have large numbers of calcium oxalate crystals in their urine, and large numbers of oxalate crystals may indicate predisposition to oxalate urolithiasis.

Sulfonamide

Sulfonamide crystals may be seen in animals being treated with sulfonamides. Sulfonamide crystals

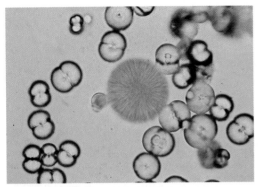

Figure 5-23. Calcium carbonate crystals, unstained. (Reprinted from Raskin RE, Meyer DJ: *Atlas of canine and feline cytology,* St Louis, 2001, Saunders.)

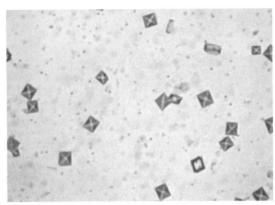

Figure 5-25. Calcium oxalate (dihydrate form) crystal in unstained canine urine. (From VanSteenhouse JL: Clinical pathology. In McCurnin DM, Bassert JM, editors: *Clinical textbook for veterinary technicians,* ed 6, St Louis, 2006, Saunders.)

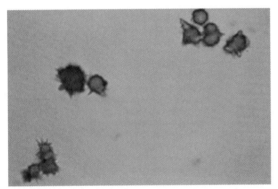

Figure 5-24. Unstained urine sediment with ammonium biurate crystals. (From VanSteenhouse JL: Clinical pathology. In McCurnin DM, Bassert JM, editors: *Clinical textbook for veterinary technicians,* ed 6, St Louis, 2006, Saunders.)

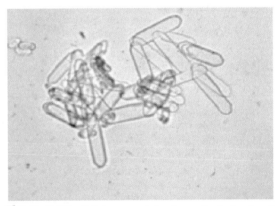

Figure 5-26. Calcium oxalate (monohydrate form) crystal in unstained canine urine. (From VanSteenhouse JL: Clinical pathology. In McCurnin DM, Bassert JM, editors: *Clinical textbook for veterinary technicians,* ed 6, St Louis, 2006, Saunders.)

are round, usually dark, with individual crystals radiating from the center. They are less likely to be observed in alkaline urine because these crystals are more soluble in alkaline urine. Prevention of precipitation of these crystals in the renal tubules is assisted by maintaining alkaline urine and encouraging the animal to drink.

Uric Acid
Uric acid crystals take on a variety of shapes but are usually diamond or rhomboid (Fig. 5-27). They

appear yellow or yellow-brown in color and are not commonly found in the dog and cat except in dalmatian dogs.

Leucine
Leucine crystals are wheel or "pincushion" shaped and are yellow or brown in color (see Fig. 5-15). Animals with liver disease may have leucine crystals in their urine.

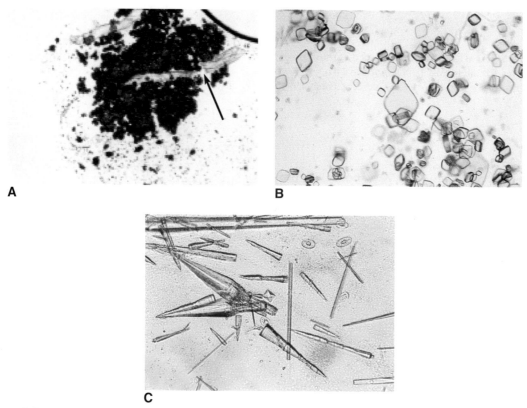

Figure 5-27. **A,** Amorphous urate crystals, unstained. A cotton fiber (contaminant) is trapped within the crystals *(arrow)*. **B,** Uric acid crystals, unstained. These are not commonly found in small animals except for Dalmatian dogs. **C,** Sodium urate crystals, unstained. May be found in association with ammonium biurate uroliths. A calcium oxalate dihyrate crystals is also present (center). (From Raskin RE, Meyer DJ: *Atlas of canine and feline cytology,* St Louis, 2001, Saunders.)

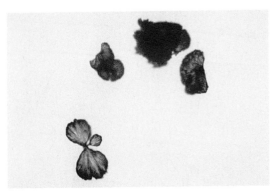

Figure 5-28. Tyrosine crystals, stained. (From Cowell RL, Tyler RD, Meinkoth JH: *Diagnostic cytology and hematology of the dog and cat,* ed 2, St Louis, 1999, Mosby.)

Tyrosine

Tyrosine crystals are dark, have needlelike projections, and are highly refractile (Fig. 5-28). They are often found in small clusters. Animals with liver disease may have tyrosine crystals in their urine. They are not a common finding in the dog and cat.

Cystine

Cystine crystals appear flat and are six-sided (hexagonal), colorless, and thin (Fig. 5-29). They can be associated with renal tubular dysfunction or cystine urolithiasis.

MICROORGANISMS

A variety of microorganisms may be found in urine sediment, including bacteria, fungi, and protozoa. Normal urine is free of bacteria but may be contaminated by bacteria residing on the epithelium of the vagina, vulva, or prepuce during urination. Normal urine collected by cystocentesis or catheterization does not contain bacteria and therefore is considered sterile. Because bacteria often proliferate in urine that has been left standing for some time, especially at room temperature, the urine must be immediately examined or refrigerated until it can be examined. Bacteria can be identified only

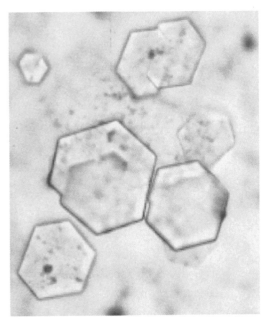

Figure 5-29. Cystine crystals, unstained. (From VanSteenhouse JL: Clinical pathology. In McCurnin DM, Bassert JM: *Clinical textbook for veterinary technicians,* ed 6, St Louis, 2006, Saunders.)

under magnification. They may be round (cocci) or rod shaped (bacilli), usually refract light, and appear to be quivering as a result of Brownian movement (see Fig. 5-11). They are reported as few, moderate, many, or too numerous to count (TNTC). A large number of bacteria accompanied by a large number of WBCs suggests infection and inflammation of the urinary tract (e.g., cystitis, pyelonephritis) or genital tract (e.g., prostatitis, metritis, or vaginitis). Bacteria in the urine sample are most significant when they are also identified within the cytoplasm of the WBCs. These samples should be submitted for bacterial culture.

Yeasts are often confused with RBCs or lipid droplets, but they usually display characteristic budding and may have double refractile walls. Yeast usually are contaminants in urine samples because yeast infections of the urinary tract are rare in domestic animals. Yeast infection of the external genitalia may cause yeast to be present in voided samples. Fungi also may be found in urine. Fungi are filamentous and usually branching. Fungal infections of the urinary tract are uncommon but are quite serious when they occur.

Parasite Ova, Microfilaria

Parasite ova may be seen in the urine sediment of animals with urinary parasites or because of fecal contamination at the time of collection of the urine sample. Some parasites of the urinary tract include *Capillaria plica,* a bladder worm of dogs and cats (Fig. 5-30), and *Dioctophyma renale,* a kidney worm of dogs. Microfilaria (e.g., *Dirofilaria immitis*) may be seen in the urine sediment of dogs with adult heartworms, and circulating microfilaria may be seen if hemorrhage into the urine occurs either from disease or as a result of trauma during collection (Fig. 5-31).

MISCELLANEOUS COMPONENTS OF URINE

Mucus Threads

Mucus threads are often confused with casts, but they do not have the well-delineated edges of casts. They resemble a twisted ribbon more than a cast (see Fig. 5-13). A large amount of mucus is normally present in equine urine because horses

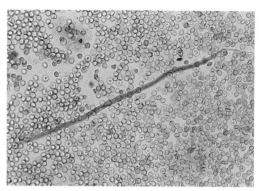

Figure 5-31. Microfilaria of *Dirofilaria immitis* in a dog with hemorrhagic cystitis, stained. (From Raskin RE, Meyer DJ: *Atlas of canine and feline cytology,* St Louis, 2001, Saunders.)

have mucus glands in the renal pelvis and ureter. In other animals, mucus indicates urethral irritation or contamination of the sample with genital secretions.

Spermatozoa

Spermatozoa are occasionally seen in the urine sediment of intact male animals (see Fig. 5-10). They are easily recognized and have no clinical significance. Sperm may also be present in recently bred females. Large amounts of sperm in urine may produce false positive results for proteins.

Fat Droplets

In urine sediment, fat droplets are lightly green-tinged, highly refractile, spherical bodies of varying sizes. Because they vary in size, they can be distinguished from RBCs and yeast, which tend to be uniform in size. If a sediment smear sits for a few moments before being examined, fat droplets rise to a plane just beneath the cover slip, whereas other formed elements settle to the top of the slide. Therefore fat droplets are often not in the plane of focus of other formed elements. Small, round structures found under the cover slip are usually fat globules. Uniformly sized, round structures found in a lower plane are usually RBCs. In sediment stained

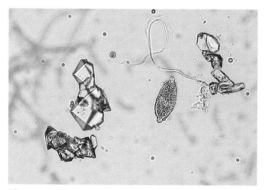

Figure 5-30. Ova of *Capillaria plica* in unstained urine sediment. (Reprinted from Raskin RE, Meyer DJ: *Atlas of canine and feline cytology,* St Louis, 2001, Saunders.)

with Sudan III stain, fat droplets appear orange or red in color. Frequently, fat droplets from catheter lubricants or from oily surfaces of collecting vials and pipettes may contaminate urine. Fat in the urine, called lipuria, is seen to some degree in most cats. Lipuria is also seen with obesity, diabetes mellitus, hypothyroidism, and rarely, after a high-fat meal.

Artifacts

Many artifacts may enter the urine sample during collection, transportation, or examination. Recognition of these structures as irrelevant and not a normal part of the sediment evaluation. These contaminants may be a source of great confusion.

Air bubbles, oil droplets (usually resulting from lubricated catheters), starch granules (from surgical gloves), hair, fecal material, plant spores, pollen, cotton fiber, dust, glass particles or chips, bacteria, and fungi may contaminate urine. Ova of intestinal parasites may be observed as a result of fecal contamination of the urine sample.

UROLITHIASIS

Uroliths are calculi (stones) composed of various minerals that are found anywhere in the urinary tract; their occurrence is termed urolithiasis. They may cause blockage of urine outflow from the bladder into the urethra; lodge in the urethra causing severe, acute inability to urinate; or remain in the bladder and cause inflammation and bleeding. Determining the composition of calculi is critical because their prevention and the animal's prognosis depend on identification of their composition. Once composition is determined, proper therapy may be initiated to remove them and prevent their reoccurrence. Urolithiasis may be a particular problem in castrated male ruminants. Lodging of calculi in the urethra obstructs the outflow of urine, which is a major problem in lambs and steers, particularly those that are fed high-concentrate rations. The most common calculi in these species are composed of calcium, magnesium, and ammonium carbonate or calcium, magnesium, and ammonium phosphate.

Analysis of the mineral composition of uroliths may be determined by submitting it intact to a reference laboratory for quantitative analysis. Occasionally, a reasonable idea about the composition of a urolith may be made by its gross and radiographic appearance and the crystal types found in the sediment. Uroliths of dogs and cats are usually struvite. Cystine and oxalate uroliths may also be observed. Urate uroliths are seen mostly in Dalmatians because this breed excretes large amounts of uric acid.

Recommended Reading

Cowell RL, Tyler RD, Meinkoth JH: *Diagnostic cytology and hematology of the dog and cat,* ed 2, St Louis, 1999, Mosby.

Graff L: *A handbook of routine urinalysis,* Philadelphia, 1983, Lippincott.

Meyer DJ, Harvey JW: *Veterinary laboratory medicine interpretation and diagnosis,* ed 3, St Louis, 2004, Saunders.

Modern urine chemistry, Elkhart, IN, 1993, Miles Laboratories.

Osborne CA, Stevens JB: *Urinalysis: a clinical guide to compassionate patient care,* Shawnee Mission, KS, 1999, Bayer.

Raskin RE, Meyer DJ: *Atlas of canine and feline cytology,* St Louis, 2001, Saunders.

CHAPTER 6

Internal Parasites

Charles M. Hendrix

KEY POINTS

- Parasites which reside that the host's body are referred to as endoparasites.
- Endoparasites of domestic animals include unicellular protozoans, trematodes (flukes), cestodes (tapeworms with their associated metacestode stages), nematodes (roundworms), and acanthocephalans (thorny-headed worms). A few arthropods (e.g., horse bots) are endoparasites.
- Endoparasites produce a parasitic infection or endoparasitism.
- The host that harbors the adult, mature, or sexual stages of a parasite is called the definitive host, whereas the one that harbors the larval, immature, or asexual stages of a parasite is called the intermediate host.
- The time elapsed between initial infection with a parasite until the infection can be detected using common diagnostic procedures is called the prepatent period.

- Because endoparasites of domestic animals vary in form, size, location within host, and means of transmission, no single diagnostic test can used to diagnose all endoparasites.
- Diagnosis of alimentary parasitism requires examination of a fecal specimen for the presence of eggs (ova), oocysts, larvae, tapeworm proglottids, and adult parasites.
- Methods to examine fecal specimens include gross examination and microscopic examination of feces.
- Microscopic examination of fecal samples may involve direct examination of concentration of material by fecal flotation or fecal sedimentation.
- Hemoparasites (blood parasites) can be identified by microscopic examination of peripheral blood smears or by using a variety of concentration techniques, such as the modified Knott's procedure.

This chapter discusses the roles that veterinary technicians play in assisting the veterinarian in diagnosing endoparasites (internal parasites) of domestic animals such as dogs, cats, cattle, horses, sheep, and poultry. Diagnosis of endoparasitism is one of the most frequently performed procedures in the veterinary clinical setting. As such, diagnoses must be performed accurately and efficiently so that the appropriate treatment may be initiated.

An accurate diagnosis of endoparasitism is based primarily on the veterinarian's and the technician's awareness of parasites that are prevalent in the immediate geographic area or ecosystem. However, because of the far-ranging mobility of owners and their pets in the twenty-first century, residence in or travel to another geographic region also should be considered when endoparasitism is among several differential diagnoses.

Heavily parasitized animals often show clinical signs suggestive of the infected organ system. Depending on the affected organ system, these signs may include diarrhea or constipation, anorexia, vomiting, blood in the stool, or fat in the stool. Parasitized animals are frequently lethargic and display an unthrifty appearance characterized by weight loss or stunted growth, dull haircoat, dehydration, or anemia. The animal also may experience coughing or labored breathing.

Internal parasites of domestic animals comprise several types of organisms that live internally in animals, feed on their tissues or body fluids, or compete directly for their food. These organisms range in size from being too small to be seen with the naked eye (microscopic) to being more than 1 m in length. Parasites also vary in their location within the host and in the means by which they are transmitted from one host to another. Because of these diverse variations, no single diagnostic test can identify all endoparasites.

The veterinary technician may be asked to perform a wide variety of diagnostic procedures to diagnose endoparasitism. These procedures usually detect the adult stages of a parasite or their eggs or larval stages in the animal's feces, urine, or blood. In addition, a variety of immunologic tests are available for confirming the presence of both metazoan and protozoan parasites infecting domestic animals. Mature parasites are seldom found because they are generally hidden within the body of the animal. The only way to detect their presence is by using an immunologic test or performing a necropsy, or postmortem dissection. An assorted battery of diagnostic procedures may not be in common use in veterinary practices but are described in this chapter because they may be useful to veterinary technicians working in research or diagnostic laboratories.

This chapter includes illustrations and brief descriptions of some of the eggs, larvae, and adult parasites that may be diagnosed in common domesticated animals. Sometimes eggs of certain groups of parasites are quite similar; differentiation of individual species or genera based on their morphologic characteristics may be difficult or impossible. Parasites with similar eggs usually are differentiated by fecal culture and larval identification.

The technician must remember that the diagnostic tests used to detect endoparasitism may be unreliable. An animal may be infected with endoparasites; however, if the infection is slight, no eggs or larvae may be observed in the specimens tested. If an inappropriate test is used, it is also possible that no parasites may be detected. Another common problem is trying to diagnose endoparasitism before the parasite completely develops. Many parasites can produce clinical disease before they become reproductively mature.

The time elapsed between initial infection with a parasite until the infection can be detected by using common diagnostic procedures is called the prepatent period. The best example of this concept is trying to diagnose hookworm disease *(Ancylostoma caninum)* in a 1-week-old puppy by observation of eggs on fecal flotation. This attempted diagnosis is a waste of time because the minimum time for infection until adult hookworms are present in the bowel and begin to produce eggs (prepatent period) is 12 days. The astute veterinary practitioner uses fecal flotation results but also the puppy's history, clinical signs, and other laboratory tests (e.g., blood values) to arrive at a specific diagnosis of ancylostomiasis (infection with hookworms).

COMMON TYPES OF PARASITES

Complete coverage of the discipline of veterinary parasitology is beyond the scope of this text. Only the general types of parasites of domestic animals and their life cycle stages that may be recovered by commonly used diagnostic procedures are described. The reference texts listed at the end of this chapter provide more detailed coverage of veterinary parasitology and specific parasites.

Internal parasites, called endoparasites, live within an animal. These parasites derive their nutrition and protection at the expense of the infected animal, which is called the host. The various internal parasites have many different life cycles. Each parasite's life cycle is distinctive and is composed of various developmental stages, all of which may occur within the same host or separately within sequential hosts.

The host that harbors the adult, mature, or sexual stages of a parasite is called the definitive host. The dog is the definitive host for *Dirofilaria immitis;* adult male and female heartworms are found in the right ventricle and pulmonary arteries of the dog's heart. The host that harbors the larval, immature, or asexual stages of a parasite is called the intermediate host. The mosquito is the intermediate host for *D. immitis;* first, second, and third larval stages of *D. immitis* are found within the mosquito intermediate host.

The life cycle of most parasites has at least one stage at which the parasite may be passed from one host to the next. Diagnostic procedures frequently detect this stage; therefore it is referred to as the diagnostic stage. The diagnostic stage of a parasite may leave the host through excreta, such as feces or urine, or it may be transmitted from the bloodstream to its next host by an arthropod, such as a mosquito. The microfilarial stage is the diagnostic stage of *D. immitis;* the female mosquito takes in the microfilariae during a blood meal.

Protozoa (Unicellular Organisms)

Protozoa are unicellular, or one-cell, organisms, some of which may be parasitic in domestic animals. These protozoans can infect a variety of tissue sites within the definitive host. The most common sites for their detection are in blood samples, in which they are called blood protozoa or hemoprotozoa, or within fecal samples, in which they are called intestinal protozoa. The protozoan's life cycle may be either simple or complex.

Most hemoprotozoa seen in the United States are found in erythrocytes (red blood cells [RBCs]) within a stained blood smear. Ticks usually serve as intermediate hosts and transmit the RBCs containing the hemoprotozoa from one animal to the next. *Babesia bigemina* is a tear-shaped or pear-shaped hemoprotozoan found within the RBCs of infected cattle. It is transmitted by *Boophilus annulatus,* a tick described in Chapter 7.

Trypanosomes are another group of hemoprotozoans occasionally found in the United States. Rather than being found within RBCs, trypanosomes are extracellular and "swim" within the blood. They are 3 to 10 times as long as an RBC is wide and are banana shaped. They have a lateral undulating membrane and a thin, whiplike tail (flagellum) that is used for swimming. These parasites are also transmitted by blood-feeding arthropods (see reduviid bugs in Chapter 7).

Trematodes (Flukes)

The trematodes (also called flukes) are flatworms with unsegmented, leaf-shaped bodies. In domestic animals in the United States, most adult flukes are found in the intestinal tract, the liver, or even the lungs. In these sites, the hermaphroditic (having male and female sex organs) flukes lay eggs that are passed in the feces. The end portion of many fluke eggs has a small cap, lid, or door; this structure is called an operculum and is common among many of the flukes.

Within each fluke egg is a larval stage known as a miracidium, which hatches and exits the egg through the operculum. This stage penetrates the first intermediate host, which is usually a snail.

Within the snail, the miracidium develops into a sporocyst, which then produces many tiny internal structures called rediae. Each redia may produce many internal cercariae. The cercaria exits the snail and may take one of three pathways to enter the definitive host: it may develop into a metacercaria and encyst upon vegetation, whereby it is ingested by the definitive host; it may be ingested by a second intermediate host and become encysted as the metacercarial stage within that host, which is subsequently ingested by the definitive host; or the cercaria may directly penetrate the skin of the definitive host.

Flukes of veterinary importance include the liver flukes of cattle and sheep (*Fasciola hepatica, Fascioloides magna, Dicrocoelium dendriticum*) and the lung fluke of dogs and cats (*Paragonimus kellicotti*).

Cestodes (Tapeworms)

Like trematodes, cestodes (tapeworms) are also flatworms. They are also hermaphroditic. They differ, however, in that cestodes are ribbonlike and divided into a long chain of proglottids, which are segments connected like train cars behind a scolex or "head," by which the tapeworm attaches to the wall of the host's intestine. Most tapeworms release their proglottids one at a time or in short chains into the feces. Proglottids in the feces can be observed with the naked eye. A few tapeworms release eggs directly from the worm's uterus.

Tapeworm proglottids have muscles that enable them to move about. Pet owners often observe these tapeworms as "little white worms" crawling on the pet's feces, haircoat, or bedding. These fresh proglottids are said to resemble "cucumber seeds." When the proglottids dry out, they resemble uncooked grains of rice.

Tapeworm proglottids often contain eggs when they are passed into the feces. These eggs contain hexacanth embryos, which are embryos with an internal structure with six hooks.

An intermediate host, usually a mammalian host, such as a rabbit, ingests these hexacanth embryos. The hexacanth embryo grows within the tissues of the intermediate host to a "bladderworm" stage, which is a fluid-filled larval stage. The definitive host becomes infected by ingesting the intermediate host, which contains the bladderworm larval stage. Examples of tapeworms that develop into the bladderworm stage in the intermediate host are the canine taeniid tapeworm (*Taenia pisiformis*) and the coenurus tapeworm (*Multiceps multiceps*). In some tapeworms (*Echinococcus granulosus, Echinococcus multilocularis*), the larval stage within the vertebrate host is a hydatid cyst.

When the intermediate host is an arthropod, such as a flea or a grain mite, the hexacanth embryo develops into a microscopic larval stage known as a cysticercoid. The cysticercoid stage is tiny and contains a small fluid-filled space. The definitive host becomes infected by ingesting the intermediate host, which contains the cysticercoid larval stage. The cysticercoid stage is associated with the fringed tapeworm of cattle (*Thysanosoma actinoides*) and the double-pore tapeworm (*Dipylidium caninum*) of dogs and cats.

Nematodes (Roundworms)

Nematodes often are referred to as roundworms and are one of the most important groups of parasites in veterinary parasitology. They may be found in almost any tissue of domestic animals, including the intestines, skin, lungs, kidneys, urinary bladder, nervous tissue, musculature, and blood.

Nematodes as a group have diverse, complicated life cycles. They have separate sexes (male nematodes and female nematodes). Their eggs or larvae are most commonly recovered from the feces. The eggs of nematodes infecting the kidney or urinary bladder may be recovered from the urine.

Examples of intestinal nematodes found in dogs include large roundworms (*Toxocara canis, Toxascaris leonina*), hookworms (*Ancylostoma caninum, Uncinaria stenocephala*), and whipworms (*Trichuris vulpis*). Urinary roundworms include canine kidney worms (*Dioctophyma renale*). Respiratory roundworms include the lungworms of cattle and sheep (*Dictyocaulus* species and *Muellerius capillaris*). Nematodes of the blood vasculature are a special group, of which the heartworm of dogs (*Dirofilaria immitis*) is an example.

Adult female heartworms give birth to small, wormlike prelarval (embryonic) stages called microfilariae. The microfilariae may be observed in a peripheral blood smear and are approximately 310 µm long. Within the mosquito, the microfilariae develop into infective third-stage larvae. These infective larvae are transmitted to other animals by the infected mosquitoes.

Acanthocephalans (Thorny-Head Worms)

Acanthocephalans (thorny-head worms) are uncommon parasites with complicated life cycles. Like the nematodes, they have separate sexes. On the cranial end of these helminths is a spiny proboscis, which is used to attach to the lining of the intestine wall. Thorny-head worms do not have a true gut; they absorb nutrients through their body wall. Acanthocephalans usually are recovered at necropsy.

The most famous acanthocephalan is *Macracanthorhynchus hirudinaceus,* a parasite of pigs. This parasite has the dubious honor of possessing the longest scientific name among the parasites of domestic animals. *Oncicola canis* is an acanthocephalan found in the small intestine of dogs.

COMMON ENDOPARASITES OF DOMESTIC ANIMALS

Following are descriptions of most of the common endoparasites in domestic animals in the United States. Information is given on the organ or organ system parasitized in the host; prepatent period, or time from initial infection until the diagnostic stage may be recovered, where appropriate; description of the diagnostic stage, or life cycle stage commonly used to make a diagnosis, such as eggs or larvae; and diagnostic stage most commonly identified.

Endoparasites of Dogs and Cats

Parasites of the Gastrointestinal Tract
Nematodes (Roundworms)
Spirocerca lupi, the esophageal worm, is a nematode that often forms nodules (granulomas) in the esophageal wall of dogs and cats. Occasionally it may be found in nodules in the stomach of cats.

Adult worms reside deep within these nodules and expel their eggs through fistulous openings in the granuloma. Eggs are passed into the lumen of the host animal's esophagus and pass out in the feces. The thick-shelled eggs are 30 to 38 µm by 11 to 15 µm and contain a larva when they are laid. These eggs have a unique paper-clip shape. Figure 6-1 shows the characteristic ovum of *S. lupi.* Eggs usually may be observed on fecal flotation and may be recovered when vomitus has been subjected to a standard fecal flotation procedure. Radiographic or endoscopic examination may reveal characteristic granulomas within the esophagus or within the stomach. The prepatent period is 6 months.

Physaloptera species are stomach worms of dogs and cats. Although they occasionally are found in the lumen of the stomach or small intestine, *Physaloptera* species usually are firmly attached to the mucosal surface of the stomach, where they suck blood. At this site, these nematodes may be viewed with an endoscope. Their diet consists of blood and tissue derived from the host's gastric mucosa. Their attachment sites continue to bleed after the parasite detaches. Vomiting, anorexia,

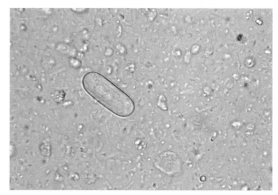

Figure 6-1. Characteristic ovum of *Spirocerca lupi.* The thick-shelled eggs contain larvae and measure 30 to 38 µm by 11 to 15 µm. Eggs usually may be observed on fecal flotation and may be recovered when vomitus has been subjected to a standard fecal flotation procedure. (From Hendrix CM, Robinson E: *Diagnostic parasitology for veterinary technicians,* ed 3, St Louis, 2006, Mosby.)

and dark, tarry stools may be observed in affected animals.

The adults are creamy white, sometimes tightly coiled, and 1.3 to 4.8 cm long. They are often recovered in the pet's vomitus and may be confused with ascarids, or roundworms. A quick way to differentiate these two parasites is to break open an adult specimen and (if that specimen happens to be female) examine the released eggs microscopically. The eggs of *Physaloptera* species are small, smooth, thick shelled, and embryonated when passed in the feces. Eggs are 30 to 34 μm by 49 to 58 μm and contain a larva when they are laid. Figure 6-2 shows the characteristic ovum of *Physaloptera* species. Eggs usually may be recovered on a standard fecal flotation by using solutions with a specific gravity greater than 1.25. The prepatent period is 56 to 83 days.

Aonchotheca putorii is commonly referred to as the gastric capillarid of cats. It was once known by a former name, *Capillaria putorii*. This capillarid frequently parasitizes mustellids, such as mink, but it also has been reported in cats. These nematodes are rarely reported in North America. The eggs of *A. putorii* are easily confused with other trichinelloid nematodes (see the section on feline whipworms). Their eggs are 53 to 70 μm by 20 to 30 μm and exhibit a netlike surface similar to that of the eggs of *Eucoleus aerophilus*, an upper respiratory capillarid. The eggs of *A. putorii* are dense, less delicate than those of *E. aerophilus*, and organized in a longitudinal formation. They have flattened sides and contain a one- or two-cell embryo, which fills the egg.

Ollulanus tricuspis is "the feline trichostrongyle." This parasite usually is associated with vomiting in cats. It is most commonly identified by examination of the cat's vomitus with a dissecting or compound microscope. Feline vomitus also may be examined by a standard fecal flotation procedure. The best flotation solution for identification is a modified Sheather's flotation solution. Adult female *O. tricuspis* are 0.8 to 1.0 mm long and have three major tail cusps, which are the origin of the name tricuspis. Adult males are 0.7 to 0.8 mm long and have a copulatory bursa. The female worms are viviparous (bear live young). The infective third-stage larvae (500 by 22 μm) mature to adults in the cat's stomach. Free-living stages are not required for completion of the life cycle. Transmission occurs through ingestion of vomitus from infected cats.

Toxocara canis, *Toxocara cati*, and *Toxascaris leonina* are the ascarids of dogs and cats. These roundworms are found in the small intestine of dogs and cats in most areas of the world. All young puppies and kittens presented to a veterinary clinic should be examined for these large, robust nematodes. Adult ascarids may vary from 3 to 18 cm in length and when passed are usually tightly coiled, much like a coiled bedspring. The eggs of *Toxocara* species are spherical, with a deeply pigmented center and a rough, pitted outer shell (Fig. 6-3). Eggs of *T. canis* are 75 to 90 μm in diameter, whereas those of *T. cati* are smaller, only 65 to 75 μm in diameter (Fig. 6-4). The eggs of *Toxascaris leonina* are spherical to ovoid, with dimensions of 75 μm by 85 μm. These eggs have a smooth outer shell and a hyaline or "ground glass" central portion. Figure 6-5 shows the characteristic ovum of *T. leonina*. The prepatent period for *T. canis* is 21 to 35 days, whereas that of *T. leonina* is 74 days.

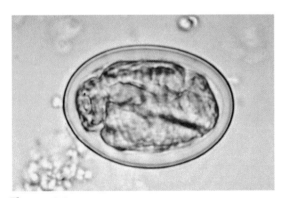

Figure 6-2. Characteristic ovum of *Physaloptera* species. The oval, thick-shelled eggs contain larvae and measure 49 to 58 μm by 30 to 34 μm. Eggs usually may be recovered on a standard fecal flotation by using solutions with a specific gravity greater than 1.25. (From Hendrix CM, Robinson E: *Diagnostic parasitology for veterinary technicians,* ed 3, St Louis, 2006, Mosby.)

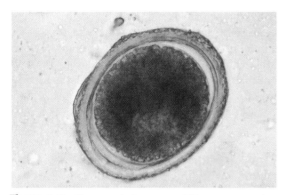

Figure 6-3. Characteristic ovum of *Toxocara* species. These eggs are spherical, with a deeply pigmented center and a rough, pitted outer shell. Eggs of *T. canis* are 75 to 90 μm in diameter. (From Hendrix CM, Robinson E: *Diagnostic parasitology for veterinary technicians,* ed 3, St Louis, 2006, Mosby.)

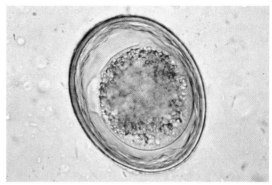

Figure 6-5. Characteristic ovum of *Toxascaris leonina.* These eggs are spherical to ovoid, with dimensions of 75 by 85 μm. They have a smooth outer shell and a hyaline or "ground glass" central portion. (From Hendrix CM, Robinson E: *Diagnostic parasitology for veterinary technicians,* ed 3, St Louis, 2006, Mosby.)

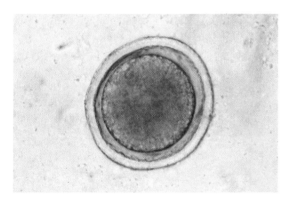

Figure 6-4. Characteristic ovum of *Toxocara cati.* These eggs are smaller than those of *T. canis,* measuring only 65 to 75 μm in diameter. (From Hendrix CM, Robinson E: *Diagnostic parasitology for veterinary technicians,* ed 3, St Louis, 2006, Mosby.)

Ancylostoma caninum, a canine hookworm; *Ancylostoma tubaeforme,* a feline hookworm; *Ancylostoma braziliense,* a canine and feline hookworm; and *Uncinaria stenocephala,* a northern canine hookworm, are small intestinal nematodes. Hookworms are found throughout the world and are common in tropical and subtropical areas of North America. Hookworm infection, which can produce severe anemia in young kittens and puppies, can be a serious problem in kennels and catteries. The prepatent period depends on the species of hookworm and the route of infection.

Eggs of all hookworm species are oval or ellipsoid, have thin walls, and contain 8 to 16 cells when passed in the pet's feces. Because these eggs larvate rapidly in the external environment (as early as 48 hours after feces are passed), fresh feces are needed for diagnosing hookworm infections. Eggs of *A. caninum* are 56 to 75 μm by 34 to 47 μm (Fig. 6-6). Those of *A. tubaeforme* are 55 to 75 μm by 34.4 to 44.7 μm. Those of *A. braziliense* are 75 μm by 45 μm and those of *U. stenocephala* are 65 to 80 μm by 40 to 50 μm. These eggs usually may be recovered on a standard fecal flotation.

Strongyloides stercoralis and *Strongyloides tumefaciens* are often referred to as "intestinal threadworms." These nematodes are unique; only a parthenogenetic female (female that can lay eggs without copulation with a male) is parasitic in the host. Parasitic males do not exist. These females produce eggs, but in dogs these eggs hatch in the intestine, releasing first-stage larvae. Figure 6-7 shows the parasitic adult females, eggs, and first-stage larvae of *Strongyloides* species. The larvae are 280 to 310 μm long and have a rhabditiform (club-shaped) esophagus, with a club-shaped cranial corpus, a narrow median isthmus, and a caudal bulb. The prepatent period is 8 to 14 days.

Trichuris vulpis, the canine whipworm, and *Trichuris campanula* and *Trichuris serrata*, the feline whipworms, reside in the cecum and colon of their respective hosts. Canine whipworms are common, but feline whipworms are rare in North America and diagnosed only sporadically throughout the world. Whipworms derive their name from the fact that the adults have a thin, filamentous cranial end (i.e., the lash of the whip) and a thick caudal end (i.e., the handle of the whip). The egg of the whipworm is described as trichinelloid or trichuroid. It has a thick, yellow-brown, symmetric shell with polar plugs at both ends. The eggs are unembryonated (not larvated) when laid. Eggs of *T. vulpis* are 70 to 89 μm by 37 to 40 μm. Figure 6-8 shows the characteristic egg of *T. vulpis*. The prepatent period for *T. vulpis* is 70 to 90 days.

The eggs of *T. campanula* and *T. serrata* may be easily confused with those of *Aonchotheca putorii*, *Eucoleus aerophilus*, and *Personema feliscati*, parasites of the feline stomach, respiratory tract, and urinary system, respectively. The eggs of *T. campanula* average 63 to 85 μm by 34 to 39 μm. When examining a cat's feces for feline trichurids, the veterinary technician should be aware of pseudoparasites; the eggs of trichurids or capillarids frequently parasitize an outdoor cat's prey: hosts such as mice, rabbits, or birds. The eggs of these trichurids or capillarids may pass unaltered through

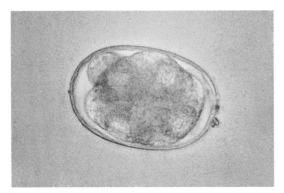

Figure 6-6. Characteristic hookworm ovum. The eggs of *Ancylostoma caninum* are 56 to 75 μm by 34 to 47 μm, those of *A. tubaeforme* are 55 to 75 μm by 34.4 to 44.7 μm, those of *A. braziliense* are 75 μm by 45 μm, and those of *U. stenocephala* are 65 to 80 μm by 40 to 50 μm. (Reprinted from Hendrix CM, Robinson E: *Diagnostic parasitology for veterinary technicians,* ed 3, St Louis, 2006, Mosby.)

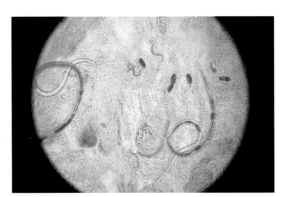

Figure 6-7. Parasitic adult females, eggs, and first-stage larvae of *Strongyloides* species. These larvae are 280 to 310 μm long and have a rhabditiform esophagus, with a club-shaped cranial corpus, a narrow median isthmus, and a caudal bulb. (Reprinted from Hendrix CM, Robinson E: *Diagnostic parasitology for veterinary technicians,* ed 3, St Louis, 2006, Mosby.)

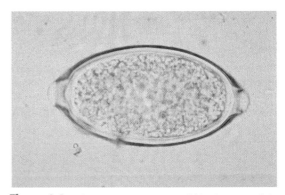

Figure 6-8. Characteristic ovum of *Trichuris vulpis.* Eggs of *T. vulpis* are 70 to 89 μm by 37 to 40 μm. (From Hendrix CM, Robinson E: *Diagnostic parasitology for veterinary technicians,* ed 3, St Louis, 2006, Mosby.)

the cat's gastrointestinal system, remaining intact and unembryonated and thus appearing to infect the feline host.

Enterobius vermicularis is the human pinworm and does not parasitize dogs or cats. Nevertheless, the family pet is often falsely incriminated by family practitioners or pediatricians as a source of pinworm infection in young children. The veterinary technician should remember this rule: Pinworms are parasites of omnivores (mice, rats, monkeys, human beings) and herbivores (rabbits, horses) but never carnivores (dogs, cats).

Cestodes (Tapeworms)

Dipylidium caninum is often called the "double-pore" or "cucumber seed" tapeworm. This tapeworm is the most common tapeworm found in the small intestine of the dog and cat because the dog or cat becomes infected by ingesting the flea intermediate host. Fleas often contain this parasite's infective cysticercoid stage. This tapeworm has motile, terminal, gravid proglottids, which usually are found on the feces (Fig. 6-9, *A*), on the pet's haircoat, or in the bedding of the host. In the fresh state, these proglottids resemble cucumber seeds. These terminal proglottids have a lateral pore located along the midpoint of each of their long edges, the origin of the tapeworm's other common name, the "double-pore" tapeworm (Fig. 6-9, *B*).

If fresh proglottids of *D. caninum* (Fig. 6-10, *A*) are teased or broken open, they may reveal thousands of unique egg packets, each containing 20 to 30 hexacanth embryos. Figure 6-10, *B*, shows the unique egg packet of *D. caninum*. The proglottids of *D. caninum* often dry out in the external environment. As they lose moisture, they shrivel up and resemble uncooked grains of rice (Fig. 6-10, *C*). If reconstituted with water, the dried proglottids usually assume their former cucumber seed appearance. The prepatent period for *D. caninum* is 14 to 21 days.

Taenia pisiformis, Taenia hydatigena, and *Taenia ovis* are the canine taeniids. As with *D. caninum, Taenia* tapeworms appear as motile, terminal, gravid proglottids on the feces, on the pet's haircoat, or in the bedding of the host. In the fresh state, these proglottids have a single lateral pore

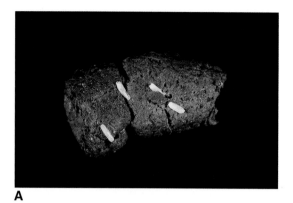

A

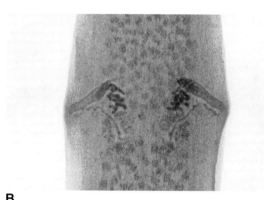

B

Figure 6-9. A, Characteristic motile, terminal, gravid proglottids of *Dipylidium caninum* on canine feces. In the fresh state, these proglottids resemble cucumber seeds; hence the common name, the "cucumber seed" tapeworm. **B,** These proglottids of *D. caninum* have a lateral pore along the midpoint of each long edge, thus the second common name, double-pored tapeworm. (From Hendrix CM, Robinson E: *Diagnostic parasitology for veterinary technicians,* ed 3, St Louis, 2006, Mosby.)

located along the midpoint of either of their long edges (as opposed to the double-pore tapeworm).

As with *D. caninum,* if these fresh proglottids are teased or broken open, they may reveal thousands of hexacanth embryos. The proglottids of *Taenia* species also dry out in the external environment and resemble uncooked grains of rice. If reconstituted with water, they too usually assume their former single-pore appearance. If gravid proglottids of *Taenia* species are recovered from a

A

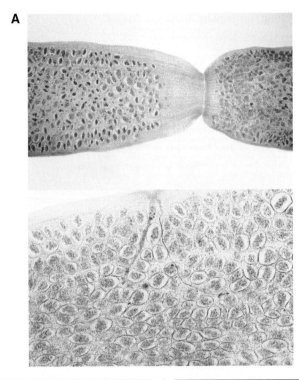

B   **C**

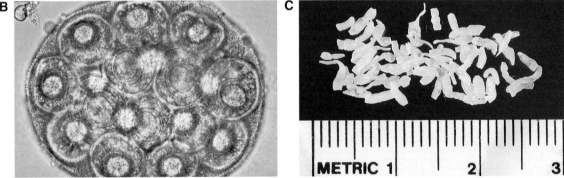

Figure 6-10. A, Gravid proglottids of *Dipylidium caninum* are filled with thousands of egg packets. **B,** Characteristic egg packet of *D. caninum.* Each egg packet may contain up to 30 hexacanth embryos. **C,** Dried proglottids of *D. caninum* resemble uncooked grains of rice. When water is added, they assume their natural state. (From Hendrix CM, Robinson E: *Diagnostic parasitology for veterinary technicians,* ed 3, St Louis, 2006, Mosby.)

dog's or cat's feces, the proglottid should be torn open or macerated in a drop of saline solution on a glass slide to reveal the characteristic eggs under the compound microscope.

The eggs of taeniid tapeworms are slightly oval and are 43 to 53 μm by 43 to 49 μm in diameter *(T. pisiformis),* 36 to 39 μm by 31 to 35 μm in diameter *(T. hydatigena),* and 19 to 31 μm by 24 to 26 μm *(T. ovis).* Eggs of *Taenia* species contain a single oncosphere with three pairs of hooks. The oncosphere is the hexacanth embryo. Figure 6-11 shows the unique features of this

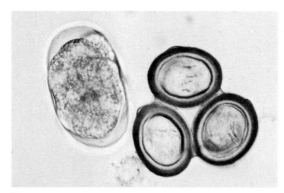

Figure 6-11. Characteristic ova of the taeniid tapeworms are slightly oval and 43 to 53 μm by 43 to 49 μm in diameter *(Taenia pisiformis),* 36 to 39 μm by 31 to 35 μm in diameter *(Taenia hydatigena),* and 19 to 31 μm by 24 to 26 μm *(Taenia ovis).* Eggs of *Taenia* species contain a single oncosphere with three pairs of hooks. The oncosphere is often called a hexacanth embryo. The eggs are similar to those of *Echinococcus* and *Multiceps* species. The dissimilar ovum is that of *A. caninum,* the hookworm. (From Hendrix CM, Robinson E: *Diagnostic parasitology for veterinary technicians,* ed 3, St Louis, 2006, Mosby.)

taeniid tapeworm. The eggs are also similar to those of *Echinococcus* and *Multiceps* species.

Taenia taeniaeformis, or *Hydatigera taeniae-formis,* is called the "feline tapeworm" or the "feline taeniid." This tapeworm is observed infrequently in cats allowed to roam and prey on house and field mice and rats. The egg of this tapeworm is 31 to 36 μm in diameter and contains a single onco-sphere with three pairs of hooks. The oncosphere is often called a hexacanth embryo. As with the eggs of the canine taeniids, the eggs are similar to those of *Echinococcus* species (see Fig. 6-11).

Multiceps multiceps and *Multiceps serialis* also are tapeworms of the small intestine of canids. The eggs of *M. multiceps* are 29 to 37 μm in diameter, whereas those of *M. serialis* are elliptic and meas-ure 31 to 34 μm by 29 to 30 μm. Both contain a single oncosphere with three pairs of hooks. As with the eggs of the canine and feline taeniids, the eggs of *Multiceps* species are similar to those of *Echinococcus* species (see Fig. 6-11).

Echinococcus granulosus and *Echinococcus multilocularis* are tapeworms associated with unilocular and multilocular hydatid disease. *E. granulosus* is the hydatid cyst tapeworm of dogs, whereas *E. multilocularis* is the hydatid cyst tapeworm of cats. These are important parasites because of their extreme zoonotic potential. The egg of *E. granulosus* is ovoid and 32 to 36 μm by 25 to 30 μm. It contains a single oncosphere with three pairs of hooks. The egg of *E. multilocularis* is ovoid and 30 to 40 μm. It contains a single oncosphere with three pairs of hooks. These eggs are very similar in appearance to those of *Taenia* and *Multiceps* species (see Fig. 6-11).

The adult *Echinococcus* is a tiny tapeworm, only 1.2 to 7.0 mm in length. The entire tapeworm has only three proglottids: one immature proglottid, one mature proglottid, and one gravid proglottid. When passed, the tiny gravid proglottids are so small that they are often overlooked by the client, the veterinary technician, and the veterinarian. Definitive diagnosis of *Echinococcus* infection is best achieved by identifying adult tapeworms taken from the host's intestinal tract. In the rare instances in which *Echinococcus* infection is suspected, antemortem diagnosis is accomplished by purging the dog or cat with arecoline hydro-bromide per os at 3.5 mg/kg and collecting the feces. This procedure usually is performed only when this infection is strongly suspected. Entire worms or their proglottids may be collected from the final clear mucus. Because of the severe zoonotic potential, all evacuated material should be handled with caution. Rubber gloves should be worn. After the feces have been examined, they should be incinerated.

Spirometra species are often referred to as "zipper" tapeworms or sparganosis tapeworms (Fig. 6-12). These tapeworms are often found in the small intestine of both the dog and cat and in pets in Florida and along the Gulf Coast of North America. This tapeworm is a clinical oddity because it produces an operculated egg. Each proglottid of *Spirometra* species has a central spiral uterus and an associated uterine pore through which eggs are released. These tapeworms characteristically release eggs until they exhaust their uterine contents.

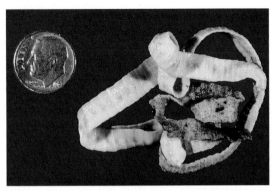

Figure 6-12. Spent proglottids of *Spirometra mansonoides,* the "zipper tapeworm." This tapeworm is unique because although it is attached to the host's jejunum, the mature proglottids often separate along the longitudinal axis for a short distance. The tapeworm appears to "unzip," which provides the origin for its common name. Spent "zipped" and "unzipped" proglottids often appear in the feces of the patient. (From Hendrix CM, Robinson E: *Diagnostic parasitology for veterinary technicians,* ed 3, St Louis, 2006, Mosby.)

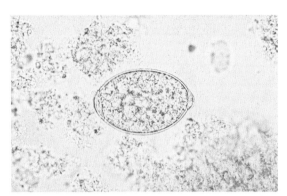

Figure 6-13. Characteristic ovum of *Spirometra mansonoides.* The egg of *Spirometra* species resembles that of a fluke (digenetic trematode). The egg has a distinct operculum at one end of the shell. The eggs are oval and yellowish-brown. They average 60 by 36 μm and have an asymmetric appearance. They tend to be rather pointed at one end. (From Hendrix CM, Robinson E: *Diagnostic parasitology for veterinary technicians,* ed 3, St Louis, 2006, Mosby.)

Gravid segments usually are not discharged into the pet's feces.

The tapeworm is unique because while it is attached to the host's jejunum, the mature proglottids often separate along the longitudinal axis for a short distance. The tapeworm appears to "unzip," which is the origin of its common name, the "zipper tapeworm." Spent "zipped" and "unzipped" proglottids often appear in the feces of the pet.

The egg of *Spirometra* species resembles that of a fluke, or digenetic trematode (Fig. 6-13). The egg has a distinct operculum at one end of the pole of the shell. The eggs are oval and yellowish-brown. They average 60 μm by 36 μm, have an asymmetric appearance, and are rather pointed at one end. When the eggs rupture, a distinct operculum is visible. The eggs are unembryonated when passed in the feces.

Diphyllobothrium species are often referred to as "broad fish" tapeworms. This tapeworm may be 2 to 12 m long; however, it probably does not grow as large as 12 m in dogs and cats. Each proglottid of this tapeworm has a central rosette-shaped uterus

and an associated uterine pore through which eggs are released. These tapeworms continually release eggs until they exhaust their uterine contents. The terminal proglottids become senile rather than gravid and detach in chains rather than individually.

The egg of *Diphyllobothrium* species also resembles that of a fluke (digenetic trematode). The egg is oval and has a distinct operculum at one end of the shell. The eggs are light brown, averaging 67 to 71 μm by 40 to 51 μm. They tend to be rounded on one end. The operculum is present on the end opposite the rounded end. The eggs are unembryonated when passed in the feces.

Trematodes (Flukes)

Platynosomum fastosum is the "lizard poisoning fluke" of cats (Fig. 6-14). The adult flukes inhabit the liver, gallbladder, bile ducts, and less commonly, the small intestine. The brownish, operculated eggs are 34 to 50 μm by 20 to 35 μm.

Nanophyetus salmincola is the "salmon poisoning fluke" of dogs in the Pacific Northwest region of North America. The adult fluke inhabits the small intestine and serves as a vector for rickettsial agents, which produce "salmon poisoning"

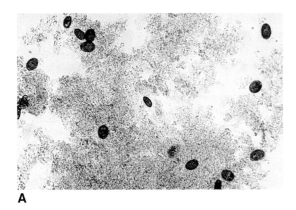

A

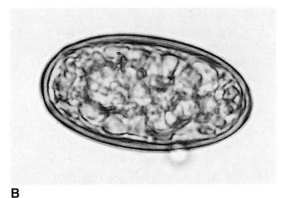

B

Figure 6-14. **A,** Characteristic ova of *Platynosomum fastosum,* the "lizard poisoning fluke" of cats. **B,** The brownish, operculated eggs are 34 to 50 µm by 20 to 35 µm. (From Hendrix CM, Robinson E: *Diagnostic Parasitology for Veterinary Technicians,* ed 3, St Louis, 2006, Mosby.)

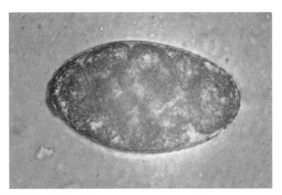

Figure 6-15. Characteristic ovum of *Nanophyetus salmincola.* The eggs are unembryonated when laid and measure 52 to 82 µm by 32 to 56 µm. They have an indistinct operculum and a small, blunt point at the end opposite the operculum. (From Hendrix CM, Robinson E: *Diagnostic parasitology for veterinary technicians,* ed 3, St Louis, 2006, Mosby.)

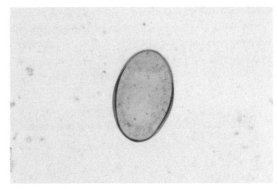

Figure 6-16. Characteristic ovum of *Alaria* species, the intestinal flukes of dogs and cats. They are found throughout the northern half of North America. The eggs are large, golden brown, and operculated. They measure 98 to 134 µm by 62 to 68 µm. (From Hendrix CM, Robinson E: *Diagnostic parasitology for veterinary technicians,* ed 3, St Louis, 2006, Mosby.)

and "Elokomin fluke fever" in dogs. The eggs are unembryonated when laid and measure 52 to 82 µm by 32 to 56 µm (Fig. 6-15). They have an indistinct operculum and a small, blunt point at the end opposite the operculum.

Alaria species are intestinal flukes of dogs and cats and are found throughout the northern half of North America. Their ova are large, golden brown, and operculated (Fig. 6-16). They are 98 to 134 µm by 62 to 68 µm.

Protozoans (Unicellular Organisms)

Isospora species (coccidians) are protozoan parasites of the small intestine of both dogs and cats. They produce a clinical syndrome known as coccidiosis, one of the most commonly diagnosed protozoan diseases in puppies and kittens. Coccidiosis is rarely a problem in mature animals. The oocyst is the diagnostic stage observed in a fecal flotation of fresh feces. It is unsporulated in fresh feces and varies in size and shape among the common *Isospora* species (Figs. 6-17 and 6-18).

The canine coccidians and their oocyst measurements are *Isospora canis,* 34 to 40 μm by 28 to 32 μm; *Isospora ohioensis,* 20 to 27 μm by 15 to 24 μm; and *Isospora wallacei,* 10 to 14 μm by 7.5 to 9.0 μm. The feline coccidians and their measurements are *Isospora felis,* 38 to 51 μm by 27 to 29 μm, and *Isospora rivolta,* 21 to 28 μm by 18 to 23 μm. The prepatent period varies among species but is usually 7 to 14 days.

Toxoplasma gondii is another intestinal coccidian of cats. Its oocysts usually are diagnosed using a standard fecal flotation. Oocysts of *T. gondii* are unsporulated in fresh feces and measure 10 μm by 12 μm. Several immunodiagnostic tests using whole blood or serum are available for diagnosis of *T. gondii* infection. The prepatent period is highly variable, ranging from 5 to 24 days, and depends on the route of infection.

Cryptosporidium is another coccidian parasite that parasitizes the small intestine of a wide variety of animals, including dogs and cats, but particularly young calves. The sporulated oocysts in the feces are oval to spherical and measure only 4 to 6 μm. Diagnosis is by a standard fecal flotation. The oocysts are extremely small and may be observed just under the cover slip, not in the same plane of focus as other oocysts and parasite ova (Fig. 6-19). Examination of fresh fecal smears with special stains (modified acid-fast stain) is also helpful. Because people may become infected with *Cryptosporidium* species, feces suspected of harboring this protozoan should be handled with great care.

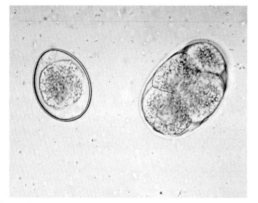

Figure 6-17. Unsporulated oocyst of *Isospora* species (left). Oocysts vary greatly in size. Also see Fig. 6-18, *Ancylostoma caninum (right).*

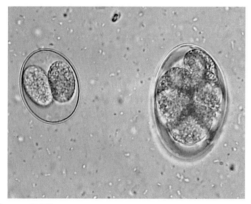

Figure 6-18. Sporulated oocyst of *Isospora* species. The canine coccidians and their measurements are *Isospora canis,* 34 to 40 μm by 28 to 32 μm; *Isospora ohioensis,* 20 to 27 μm by 15 to 24 μm; and *Isospora wallacei,* 10 to 14 μm by 7.5 to 9.0 μm. The feline coccidians and their measurements are *Isospora felis,* 38 to 51 μm by 27 to 29 μm, and *Isospora rivolta,* 21 to 28 μm by 18 to 23 μm. *Ancylostoma caninum (right).*

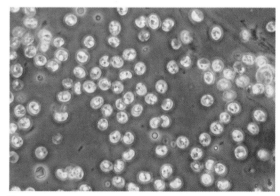

Figure 6-19. Oocysts of *Cryptosporidium* species. (From Hendrix CM, Robinson E: *Diagnostic parasitology for veterinary technicians,* ed 3, St Louis, 2006, Mosby.)

Sarcocystis is another coccidian parasite found in the small intestine. Several species infect dogs and cats. Identification of an individual species may be quite difficult. The oocysts of *Sarcocystis* species are sporulated when passed in the feces. Each oocyst contains two sporocysts, each with four sporozoites. These individual oocysts measure 12 to 15 µm by 8 to 12 µm and may be recovered in a standard fecal flotation of fresh feces.

Giardia species are flagellated protozoans often recovered from the feces of dogs and cats with diarrhea, but they also may be recovered from animals with normal stools. This parasite occurs in two morphologic forms: a motile feeding stage the trophozoite, (Fig. 6-20) and a resistant cyst stage. The motile stage is pear shaped and dorsoventrally flattened and contains four pairs of flagella. It measures 9 to 21 µm by 5 to 15 µm. Two nuclei and a prominent adhesive disk are present on the cranial portion of the cell, resembling a pair of eyes staring back at the observer.

The mature cysts are oval and are 8 to 10 µm by 7 to 10 µm. They have a refractile wall and four nuclei. Immature cysts, which represent recently encysted motile forms, contain only two nuclei (Fig. 6-21). In dogs, diarrhea may begin as early as 5 days after exposure to *Giardia*, with cysts first appearing in the feces at 1 week.

Diagnosis is by a standard fecal flotation. Zinc sulfate (specific gravity 1.18) is considered the best

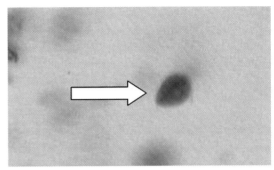

Figure 6-21. Cysts of *Giardia* species. The mature cysts are oval and measure 8 to 10 µm by 7 to 10 µm. They have a refractile wall and four nuclei. Immature cysts, which represent recently encysted motile forms, contain only two nuclei. (From Hendrix CM, Robinson E: *Diagnostic parasitology for veterinary technicians,* ed 3, St Louis, 2006, Mosby.)

flotation medium for recovering cysts. Cysts are often distorted, with a semilunar appearance. The motile trophozoite occasionally may be found on a direct smear of fresh feces with isotonic saline. Lugol's iodine may be used to visualize the internal structures of cysts and trophozoites. Fecal immuno-diagnostic tests are also commonly used.

Parasites of the Circulatory System
Nematodes (Roundworms)

Dirofilaria immitis is often referred to as the canine heartworm; however, this nematode also has been known to parasitize cats and ferrets. Adult heartworms are found within the right ventricle, the pulmonary artery, and the fine branches of that artery. This parasite is often recovered in a variety of aberrant sites, such as the brain, the anterior chamber of the eye, and subcutaneous sites. The prepatent period in dogs is approximately 6 months.

In microfilaremic dogs, diagnosis is by observing microfilariae in blood samples using one of several concentration techniques (modified Knott's test) or the commercially available filter techniques (Figs. 6-22 and 6-23). For infected dogs and cats with no circulating microfilariae, infection also may be diagnosed by commercially available immuno-diagnostic tests.

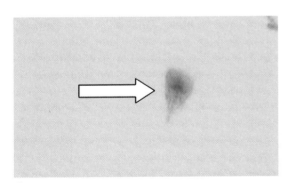

Figure 6-20. Motile trophozoite of *Giardia* species. (From Hendrix CM, Robinson E: *Diagnostic parasitology for veterinary technicians,* ed 3, St Louis, 2006, Mosby.)

A subcutaneous filariid of dogs, *Dipetalonema reconditum,* also produces microfilariae in the peripheral blood. The microfilariae of this non-pathogenic nematode must be differentiated from those of *D. immitis* (see Figs. 6-22 and 6-23).

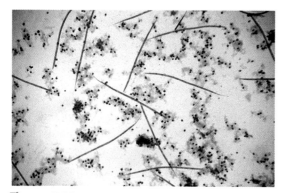

Figure 6-22. Microfilariae of *Dirofilaria immitis* from a peripheral blood sample subjected to the modified Knott's test. The microfilariae of *D. immitis* average 310 μm long. In contrast, the microfilariae of *Dipetalonema reconditum* average 285 μm long. (From Hendrix CM, Robinson E: *Diagnostic parasitology for veterinary technicians,* ed 3, St Louis, 2006, Mosby.)

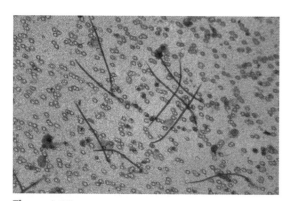

Figure 6-23. An individual microfilaria of *Dirofilaria immitis* from a peripheral blood sample subjected to the modified Knott's test. Note the tapered cranial end and straight tail. Microfilariae of *Dipetalonema reconditum* have a blunt (rounded) cranial end and may exhibit a shepherd's crook (hooked) tail. (From Hendrix CM, Robinson E: *Diagnostic parasitology for veterinary technicians,* ed 3, St Louis, 2006, Mosby.)

Trematodes (Flukes)

Heterobilharzia americanum, the canine schistosome, is a blood fluke that parasitizes the mesenteric veins of the small and large intestines and portal veins of the dog. This fluke is enzootic in the Mississippi delta and the coastal swampland of Louisiana. Although this fluke inhabits the vasculature, its presence is manifested by bloody diarrhea. Infected dogs also exhibit emaciation and anorexia. Diagnosis is by identification of the thin-shelled egg, approximately 80 μm by 50 μm, which contains a miracidium. Figure 6-24 shows the morphologic features of the egg of *H. americanum.* The prepatent period is approximately 84 days.

Protozoans (Unicellular Organisms)

Babesia canis is an intracellular parasite found within the erythrocytes of dogs, also referred to as a piroplasm (pear-shaped body) (Fig. 6-25). Diagnosis is by observing basophilic, pear-shaped trophozoites in RBCs on stained blood smears.

Cytauxzoon felis is another intracellular parasite sporadically reported in the RBCs of cats in various locales (Missouri, Arkansas, Georgia, Texas) throughout the United States. It also produces piroplasms,

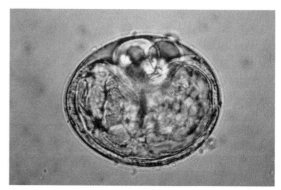

Figure 6-24. Characteristic thin-shell ovum of *Heterobilharzia americanum.* These ova are approximately 80 by 50 μm and contain a miracidium. (From Hendrix CM, Robinson E: *Diagnostic parasitology for veterinary technicians,* ed 3, St Louis, 2006, Mosby.)

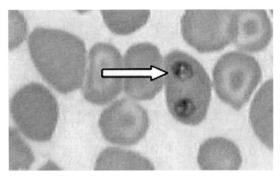

Figure 6-25. Basophilic, pear-shaped trophozoites of *Babesia canis* within canine RBCs in a stained blood smear. (From Hendrix CM, Robinson E: *Diagnostic parasitology for veterinary technicians,* ed 3, St Louis, 2006, Mosby.)

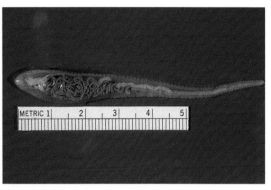

Figure 6-26. Adult female *Linguatula serrata,* the "canine pentastome" or "canine tongueworm." This parasite of the nasal and respiratory passages of dogs resembles a helminth, but it is actually a type of arthropod (it has a mitelike larval stage). (From Hendrix CM, Robinson E: *Diagnostic parasitology for veterinary technicians,* ed 3, St Louis, 2006, Mosby.)

which have been described as shaped like a "bejeweled ring" and are referred to as the ring form in stained blood smears. Cytauxzoonosis is a rapidly fatal disease, and its prognosis is poor.

Hepatozoon canis and *Hepatozoon americanum* are intracellular, malaria-like parasites affecting dogs. The blood forms of the parasites (the gamonts) of these protozoan parasites are found in the leukocytes. Leukocytes containing gamonts of *H. canis* are common in peripheral blood smears, whereas those of *H. americanum* are rare. Schizonts are found in endothelial cells of the spleen, bone marrow, and liver. The gamonts are surrounded by a delicate capsule and stain pale blue with a dark, reddish-purple nucleus. Numerous pink granules are found in the cytoplasm of the leukocyte. The "onion skin" tissue cysts of *H. americanum* are found in the skeletal muscle of dogs. (For cystic stages of this parasite, see Parasites of the Musculoskeletal System.) This is an unusual parasite in that the dog becomes infected by ingestion of an infected tick, *Amblyomma americanum*. *H. canis* is well adapted to its canine host and varies from producing a subclinical to a mild disease. *H. americanum* produces a violent and frequently fatal course of disease; it is theorized to have crossed the species barrier from a wild animal host to the domestic dog.

Parasites of the Respiratory System
Pentastomids (Tongueworms)

Pentastomids (tongueworms) resemble helminths but are actually related to the arthropods. *Linguatula serrata* is the "canine pentastome" or the "canine tongueworm" (Fig. 6-26). Pentastomes are usually parasites of snakes and reptiles, but this tongueworm parasitizes the nasal and respiratory passages of dogs. It resembles a helminth but is classified as a type of arthropod because it has a mitelike larval stage. The pentastome eggs measure 70 µm by 90 µm (Fig. 6-27). On the inside of the egg, the mitelike larval stage with its jointed claws is often visible.

Nematodes (Roundworms)

Aelurostrongylus abstrusus is the feline lungworm. The adults live in the terminal respiratory bronchioles and alveolar ducts, where they form small egg nests or nodules. The eggs of this parasite are forced into the lung tissue, where they hatch to form characteristic first-stage larvae, approximately 360 µm long. Each larva has a tail with an S-shaped bend and a dorsal spine (Fig. 6-28). Characteristic larvae on fecal flotation or the Baermann technique can determine their presence. Recovering the larvae

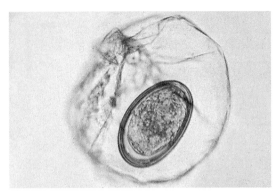

Figure 6-27. Characteristic ovum of *Linguatula serrata.* The pentastome eggs measure 70 by 90 µm. In the interior of many pentastome eggs, a mitelike larval stage with jointed claws can be observed. (From Hendrix CM, Robinson E: *Diagnostic parasitology for veterinary technicians,* ed 3, St Louis, 2006, Mosby.)

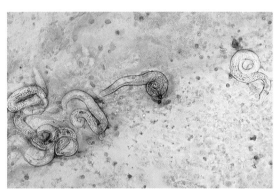

Figure 6-29. Numerous first-stage larvae of *Aelurostrongylus abstrusus* recovered on tracheal washing. (From Hendrix CM, Robinson E: *Diagnostic parasitology for veterinary technicians,* ed 3, St Louis, 2006, Mosby.)

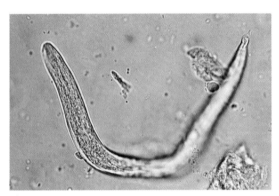

Figure 6-28. Characteristic first-stage larva of *Aelurostrongylus abstrusus,* the feline lungworm. The larva is approximately 360 µm long and has a tail with an S-shaped bend and a dorsal spine. Diagnosis is accomplished by finding these characteristic larvae on fecal flotation or by using the Baermann technique. (From Hendrix CM, Robinson E: *Diagnostic parasitology for veterinary technicians,* ed 3, St Louis, 2006, Mosby.)

on tracheal washing is also possible (Fig. 6-29). The prepatent period is approximately 30 days.

Filaroides (Oslerus) osleri, Filaroides birthi, and *Filaroides milksi,* the canine "lungworms," are found in the trachea, the lung parenchyma, and the bronchioles of canids, respectively. The larva is

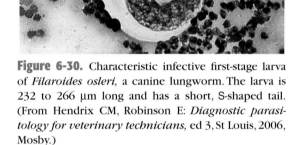

Figure 6-30. Characteristic infective first-stage larva of *Filaroides osleri,* a canine lungworm. The larva is 232 to 266 µm long and has a short, S-shaped tail. (From Hendrix CM, Robinson E: *Diagnostic parasitology for veterinary technicians,* ed 3, St Louis, 2006, Mosby.)

232 to 266 µm long and has a short, S-shaped tail. *Filaroides* species are unique among the nematodes in that their first-stage larvae are immediately infective for the canine definitive host. No period of development is required outside the host. Diagnosis is by finding these characteristic larvae on fecal flotation or by using the Baermann technique. Figure 6-30 shows the unique infective larvae of *F. osleri.* Nodules of *F. osleri* are usually found at the bifurcation of the trachea, where they can be

observed by endoscopic examination. The prepatent period for *F. osleri* is approximately 10 weeks.

Eucoleus aerophilus (*Capillaria aerophila*) is a capillarid nematode found in the trachea and bronchi of both dogs and cats. The prepatent period is approximately 40 days. In standard fecal flotations, eggs of *Eucoleus* species are often confused with those of *Trichuris* (whipworms). Eggs of *E. aerophilus* are smaller than whipworm eggs (59 to 80 μm by 30 to 40 μm), more broadly barrel shaped, and lighter in color. The egg also has a rough outer surface with a netted appearance.

Eucoleus böehmi is found in the nasal cavity and frontal sinuses of dogs. Its eggs are smaller and have a smoother outer surface than those of *E. aerophilus*. Its shell has a pitted appearance. This parasite can be detected by standard fecal flotation.

Trematodes (Flukes)

Paragonimus kellicotti is the "lung fluke" of dogs. Hermaphroditic adult flukes occur in cystic spaces within the lung parenchyma of both dogs and cats. These cystic spaces connect to the terminal bronchioles. The eggs are found in sputum or feces. The egg is yellowish-brown with an operculum and measures 75 to 118 μm by 42 to 67 μm (Fig. 6-31). Fluke eggs usually are recovered by fecal sedimentation techniques; however, the eggs of *P. kellicotti* may be recovered by standard fecal flotation solutions. The eggs of *P. kellicotti* also may be recovered in the sputum collected by tracheal washing. The adult flukes within the cystic spaces of the lung parenchyma can also be observed in thoracic radiographs. This fluke's prepatent period is 30 to 36 days.

Parasites of the Urogenital System
Nematodes (Roundworms)

Dioctophyma renale is the "giant kidney worm" of dogs. This largest of parasitic nematodes frequently infects the right kidney of dogs and gradually ingests the renal parenchyma, leaving only the capsule of the kidney. Eggs may be recovered by centrifugation and examination of the urine sediment. They are characteristically barrel shaped, bipolar, and yellow brown. The egg's shell has a pitted appearance. Eggs measure 71 to 84 μm by 46

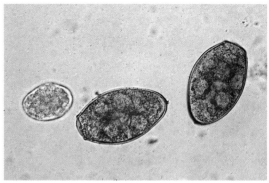

Figure 6-31. Characteristic ovum of *Paragonimus kellicotti,* the lung fluke of dogs recovered by standard fecal flotation. The eggs may be found in either sputum or feces but often are recovered on fecal flotation. The yellowish-brown, operculated eggs measure 75 to 118 μm by 42 to 67 μm. *Ancylostoma caninum egg (left).* (From Hendrix CM, Robinson E: *Diagnostic parasitology for veterinary technicians,* ed 3, St Louis, 2006, Mosby.)

to 52 μm. Figure 6-32 shows the characteristic ovum of *D. renale. D. renale* also may occur freely within the peritoneal cavity. When it is in this location, eggs are not passed to the external environment. The prepatent period is approximately 18 weeks.

Capillaria plica and *Capillaria (Personema) feliscati* are nematodes of the urinary bladder of dogs and cats, respectively. Their eggs may be found in urine or in feces contaminated with urine. Eggs are clear to yellow in color, measure 63 to 68 μm by 24 to 27 μm, and have flattened bipolar end plugs. Their outer surface is roughened. These eggs may be confused with those of the respiratory and gastric capillarids and with those of the whipworms.

Parasites of the Eye and Adnexa
Nematodes (Roundworms)

Thelazia californiensis is the "eyeworm" of dogs and cats. Adult parasites can be recovered from the conjunctival sac and lachrymal duct. Examination of the lachrymal secretions may reveal eggs or first-stage larvae. As mentioned previously, *D. immitis* may be recovered from a variety of aberrant sites, such as the anterior chamber of the eye.

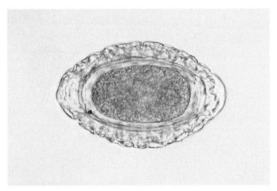

Figure 6-32. Characteristic ovum of *Dioctophyma renale* recovered from urine sediment. These eggs are characteristically barrel shaped, bipolar, and yellow brown. The egg shell has a pitted appearance. Eggs measure 71 to 84 μm by 46 to 52 μm. (From Hendrix CM, Robinson E: *Diagnostic parasitology for veterinary technicians,* ed 3, St Louis, 2006, Mosby.)

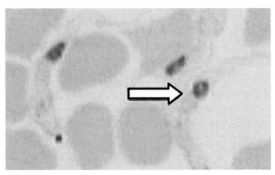

Figure 6-33. The "onion skin" tissue cysts of *Hepatozoon americanum* are found in skeletal muscle of dogs. (From Hendrix CM, Robinson E: *Diagnostic parasitology for veterinary technicians,* ed 3, St Louis, 2006, Mosby.)

Parasites of the Musculoskeletal System
Protozoans (Unicellular Parasites)

In the United States, canine hepatozoonosis is most commonly diagnosed by muscle biopsy rather than by examination of peripheral blood smears for infected leukocytes. Muscle lesions consist of large cysts, pyogranulomas, and myositis. The cysts produced are round to ovoid and range from 250 to 500 μm in diameter. The center of the cyst demonstrates a basophilic nucleus surrounded by small basophilic bodies. Surrounding the nucleus and the basophilic bodies are concentric layers of fine multilaminated membranes, giving an "onion skin" appearance. In most cases, no inflammatory response is associated with the cyst (Fig. 6-33).

Endoparasites of Cattle and Other Ruminants

Parasites of the Gastrointestinal Tract
Nematodes (Roundworms)

The bovine trichostrongyles are composed of several genera of nematodes within the abomasum and small and large intestine of cattle and other ruminants. Genera that produce trichostrongyle-type eggs are *Bunostomum, Cooperia, Chabertia,* *Haemonchus, Oesophagostomum, Ostertagia,* and *Trichostrongylus.* These seven genera (and others) produce oval, thin-shelled eggs. They contain four or more cells and are 70 to 120 μm long. Some of these ova may be identified to their respective genera; however, identification is usually difficult because mixed infections of bovine trichostrongyles are quite common.

Upon identification of the characteristic eggs, the veterinary technician should record the finding as a trichostrongyle-type egg (Fig. 6-34). They should never be recorded as individual genus names. Identification of genus and species usually can be performed only by fecal culture and larval identification.

Nematodirus species and *Marshallagia* species are also bovine trichostrongyles; however, their eggs are much larger than those of the genera mentioned previously. Their eggs are the largest in the trichostrongyle family. Figure 6-35 shows the large eggs of *Nematodirus* species. In a standard fecal flotation, the eggs of *Nematodirus* species are large (150 to 230 μm by 80 to 100 μm) and have tapering ends and four to eight cells. The eggs of *Marshallagia* species also are large (160 to 200 μm by 75 to 100 μm), have parallel sides and rounded ends, and contain 16 to 32 cells.

Strongyloides papillosus is often referred to as the "intestinal threadworm." These nematodes

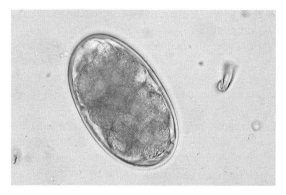

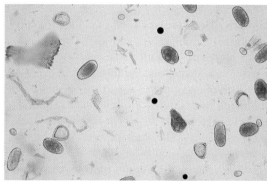

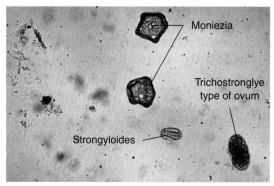

Moniezia

Trichostronglye type of ovum

Strongyloides

Figure 6-34. Characteristic trichostrongyle-type ova of the bovine trichostrongyles. These oval, thin-shelled eggs contain four or more cells. They measure 70 to 120 μm long. Some of these ova can be identified by their respective genus; however, identification is usually difficult because mixed infections are common. (From Hendrix CM, Robinson E: *Diagnostic parasitology for veterinary technicians,* ed 3, St Louis, 2006, Mosby.)

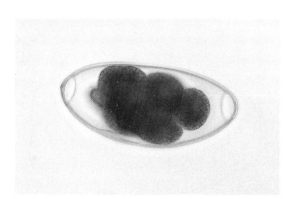

Figure 6-35. Characteristic large ova of *Nematodirus* species. In standard fecal flotation, the eggs of *Nematodirus* species are larger than those of other bovine trichostrongyles (150 to 230 μm by 80 to 100 μm), have tapering ends, and have four to eight cells. (From Hendrix CM, Robinson E: *Diagnostic parasitology for veterinary technicians,* ed 3, St Louis, 2006, Mosby.)

are unique in that only a parthenogenetic female (female that lays eggs without copulating with a male) is parasitic in the host. Parasitic males do not exist. These females produce larvated eggs measuring 40 to 60 μm by 20 to 25 μm. Eggs usually are recovered in flotation of fresh feces. The prepatent period is 5 to 7 days. (See Fig. 6-7 for the parasitic adult females, eggs, and first-stage larvae of *Strongyloides* species.)

Trichuris ovis is commonly called the whipworm, infecting the cecum and colon of ruminants. The previous section on nematode parasites of the gastrointestinal tract of dogs and cats contains details regarding the gross morphologic characteristics of adult whipworms. The egg of the whipworm is described as trichinelloid or trichuroid. It has a thick, yellow-brown, symmetric shell with plugs at both ends. The eggs are unembryonated (not larvated) when laid. Eggs of bovine whipworms measure 50 to 60 μm by 21 to 25 μm.

Cestodes (Tapeworms)

Moniezia species are tapeworms found in the small intestine of cattle, sheep, and goats. These tapeworms produce eggs with a characteristic cuboidal or pyramidal shape; under the compound microscope these eggs appear square or triangular in silhouette. Two species are common, *Moniezia benedini* in cattle and *Moniezia expansa* in cattle, sheep, and goats. The eggs of both species can be easily differentiated by standard fecal flotation procedures. Figure 6-36 shows representative eggs of *Moniezia* species. The eggs of *M. expansa* appear triangular and measure 56 to 67 μm in diameter. The eggs of *M. benedini* appear square and are approximately 75 μm in diameter. The prepatent period for these tapeworms is approximately 40 days.

Thysanosoma actinoides is the "fringed tapeworm" found in the bile ducts, pancreatic ducts, and small intestine of ruminants. Eggs of this tapeworm occur in packets of 6 to 12 eggs, with individual eggs measuring 19 by 27 μm.

Trematodes (Flukes)

"Rumen flukes" are composed of two genera, *Paramphistomum* and *Cotylophoron*. These adult flukes reside in the rumen and reticulum of cattle, sheep, goats, and many other ruminants. The eggs of *Paramphistomum* species measure 114 to 176 μm by 73 to 100 μm, whereas the eggs of *Cotylophoron* species measure 125 to 135 μm by 61 to 68 μm. The prepatent period of *Paramphistomum* species is 80 to 95 days.

Fasciola hepatica is the "liver fluke" of cattle, sheep, and other ruminants. The hermaphroditic adult flukes are found in the bile ducts of the liver. The eggs measure 140 μm by 100 μm and are yellowish-brown, oval, and operculated (Fig. 6-37). The prepatent period for *F. hepatica* is approximately 56 days.

Dicrocoelium dendriticum is the "lancet fluke" of sheep, goats, and oxen. These tiny flukes reside within the fine branches of the bile ducts. The brown eggs have an indistinct operculum and measure 36 to 45 μm by 20 to 30 μm. Eggs of this and the aforementioned trematodes may be recovered from feces by fecal sedimentation or a commercially available fluke egg recovery test.

Protozoans (Unicellular Organisms)

Ruminants serve as host to many species of *Eimeria*. Identification of individual species of

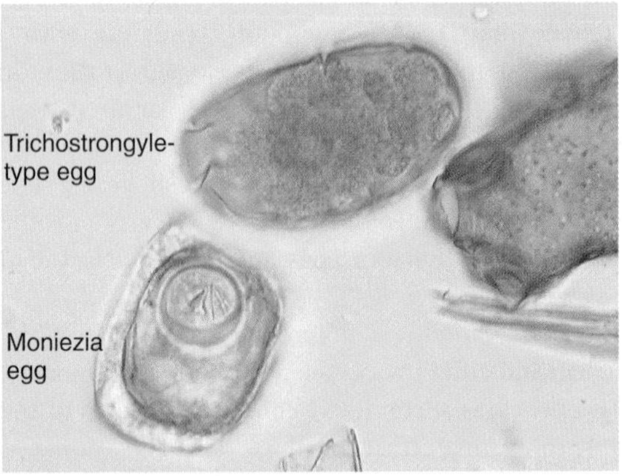

Figure 6-36. Characteristic ova of *Moniezia* species. The eggs of *Moniezia expansa* are triangular or pyramidal and 56 to 67 μm in diameter. The eggs of *Moniezia benedini* are square or cuboidal and approximately 75 μm in diameter. (From Hendrix CM, Robinson E: *Diagnostic parasitology for veterinary technicians,* ed 3, St Louis, 2006, Mosby.)

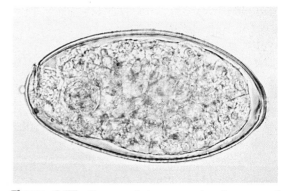

Figure 6-37. Characteristic operculated ovum of *Fasciola hepatica,* the liver fluke of cattle, sheep, and other ruminants. The eggs measure 140 by 100 μm and are yellowish-brown and oval. (From Hendrix CM, Robinson E: *Diagnostic parasitology for veterinary technicians,* ed 3, St Louis, 2006, Mosby.)

coccidia is often difficult because their oocysts are so similar in size and shape. The two most common species of coccidia in cattle, *Eimeria bovis* and *Eimeria zurnii*, can be differentiated on a standard fecal flotation. Oocysts of *E. bovis* are oval, have a micropyle, and measure 20 μm by 28 μm, whereas those of *E. zurnii* are spherical, lack the micropyle, and measure 15 to 22 μm by 13 to 18 μm. When oocysts are recovered on fecal flotation, the observation is usually noted as "coccidia."

Cryptosporidium is another coccidian parasite that parasitizes the small intestine of a variety of animals, including cattle, sheep, and goats. The sporulated oocysts in the feces are colorless and transparent and are extremely tiny, only 4.5 to 5.0 μm in diameter. Diagnosis is by standard fecal flotation and stained fecal smears. Because human beings may become infected with *Cryptosporidium* species, feces suspected of harboring this protozoan should be handled with great care (see Fig. 6-19).

Parasites of the Circulatory System
Nematodes (Roundworms)

Elaeophora schneideri, the "arterial worm," is found in the common carotid arteries of sheep in the western and southwestern United States. Microfilariae are 270 μm long and 17 μm thick, bluntly rounded cranially, and tapering caudally. They are found in the skin, usually in the capillaries of the forehead and face. Filarial dermatitis is seen on the face, poll region, and feet of sheep.

Diagnosis is by observation of characteristic lesions and identification of microfilariae in the skin. The most satisfactory means of diagnosis is to macerate a piece of skin in warm saline and examine the material for microfilariae after approximately 2 hours. In sheep, microfilariae are rare and may not be found in the skin of infected animals. Postmortem examination may be necessary to confirm the diagnosis. The prepatent period is 18 weeks or longer.

Protozoans (Unicellular Organisms)

Babesia bigemina is an intracellular parasite found within the RBCs of cattle. This parasite is a large piroplasm, 4 to 5 μm long by approximately 2 μm wide. It is characteristically pear shaped and occurs in pairs, forming an acute angle within the erythrocyte. The intermediate host for this protozoan parasite is the tick *Boophilus annulatus*.

Parasites of the Respiratory System
Nematodes (Roundworms)

Dictyocaulus species are lungworms of cattle (*Dictyocaulus viviparus*), sheep, and goats (*Dictyocaulus filaria*). Adults are found in the bronchi. The prepatent period varies with the species but is approximately 28 days. Eggs usually are coughed up and swallowed and hatch in the intestine, producing larvae that may be recovered in the feces.

Larvae of *D. filaria* have brownish food granules in their intestinal cells, a blunt tail, and a cranial cuticular knob. They are 550 to 580 μm long. Larvae of *D. viviparus* also have brownish food granules in their intestinal cells but have a straight tail; they lack the cranial cuticular knob. These larvae are 300 to 360 μm in length (Fig. 6-38).

Muellerius capillaris often is called the "hair lungworm." Adults are found within the bronchioles, mostly in nodules in the lung parenchyma of sheep and goats. The eggs develop in the lungs of the definitive host and the first-stage larvae are coughed up, swallowed, and passed out with the feces. They are 230 to 300 μm long. The larval tail has an undulating tip and a dorsal spine (Fig. 6-39).

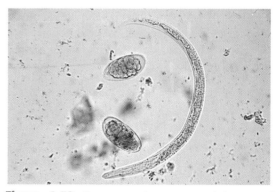

Figure 6-38. Representative eggs and larvae of *Dictyocaulus* species, or cattle lungworms. (From Hendrix CM, Robinson E: *Diagnostic parasitology for veterinary technicians,* ed 3, St Louis, 2006, Mosby.)

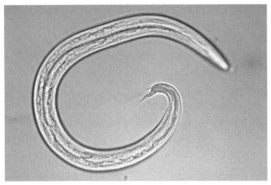

Figure 6-39. First-stage larva of *Muellerius capillaris,* the "hair lungworm" of sheep and goats. First-stage larvae are 230 to 300 μm long. The larval tail has an undulating tip and a dorsal spine. (From Hendrix CM, Robinson E: *Diagnostic parasitology for veterinary technicians,* ed 3, St Louis, 2006, Mosby.)

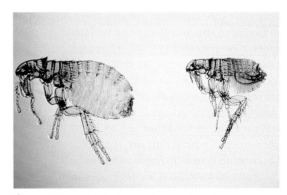

Figure 6-40. Adult *Thelazia* species, the eyeworm, from the conjunctival sac of a cow.

Adult *Protostrongylus* species occur in the small bronchioles of sheep and goats. Again, the eggs develop in the lungs of the definitive host and the first-stage larvae are coughed up, swallowed, and passed out with the feces. These larvae are 250 to 320 μm long. This nematode's larval tail has an undulating tip but lacks the dorsal spine. The Baermann technique is used to diagnose lungworm infection in ruminants.

Parasites of the Eye and Adnexa
Nematodes (Roundworms)
Thelazia rhodesii and *Thelazia gulosa* are the "eyeworms" of cattle, sheep, and goats. Adult parasites may be recovered from the conjunctival sac and lachrymal duct. Examination of the lachrymal secretions may reveal eggs or first-stage larvae. Figure 6-40 shows adult *Thelazia* in the conjunctival sac of a cow.

Parasites of the Abdominal Cavity
Setaria cervi is the "abdominal worm" of cattle. Adults are found free within the peritoneal cavity. The sheathed microfilariae are approximately 250 μm by 7 μm. Diagnosis is by demonstration of microfilariae in blood smears. Cysticercus tenuicollis, the bladderworm (larval or metacestode stage) of *Taenia hydatigena,* may be found

attached to the greater omentum within the abdominal cavity of many ruminants. These cysticerci are usually diagnosed on postmortem examination.

Parasites of the Musculoskeletal System
Cysticercus bovis, the bladderworm (larval or metacestode stage) of *Taenia saginata,* the beef tapeworm of human beings, may be found within the musculature of the bovine intermediate host. These cysticerci are colloquially referred to as "beef measles" and are usually diagnosed during postmortem meat inspection. Human beings become infected with the adult tapeworm by eating poorly cooked beef.

Endoparasites of Horses

Parasites of the Gastrointestinal Tract
Arthropods (Larval Flies)
These parasites are unusual; their adult form is an ectoparasite and their larval form is an endoparasite. Larval *Gasterophilus* species, or "horse bots," parasitize the stomach of horses. Because these stages are larval or immature stages of nonparasitic adult flies, no demonstrable egg stage may be recovered from horse feces; however, adult flies do deposit eggs on the hairs of the legs of horses (Figs. 6-41 and 6-42). The third larval stage exits the gastrointestinal tract by the feces; therefore this stage may be recovered from the feces. The brown larvae are up to 20 mm in length and have dense

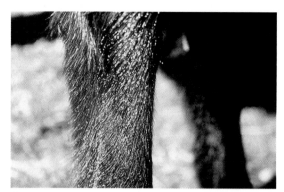

Figure 6-41. Numerous eggs cemented to forelimb of a horse. (From Hendrix CM, Robinson E: *Diagnostic parasitology for veterinary technicians,* ed 3, St Louis, 2006, Mosby.)

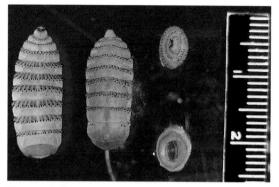

Figure 6-43. Final larval stage of *Gasterophilus* species is often found within feces of equine host. Note the presence of an anterior hook, with larva attached to gastric mucosa. (From Hendrix CM, Robinson E: *Diagnostic parasitology for veterinary technicians,* ed 3, St Louis, 2006, Mosby.)

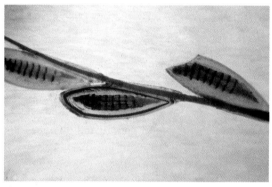

Figure 6-42. Individual egg of *Gasterophilus* species cemented by adult female fly to hairs on a horse's leg. Friction and moisture of horse's licking cause the egg to hatch. Note emergence of larval bot. (From Hendrix CM, Robinson E: *Diagnostic parasitology for veterinary technicians,* ed 3, St Louis, 2006, Mosby.)

Habronema microstoma and *H. muscae* occur on the stomach mucosa, just beneath a thick layer of mucus; *D. megastoma* is often associated with large, thickened fibrous nodules within the stomach mucosa. Larvae of both may parasitize skin lesions, causing a condition known as "summer sores" (see Chapter 7). The prepatent period is approximately 60 days. Larvated eggs or larvae may be recovered on a standard fecal flotation. The eggs of both genera are elongated, have thin walls, and measure 40 to 50 μm by 10 to 12 μm (Fig. 6-44).

Trichostrongylus axei is another nematode that may infect the stomach of horses. They are unusual in that they also can infect cattle and sheep. Their eggs are classified as strongyle-type eggs.

Parascaris equorum often is called the "equine ascarid" or "equine roundworm." It is found in the small intestine of horses, particularly young foals. The prepatent period is 75 to 80 days. Eggs recovered from the feces of young horses are oval and brown. The shell is thickened, with a finely granular surface. The eggs measure 90 to 100 μm in diameter. The center of the egg contains one or two cells (Fig. 6-45). Eggs may be recovered easily on standard fecal flotation.

Strongyles are nematodes that parasitize the large intestine of horses and are typically divided into two types: large strongyles and small strongyles.

spines on the cranial border of each segment. A pair of distinct mouth hooks is found on the cranial end of the first segment and a spiracular plate on the caudal end (Fig. 6-43). The veterinary technician should be able to identify horse bots grossly as *Gasterophilus* species.

Nematodes (Roundworms)

Habronema species and *Draschia megastoma* are nematodes found in the stomach of horses.

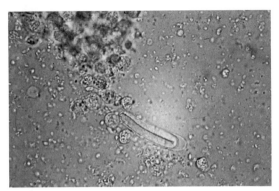

Figure 6-44. Larvated eggs or larvae of *Habronema* and *Draschia* species may be recovered on standard fecal flotation. Eggs of both genera are elongated, have thin walls, and often contain first-stage larvae. (From Hendrix CM and Robinson E: *Diagnostic parasitology for veterinary technicians,* ed 3, St Louis, 2006, Mosby.)

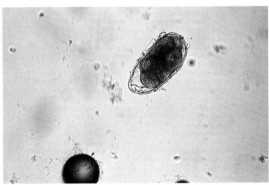

Figure 6-46. Strongyle-type ovum of horses. These eggs contain an 8- to 16-cell morula and measure approximately 70 to 90 μm by 40 to 50 μm. When these characteristic eggs are found on fecal flotation, the observation is recorded as strongyle-type ova rather than as a particular species of strongyle. (From Hendrix CM, Robinson E: *Diagnostic parasitology for veterinary technicians,* ed 3, St Louis, 2006, Mosby.)

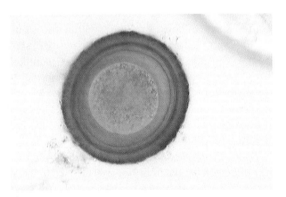

Figure 6-45. Characteristic ovum of *Parascaris equorum,* the equine ascarid or the equine round-worm. The shell is thickened, with a finely granular surface. The eggs measure 90 to 100 μm in diameter. The center of the egg contains one or two cells. (From Hendrix CM, Robinson E: *Diagnostic parasitology for veterinary technicians,* ed 3, St Louis, 2006, Mosby.)

The small strongyles comprise several genera that vary in pathogenicity. The large strongyles are the most pathogenic of the strongyles. *Strongylus vulgaris, Strongylus edentatus,* and *Strongylus equinus* are the large strongyles (Fig. 6-46).

Regardless of whether these endoparasites are a small strongyle or a large strongyle, their eggs are virtually identical. Identification to the species level is accomplished by fecal culture and identification of larvae. Strongyle eggs are most often observed in a standard fecal flotation. They contain an 8- to 16-cell morula and measure approximately 70 to 90 μm by 40 to 50 μm. When these characteristic eggs are found on fecal flotation, the observation is recorded as strongyle-type ova rather than as a particular species of strongyles.

Strongyloides westeri is often referred to as the "intestinal threadworm" of horses. These nematodes are unique; only a parthenogenetic female (one that can lay eggs without copulating with a male) is parasitic in the host. Parasitic males do not exist. These females produce larvated eggs measuring 40 to 52 μm by 32 to 40 μm. Eggs usually are recovered on flotation of fresh feces. The prepatent period is 5 to 7 days (see Fig. 6-7).

Oxyuris equi is the pinworm of horses. The adult worms are found in the cecum, colon, and rectum. Adult worms are often observed protruding from the horse's anus. The adult female worms attach their eggs to the anus with a sticky, gelatinous material that produces anal pruritus in infected horses. Eggs also may be recovered from the feces. The eggs are 90 μm by 40 μm, with a smooth, thick shell. They are operculated, slightly flattened on one side, and may be larvated (Fig. 6-47). The prepatent period is approximately 4 to 5 months. Diagnosis is by finding the characteristic eggs on microscopic examination of cellophane tape impressions or by scraping the surface of the anus.

Cestodes (Tapeworms)

Anoplocephala perfoliata, Anoplocephala magna, and *Paranoplocephala mamillana* are the equine tapeworms. *A. perfoliata* is found in the small and large intestine and cecum. *A. magna* is found in the small intestine and occasionally the stomach. *P. mamillana* also is found in the small intestine and occasionally the stomach. The eggs of *A. perfoliata* have thick walls, with one or more flattened sides, and measure 65 to 80 μm in diameter. Those of *A. magna* are similar but slightly smaller, measuring 50 to 60 μm. The eggs of *P. mamillana* are oval and have thin walls, measuring 51 to 37 μm. Eggs of all three species have a three-layer egg shell, with the innermost lining called the pyriform apparatus, which is pear shaped. Eggs of all equine tapeworms

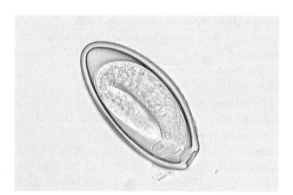

Figure 6-47. Characteristic ovum of *Oxyuris equi,* the pinworm of horses. The eggs are 90 by 40 μm, with a smooth, thick shell. They are operculated and slightly flattened on one side. The eggs may be larvated. (From Hendrix CM, Robinson E: *Diagnostic parasitology for veterinary technicians,* ed 3, St Louis, 2006, Mosby.)

can be recovered by standard fecal flotation. The prepatent period of all three species ranges from 28 to 42 days.

Protozoans (Unicellular Organisms)

Eimeria leuckarti is a coccidian found in the small intestine of horses. This protozoan demonstrates unique, large oocysts (80 to 87 μm by 55 to 60 μm) with a thick wall, a distinct micropyle, and a dark brown color. These oocysts can be recovered on fecal flotation and are the largest coccidian oocysts. They are frequently observed on histopathologic examination. The prepatent period ranges from 15 to 33 days.

Parasites of the Circulatory System
Protozoans (Unicellular Organisms)

Babesia equi and *Babesia caballi* are intracellular parasites found within the RBCs of horses. They are also referred to as the equine piroplasms. Diagnosis is by observing basophilic, pear-shaped trophozoites in RBCs on stained blood smears. Trophozoites of *B. equi* may be round, amoeboid, or pyriform. Four organisms may be joined, giving the effect of a Maltese cross. Individual organisms are 2 to 3 μm long. Trophozoites of *B. caballi* are pyriform, round or oval, and 2 to 4 μm long. They occur characteristically in pairs at acute angles to each other.

Parasites of the Respiratory System
Nematodes (Roundworms)

Dictyocaulus arnfieldi, the equine lungworm, is found in the bronchi and bronchioles of horses, mules, and donkeys. Its eggs are ellipsoid and embryonated, measuring approximately 80 to 100 μm by 50 to 60 μm. Eggs can be recovered on fecal flotation of fresh (less than 24 hours old) feces. Larvae hatch from the eggs within a few hours after feces are passed. The prepatent period for the equine lungworm is 42 to 56 days.

Parasites of the Eye and Adnexa

Thelazia lacrymalis is the eyeworm of horses throughout the world. Adult parasites may be recovered from the conjunctival sac and lachrymal duct. Examination of the lachrymal secretions may reveal eggs or first-stage larvae.

The unsheathed microfilariae of *Onchocerca cervicalis* have been incriminated as causing periodic ophthalmia and blindness in horses. These may be detected by ophthalmic examination.

Parasites of the Abdominal Cavity

Setaria equina is the abdominal worm of horses. Adults are found free within the peritoneal cavity. The sheathed microfilariae are 240 to 256 μm long. Diagnosis is by demonstration of microfilariae in blood smears.

Endoparasites of Swine

Parasites of the Gastrointestinal Tract

Nematodes (Roundworms)

Ascarops strongylina and *Physocephalus sexalatus* are the "thick stomach worms" of the porcine stomach. Both of these nematodes produce thick-walled, larvated eggs that may be recovered on fecal flotation. The eggs of both species are similar. The eggs of *A. strongylina* are 34 to 39 μm by 20 μm and have thick shells surrounded by a thin membrane that produces an irregular outline. The eggs of *P. sexalatus* are 34 to 39 μm by 15 to 17 μm. The prepatent period for both species is approximately 42 days.

Hyostrongylus rubidus is referred to as the "red stomach worm" of swine. The eggs are trichostrongyle type; that is, they are oval, thin-shelled eggs. They contain four or more cells and measure 71 to 78 μm by 35 to 42 μm. These eggs may be recovered on fecal flotation. As with bovine trichostrongyles, definitive diagnosis can be made only by fecal culture and larval identification. The prepatent period is approximately 20 days.

Ascaris suum, the swine ascarid or the large intestinal roundworm, is the largest nematode found within the small intestine of pigs. The eggs may be recovered on standard fecal flotation. They are oval and golden brown, with a thick albuminous shell bearing prominent projections. These eggs measure 70 to 89 μm by 37 to 40 μm (Fig. 6-48).

Strongyloides ransomi, the intestinal thread-worm of pigs, is found within the small intestine of pigs. This parasite is unique in that only a partheno-genetic female is parasitic in the host. Parasitic

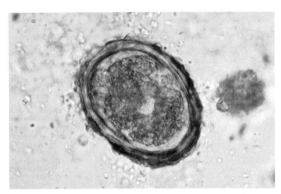

Figure 6-48. Characteristic ovum of *Ascaris suum*, the swine ascarid or the large intestinal roundworm of pigs. The eggs are oval and golden brown, with a thick, albuminous shell bearing prominent projections. They measure 70 to 89 μm by 37 to 40 μm. (From Hendrix CM, Robinson E: *Diagnostic parasitology for veterinary technicians,* ed 3, St Louis, 2006, Mosby.)

males do not exist. These females produce larvated eggs measuring 45 to 55 μm by 26 to 35 μm. Eggs are usually recovered in flotation of fresh feces. The prepatent period is 3 to 7 days (see Fig. 6-7).

Trichinella spiralis occurs in the small intestine of many hosts, most notably the pig. Swine become infected with *T. spiralis* when they ingest infective larval stages (juveniles) in undercooked meat. The larvae mature into adults in the host's small intestine in a few weeks, and the female worms give birth to larvae. The males die after fertilizing the females, and the females die after producing larvae. The larvae enter the bloodstream of the host and, eventually, end up in the pig's musculature.

Oesophagostomum dentatum, the "nodular worm of swine," is found in the large intestine of swine. The prepatent period is 50 days. Their eggs are trichostrongyle type; that is, they are oval, thin-shelled eggs. They contain 4 to 16 cells and measure 40 by 70 μm. These eggs may be recovered on a standard fecal flotation. As with bovine trichostrongyles, definitive diagnosis is made only by fecal culture and larval identification.

Trichuris suis is commonly called the whip-worm, infecting the cecum and colon of swine. See the section on nematode parasites of the gastrointestinal tract of dogs and cats for details on gross morphology of adult worms. The egg of the whipworm is described as trichinelloid or trichuroid. It has a thick, brown, barrel-shaped shell with plugs at both ends. The eggs are unembryonated (not larvated) when laid. Eggs of porcine whipworms measure 50 to 60 μm by 21 to 25 μm. The prepatent period is 42 to 49 days.

Acanthocephalans (Thorny-Head Worms)

Macracanthorhynchus hirudinaceus is the "thorny-head worm" of the small intestine of swine. "Thorny head" describes the spiny proboscis, which it embeds as an anchor into the small intestinal mucosa of the host. The eggs have a triple-layer shell, are oval, and measure 67 to 100 μm by 40 to 65 μm (Fig. 6-49). The eggs may be recovered on a standard fecal flotation. The prepatent period is 60 to 90 days.

Protozoans (Unicellular Organisms)

Balantidium coli is the ciliated protozoan found in the large intestine of swine. Although commonly observed during microscopic examination of fresh diarrheic feces, it is generally considered non-pathogenic. Two morphologic stages may be found in feces: the cyst stage and the motile trophozoite stage. Both stages may vary in size. This is a large protozoan parasite. The trophozoites may be 150 μm by 120 μm, with a sausage- to kidney-shaped macronucleus. It is covered with numerous rows of cilia and moves about the microscopic field with lively motility. The cyst is spherical to ovoid and 40 to 60 μm in diameter, with a slight greenish-yellow color. Both of these stages may be easily recognized by microscopic examination of the intestinal contents or fresh, diarrheic feces. Figure 6-50 shows the trophozoite stage of *B. coli* recovered on fecal flotation. Figure 6-51 shows *B. coli* in histopathologic section.

Cryptosporidium is a coccidian that parasitizes the small intestine of a wide variety of animals, including swine. The sporulated oocysts in the feces are colorless and transparent and measure only 4.5 to 5.0 μm. Diagnosis is by standard fecal flotation and stained fecal smears. Because people may become infected with *Cryptosporidium* species,

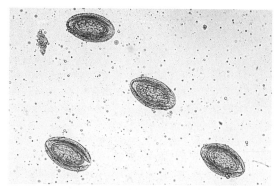

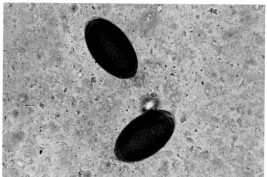

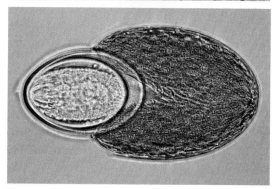

Figure 6-49. Ova of *Macracanthorhynchus hirudinaceus,* the "thorny-head worm" of the small intestine of swine. The eggs have a triple-layered shell, are oval, and measure 67 to 100 μm by 40 to 65 μm. (From Hendrix CM and Robinson E: *Diagnostic Parasitology for Veterinary Technicians,* ed 3, St Louis, 2006, Mosby.)

feces suspected of harboring this protozoan should be handled with great care (see Fig. 6-19).

Isospora suis is the coccidian that parasitizes the small intestine of swine, especially young

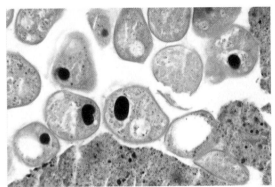

Figure 6-50. Trophozoite stage of *Balantidium coli,* the "ciliated protozoan" found in the large intestine of swine. The trophozoites may be 150 by 120 μm, with a sausage- to kidney-shaped macronucleus. They are covered with numerous rows of cilia and move about the microscopic field with lively motility. The cyst is spherical to ovoid and 40 to 60 μm in diameter, with a slight greenish-yellow color. (From Hendrix CM, Robinson E: *Diagnostic parasitology for veterinary technicians,* ed 3, St Louis, 2006, Mosby.)

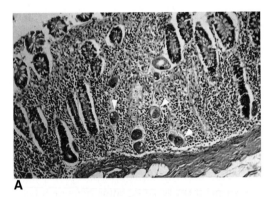

A

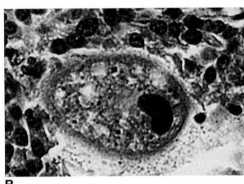

B

Figure 6-51. **A,** *Balantidium coli* of swine in histopathologic section. This photomicrograph was taken at low magnification. Note that *B. coli* is quite large and easily visible *(arrows).* **B,** *B. coli* of swine in histopathologic section. This photomicrograph was taken at higher magnification than **A.** (From Hendrix CM, Robinson E: *Diagnostic parasitology for veterinary technicians,* ed 3, St Louis, 2006, Mosby.)

piglets. Oocysts are usually found on flotation of fresh feces. They are subspherical, lack a micropyle, and measure 18 to 21 μm (Fig. 6-52). Postmortem diagnosis in piglets exhibiting clinical signs, but not shedding oocysts, can be achieved by direct smear of the jejunum stained with Diff-Quik. Diagnosis is by observation of the banana-shaped merozoites. The prepatent period is 4 to 8 days.

Parasites of the Respiratory System
Nematodes (Roundworms)

Metastrongylus apri, the swine lungworm, is found within the bronchi and bronchioles of pigs. The oval, thick-walled eggs measure 60 μm by 40 μm and contain larvae. Eggs can be recovered on fecal flotation using a flotation medium with a specific gravity greater than 1.25 or by the fecal sedimentation technique. The prepatent period is approximately 24 days.

Parasites of the Urinary System
Nematodes (Roundworms)

Stephanurus dentatus, the swine kidney worm, is found in the kidney, ureters, and perirenal tissues

of pigs (Fig. 6-53). Their eggs are strongyle type; that is, they are oval, thin-shelled eggs containing 4 to 16 cells and measuring 90 to 120 μm by 43 to 70 μm. Eggs may be recovered from the urine by urine sedimentation. The prepatent period is extremely long, approximately 9 to 24 months.

Parasites of the Musculoskeletal System

Cysticercus cellulosae, the bladderworm (larval or metacestode stage) of *Taenia solium,* the pork tapeworm of human beings, may be found within the musculature of the porcine intermediate host. These cysticerci are colloquially referred to as "pork measles" and are usually diagnosed during

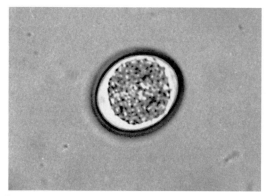

Figure 6-52. Oocyst of *Isospora suis.* (From Hendrix CM, Robinson E: *Diagnostic parasitology for veterinary technicians,* ed 3, St Louis, 2006, Mosby.)

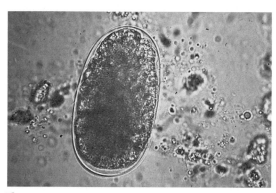

Figure 6-53. Egg of *Stephanurus dentatus,* the swine kidney worm. These eggs are strongyle type; that is, they are oval, thin-shelled eggs containing 4 to 16 cells and measuring 90 to 120 μm by 43 to 70 μm. Eggs can be recovered Reprinted from the urine by urine sedimentation. (From Hendrix CM, Robinson E: *Diagnostic parasitology for veterinary technicians,* ed 3, St Louis, 2006, Mosby.)

postmortem meat inspection. Human beings become infected with the adult tapeworm *Taenia solium* by eating poorly cooked pork containing cysticerci. Human beings may become infected with Cysticercus cellulosae in the muscles or within nervous tissue such as the brain or the eye by ingesting the eggs of *T. solium.*

Trichinella spiralis is found in many species of carnivores and omnivores but is often associated with raw or undercooked pork. Animals (including human beings) become infected with *T. spiralis* when they ingest infective larval stages (juveniles) in meat. The larvae mature into adults in the host's small intestine in a few weeks, and the female worms give birth to larvae. The males die after fertilizing the females, and the females die after producing larvae. The larvae enter the bloodstream of the host and, eventually, end up in the pig's musculature. Within the muscles, the larvae mature into infective encysted larvae. The next host becomes infected when it eats these larvae. Trichinosis is probably best known as a parasite that human beings contract from eating raw or undercooked pork. It is usually detected by proper meat inspection. Most recent outbreaks of trichinosis in the United States have been traced to pork products from pigs that have not been inspected and that have been privately slaughtered.

DIAGNOSIS OF ALIMENTARY PARASITISM

Parasites can infect the oral cavity, esophagus, stomach, small and large intestines, and other internal organs of animals. Detection of these parasites involves collection and microscopic examination of feces. Diagnosis is usually by finding life cycle stages of the parasite within the feces. These stages include eggs, oocysts, larvae, segments (tapeworms), and adult organisms. Veterinary technicians may perform the following procedures to detect parasitic infections.

Collection of Fecal Samples

Fecal samples collected for routine examination should be as fresh as possible. Specimens that cannot be examined within a few hours of excretion should be refrigerated or mixed with an equal part of 10% formalin. The need for fresh feces stems from the fact that eggs, oocysts, and other life cycle stages may be altered by development, making diagnosis extremely difficult.

Small Animal Fecal Samples
Several methods are used for collecting feces from companion animals. An owner may collect a fecal

sample immediately after the animal has defecated. The feces can be stored in any type of container, such as a zippered plastic bag or a clean, small jar. Veterinary hospitals may dispense containers to their clients for this purpose. In either case, only a small amount of feces (1 teaspoon) is required for proper examination. All specimens should be properly identified with the owner's name, animal's name, and species of animal.

Fecal samples also may be collected directly from the animal at the veterinary hospital by using a gloved finger or fecal loop. If a glove is used, the feces may remain in the glove, with the glove turned inside out, tied, and labeled. Samples collected with a fecal loop should be used for direct examination only because the amount collected is relatively small.

Large Animal Fecal Samples

Fecal specimens collected from livestock may be obtained either directly from an individual animal's rectum or from a number of animals to make up a pooled sample. Samples collected directly from an individual animal with a gloved hand can remain in the glove, with the glove turned inside out, tied, and labeled.

Pooled samples are collected from a number of animals housed together and then commingled in a single container. These samples are used to get an idea of the degree of infection within the group. Pooled samples can be collected in any type of container as long as it is clean and can be tightly sealed. These samples should be labeled with the species, pen or group number, owner, and time of collection.

Examination of Fecal Samples

The following precautions should be taken during fecal examination:

- Fecal samples are handled with care. The feces may contain parasites, bacteria, or viruses that are zoonotic (i.e., animal diseases that can be transmitted to people). Appropriate clothing, such as a clean laboratory coat or jacket and latex gloves, should be worn. If gloves are not

worn, hands should be frequently washed with soap and water. No food or drink should be allowed in the examination area. Likewise, workers should refrain from applying makeup or adjusting contact lenses. Laboratory coats should never be worn outside the veterinary clinic to reduce the chances of spreading any infections.
- The laboratory area is cleaned thoroughly after the fecal examinations are completed. Spilled materials create a hazardous area in which to work and could pose a serious threat to staff members' health.
- Accurate and thorough records are maintained. Records should contain the date, owner's name, and any parasites found in the sample. If the sample is negative, it should be recorded as such.

Gross Examination of Feces

The following characteristics of the feces should also be recorded and reported to the veterinarian:

- Consistency: Fresh feces should be somewhat formed depending on the species of animal. Diarrhea or constipation could be the result of a parasitic infection.
- Color: Fecal color may be affected by the food an animal eats. Malabsorption or a parasitic infection also may alter the color of feces.
- Blood: Blood may impart a dark reddish-brown color to feces or it may appear as bright red streaks in the feces. In either case, blood may indicate a severe parasitic infection or other serious intestinal disease. Blood in the feces is an important clinical finding and should be brought to the attention of the veterinarian. Digested blood has a dark, tarry appearance.
- Mucus: Mucus in the feces can be a result of digestive disorders or a parasitic infection. In either case, its presence should be reported to the veterinarian.
- Parasites: Adult parasites or tapeworm segments can be found in the feces. Adult roundworms resemble strings of spaghetti, and tapeworm segments look more like pieces of cooked rice. Tapeworm segments may be identified by

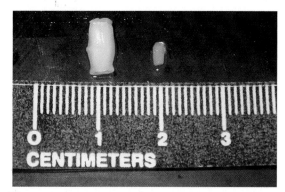

Figure 6-54. Mature segments of the most common tapeworms of dogs and cats. *Left, Taenia* species. *Right, Dipylidium caninum.* (From Hendrix CM, Robinson E: *Diagnostic parasitology for veterinary technicians,* ed 3, St Louis, 2006, Mosby.)

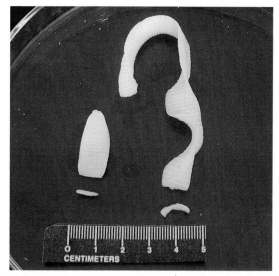

Figure 6-55. Chains and individually mature segments of tapeworms of cattle, *Moniezia (right)* and horses, *Anoplocephala (left).* (From Hendrix CM, Robinson E: *Diagnostic parasitology for veterinary technicians,* ed 3, St Louis, 2006, Mosby.)

microscopic examination (Procedure 6-1). The segments of two common tapeworms infecting dogs and cats are shown in Figure 6-54. Figure 6-55 shows common tapeworm segments, *Moniezia* species, found in cattle feces, and *Anoplocephala* species, found in horse feces.

Occasionally, a client may submit a dried tapeworm segment. To identify the tapeworm species, the dried segments must be soaked in saline for 1 to 4 hours. Once the segments are rehydrated, they may be identified by size, shape, and the eggs contained within.

Segments of some tapeworm species do not contain eggs, and some segments may have expelled their eggs before the examination was conducted. In either case, a tapeworm segment may be identified as such by finding small mineral deposits (calcareous bodies) within the segment (Fig. 6-56). This is done by crushing the tapewormlike segment between two glass slides and examining the material with a microscope.

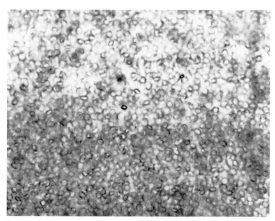

Figure 6-56. Microscopic calcium deposits (calcareous bodies) in tapeworm tissue. (From Hendrix CM, Robinson E: *Diagnostic parasitology for veterinary technicians,* ed 3, St Louis, 2006, Mosby.)

Microscopic Examination of Feces

Microscopic examination of feces is the most reliable method to detect parasitic infections. A microscope with 4×, 10×, and 40× objectives are required for proper examination of a fecal speci-men (see Chapter 1). A mechanical stage is helpful. A micrometer is also recommended but is not required.

Fecal specimens should be examined routinely with the 10× objective. The examination should

PROCEDURE 6-1

Examining Tapeworm Segments

Materials
  Thumb forceps
  Dissection needles (e.g., hypodermic needles)
  Microscope slides and cover slips
  Saline
  Wooden applicator sticks

Procedure
1. Remove the segment from the feces with thumb forceps and place a drop of saline on a slide.
2. Using the dissection needles, pull the segment into several small pieces. Crush the pieces with a wooden applicator stick.
3. Remove the large pieces. Add more saline, if needed, and place a cover slip on the slide.
4. Examine the slide with the microscope for tapeworm eggs.

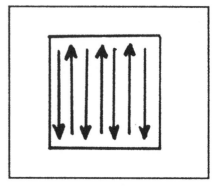

Figure 6-57. A scheme of movement of the microscopic field to examine the area under the cover slip thoroughly. (From Hendrix CM, Robinson E: *Diagnostic parasitology for veterinary technicians,* ed 3, St Louis, 2006, Mosby.)

begin at one corner of the slide and end at the opposite corner, moving over the slide in a systematic pattern (Fig. 6-57). The microscope should be continually focused with the fine-tuning knob during the examination. The initial plane of focus should be that of air bubbles because most eggs are found in this plane. Any material found during the initial scan, including parasite eggs, may be more closely examined using the more powerful objectives.

Calibration of the Microscope
The size of the various stages of many parasites is often important for correct identification. Some examples are *Trichuris* versus *Capillaria* eggs and *Dipetalonema* versus *Dirofilaria* microfilariae. Accurate measurements are easily obtained with the use of a calibrated eyepiece on the microscope. Calibration must be performed on every microscope to be used. Each objective (lens) of the microscope must be individually calibrated. Calibration of the

microscope is described in Chapter 1. Once the calibration procedure has been completed for all magnifications, the information is recorded on a label and attached to the calibrated microscope, such as in the following example:

Objective	Distance Between Hash Marks (μm)
10×	12.5
40×	2.5
100×	1.0

To measure an object such as a parasite egg, one end of the egg is placed on the zero mark and the number of divisions to the other end of the egg is counted. The number of divisions counted is multiplied by the calibration factor for the objective being used. For example, a trichostrongyle egg is 24 divisions long and 13.5 divisions wide when measured with the 40× objective. The calibration factor for the 40× objective is 2.5. Therefore the egg is:

$24 \times 2.5 = 60$ μm long
and
$13.5 \times 2.5 = 33.75$ μm wide

To measure a microfilaria, the head (the anterior end) is aligned with the zero mark and the number of divisions to the end of the tail (the posterior end) is counted. To measure round parasite eggs, the technician should measure through the middle of the egg. For more accurate measurements, the higher objective is used (40× instead of 10×).

Examination of Direct Smears

A direct smear of feces is used to estimate an animal's parasite burden rapidly. This procedure also is used to detect some of the motile protozoa found in feces.

Advantages of direct smears include short preparation time and minimal equipment required to run the procedure. Disadvantages include the small amount of feces examined, which may not be sufficient enough to detect a low parasite burden, and the amount of extraneous fecal debris on the slide, which could be confused with parasitic material.

A fecal sample for a direct smear preparation may be obtained from an animal using a fecal loop or a rectal thermometer (after measuring the animal's temperature). Either way, only a very small amount of feces is needed (Procedure 6-2).

Concentration Methods for Fecal Examination

The following methods are used to concentrate parasitic material in feces. A concentration technique makes examination of a large amount of feces possible in a relatively short time. Also, a low parasite burden can easily be identified. Two types of procedures are most often used in veterinary hospitals: flotation and sedimentation.

Flotation Solutions

Fecal flotation methods are based on the specific gravity of parasitic material and fecal debris. Specific gravity refers to the weight of an object compared with the weight of an equal volume of water. The specific gravity of most parasite eggs is between 1.100 and 1.200 g/mL, whereas the specific gravity of water is 1.000.

To allow for flotation of parasite eggs, oocysts, and other life cycle stages, the flotation solution must have a higher specific gravity than that of the parasitic material (Fig. 6-58). Several salt and sugar solutions work well for flotation (Procedure 6-3). Most have a specific gravity of 1.200 to 1.250. In this range, heavy fecal debris sinks to the bottom of the container, whereas parasitic material rises to the top of the solution.

PROCEDURE 6-2

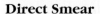

Direct Smear

Materials
> Microscope slide and cover slip
> Applicator stick or toothpick
> Optional: Lugol's iodine or new methylene blue

Procedure
1. Place a drop of saline or water on the microscope slide with an equal amount of feces. A drop of stain may be added at this time.
2. Thoroughly mix the feces and saline or water with the applicator stick to form a homogeneous emulsion.
3. Make a smear on the slide. Be sure the smear is thin enough to see newspaper print through it.
4. Remove any large pieces of feces. Add more saline or water if needed and apply a cover slip.
5. Examine the smear using the 10× objective for parasite eggs and larvae or the 40× objective for motile protozoal organisms.

Sodium nitrate solution is the most common fecal flotation solution used in veterinary hospitals today. This solution is efficient for floating parasite eggs, oocysts, and larvae. It may be purchased with commercial diagnostic test kits or in individual aliquots. The major disadvantage of using sodium nitrate is the expense. Sodium nitrate also forms crystals and distorts eggs if allowed to sit longer than 20 minutes.

Another solution commonly used for flotation is sugar solution. Sugar solution is inexpensive and does not crystallize or distort eggs. Sugar solution may be made anywhere and has a long shelf life. Although sticky to work with, spilled sugar solution may be removed with warm, soapy water.

Zinc sulfate solution is more commonly used in diagnostic laboratories. Zinc sulfate floats protozoal organisms with the least amount of distortion. It

PROCEDURE 6-3

Preparing Flotation Solutions

Sugar Solution (Sheather's Solution)

1. Pour 355 ml of warm water into a beaker. Add a stir bar and place on a hot plate. Heat the water on high but not to the boiling point.
2. Slowly add 1 lb of granulated sugar to the water, stirring constantly. Allow the sugar to dissolve completely before removing from the heat source.
3. Add 6 ml of 40% formalin or liquid phenol after the solution has completely cooled.
4. Check the specific gravity of the solution with a hydrometer before using (see Fig. 6-58). (Hydrometers are available from scientific supply houses.)
   a. If the specific gravity is below the desired range, heat the solution and add more sugar.
   b. If the specific gravity is above the desired range, add water and stir.

Sodium Nitrate Solution

1. Add approximately 315 g of sodium nitrate to 1 L of water while stirring. Heating is not necessary, but it hastens the dissolution process.
2. Check the specific gravity and adjust as needed.

Zinc Sulfate Solution

1. Add approximately 386 g of zinc sulfate to 1 L of water while stirring. Heating is not necessary, but it hastens the dissolution process.
2. Check the specific gravity and adjust as needed.

Saturated Sodium Chloride Solution

1. Add table salt to water until the salt no longer dissolves but tends to settle to the bottom of the container. The specific gravity of this solution cannot go any higher than 1.200.

generally is used in combination with one of the previously mentioned solutions.

The least desirable solution used is saturated sodium chloride solution. This solution corrodes laboratory equipment, forms crystals, and severely distorts parasite eggs. Saturated sodium chloride solution is also a poor flotation medium because the maximum specific gravity obtainable is 1.200, allowing heavier eggs to remain submerged.

Standard Fecal Flotation

The standard or simple fecal flotation is one of the most common flotation techniques used in veterinary hospitals (Procedure 6-4). This technique uses a test tube or vial in which feces and flotation solution are mixed (Fig. 6-59). A cover slip or microscope slide is placed on top of the test tube and the unit is allowed to sit undisturbed. Any parasite eggs in the feces float to the top and adhere to the underside of the cover slip or microscope slide. The cover slip or slide is then removed and micro-

scopically examined for parasitic material. Although the standard flotation technique is easy to perform, it is less efficient at floating parasitic material than the centrifugal technique, described later.

Commercial flotation kits use the same principle as the standard flotation technique. These kits contain a vial with a filter; some also include prepared flotation solution. Examples of commercial flotation kits include Fecalyzer (EVSCO Pharmaceuticals, Buena, NJ), Ovassay Plus (Synbiotics, San Diego, CA), and Ovatector (BGS Medical Products, Venice, FL) (Fig. 6-60). These kits are simple to use but expensive when compared with the simple flotation technique. Some practices reduce the expense by washing and reusing the vials and filters; this practice should be discouraged.

Centrifugal Flotation

Centrifugal flotation for parasite eggs, oocysts, and other parasitic material is the most efficient method available. It requires less time to perform than the

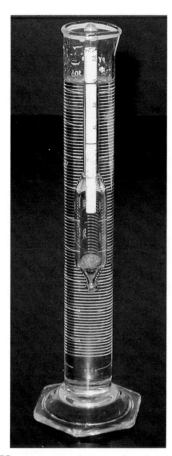

Figure 6-58. Measuring the specific gravity of a flotation solution with a hydrometer. (From Hendrix CM, Robinson E: *Diagnostic parasitology for veterinary technicians,* ed 3, St Louis, 2006, Mosby.)

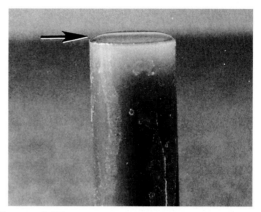

Figure 6-59. Vial filled with flotation solution, showing appearance of the meniscus. (From Hendrix CM, Robinson E: *Diagnostic parasitology for veterinary technicians,* ed 3, St Louis, 2006, Mosby.)

standard flotation method. The only drawback to this procedure is that it requires a centrifuge with a rotor that can hold 15-ml centrifuge tubes (see Chapter 1). If such a centrifuge is available, centrifugal flotation is preferred because it is easy to perform and samples can be run individually or in batches.

If testing multiple samples, the veterinary technician may want to use a numbering system to keep the samples in order. A number is assigned to the patient and that number is written on the corresponding centrifuge tube with a marking pen. This minimizes the chances of error (Procedure 6-5).

Fecal Sedimentation

Fecal sedimentation concentrates parasite eggs, oocysts, and other parasitic material by allowing them to settle to the bottom of a tube of liquid, usually water. A disadvantage of this technique is the amount of fecal debris that mixes with the parasitic material, which makes microscopic examination somewhat difficult.

This procedure is used to detect heavy eggs that would not float in flotation solution or eggs that would become distorted by the flotation solution. Trematode (fluke) eggs are often considered too heavy for flotation and are often found with fecal sedimentation. Although some flotation solutions can be adjusted to a specific gravity of 1.300 to float these eggs, such solutions are not routinely used because some distortion may occur (Procedure 6-6).

Quantitative Fecal Examination

Quantitative procedures are used to determine the number of eggs or oocysts present in each gram of feces. These procedures are used as a rough indication of the number of parasites present within a host. Their usefulness is limited, however, by the fact that the various parasite species produce different numbers of eggs. Also, egg production by

PROCEDURE 6-4

Standard Flotation

Materials

Flotation solution
Shell vial or test tube and test tube rack
Waxed paper cups
Cheesecloth cut into 6-in × 6-in squares
Wooden tongue depressor
Microscope slides and cover slips

Procedure

1. Take approximately 2 g (½ tsp) of feces and place it in the cup. Add 20 ml of flotation solution. With a tongue depressor, mix the feces and flotation solution until no large fecal pieces remain.
2. Wrap cheesecloth around the lip of the cup while bending the cup to form a spout. Pour the mixture through the cheesecloth into a vial. Fill the vial so that a meniscus is formed (see Fig. 6-60). If the cup does not have enough fluid, fill the vial with as much mixture as is available and then fill the remainder with flotation solution.
3. Gently place a cover slip on top of the vial.
4. Allow the unit to remain undisturbed for 10 to 20 minutes (sugar solution requires a longer waiting time than does sodium nitrate). If the preparation is not allowed to sit this long, some eggs will not have time to float to the surface. If allowed to sit for more than an hour, some eggs may become waterlogged and sink, or the eggs may become distorted.
5. Carefully remove the cover slip by picking it straight up and placing it on a microscope slide, with the wet side adjacent to the slide.
6. Examine the area of the slide under the cover slip, with the 10× objective. Record any parasitic material found in the sample.

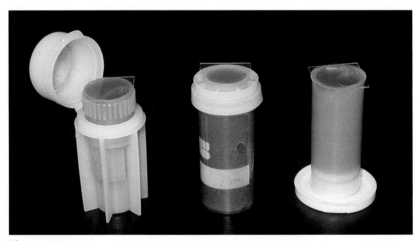

Figure 6-60. Three examples of commercial fecal flotation kits. From *left to right,* Fecalyzer, Ovassay, and Ovatector. (From Hendrix CM, Robinson E: *Diagnostic parasitology for veterinary technicians,* ed 3, St Louis, 2006, Mosby.)

PROCEDURE 6-5

Centrifugal Flotation

Materials
- Same as for standard flotation, but omit the vials
- 15-ml centrifuge tube
- Microscope slides and cover slips

Procedure
1. Prepare the fecal mixture as described in the standard flotation procedure.
2. Strain the mixture through cheesecloth into the 15-ml centrifuge tube. Fill the tube to the top. (If using a fixed-rotor centrifuge, the tube should be filled halfway and a cover slip should not be used.) Apply a cover slip to the top of the tube. Always balance the centrifuge with a 15-ml tube filled with flotation solution and a cover slip placed on top. Be sure all tubes are marked with patient identification information after centrifugation.
3. Centrifuge the tubes for 3 to 5 minutes at 1300 to 1500 rpm (400 to 650 G).
4. Remove the cover slip or use a wire loop or glass rod to remove the top part of fluid in the tube and place on a microscope slide. Microscopically examine the sample with the 10× objective.

PROCEDURE 6-6

Fecal Sedimentation

Materials
- Waxed paper cups
- Cheesecloth cut in 6-in × 6-in squares
- Wooden tongue depressors
- Centrifuge and 15-ml tubes
- Pasteur pipettes with bulbs
- Microscope slides and cover slips

Procedure
1. Mix approximately 2 g of feces with tap water in a waxed paper cup. Strain the mixture through cheesecloth into a centrifuge tube, filling the tube half full.
2. Balance the centrifuge with tubes filled with equal amounts of water. Centrifuge for 3 to 5 minutes at 1300 to 1500 rpm. If a centrifuge is unavailable, allow the tube to sit undisturbed for 20 to 30 minutes.
3. Slowly pour the liquid off the top without disturbing the sediment layer (including the fine, silty material) on the bottom.
4. Using a pipette, transfer a small amount of the fine sediment to a microscope slide. Apply a coverslip to the drop of sediment and examine microscopically. Lugol's iodine may be mixed with the drop of sediment before a coverslip is applied; this facilitates identification of protozoal cysts or trophozoites.

the parasites may be sporadic, and the number of eggs may not correlate with the number of parasites present. The last item is the most significant disadvantage because, in some cases, clinical signs of disease are caused by immature parasites that have not yet begun producing eggs or larvae.

Several quantitative procedures can be performed in veterinary hospitals. These include the Stoll egg count technique, the modified Wisconsin double centrifugation technique, and the McMaster technique. These procedures are fairly easy to perform; each requires its own specialized equipment.

Two quantitative techniques are described in Procedures 6-7 and 6-8. Other quantitative procedures may be found in the references listed at the end of this chapter.

Examination of Feces for Protozoa and Coccidia
Protozoal Trophozoites

All the previously described procedures can be used to detect protozoal cysts. However, some protozoans do not form cysts and pass out of the

PROCEDURE 6-7

Wisconsin Double Centrifugation Technique

1. Weigh a fecal sample (5 g for cattle, 2 g for horses or swine).
2. Place 12 ml of water in a small cup and add the feces to it.
3. Stir well with a wooden tongue depressor and mash the material until it is completely broken up.
4. Pour the mixture through an ordinary tea strainer into another cup, stirring the material while pouring.
5. Press the remaining material with the tongue depressor until nearly dry.
6. Squirt 2 to 3 ml of water into the small cup just emptied and rinse down the sides. Pour this rinsing fluid through the material in the strainer.
7. Press the material in the strainer until dry again and discard.
8. Stir the mixture in the second cup and immediately pour it into a 15-ml centrifuge tube.
9. Centrifuge the tube at 1500 rpm for 10 minutes.
10. Decant the supernatant from the tube, being careful not to pour off the fine material on the surface of the sediment.
11. Fill the tube half full of sugar solution (specific gravity 1.27) and mix the sediment and sugar solution with a wooden applicator stick, being careful to scrape the sides and bottom of the tube while mixing.
12. Finish filling the tube with sugar solution and place in the centrifuge.
13. With a pipette, add sugar solution to the tube until it is full enough to place a cover slip on top. No air bubbles should be under the cover slip and the material should not overflow so that it runs down the sides of the tube.
14. Centrifuge at 1500 rpm for 10 minutes.
15. Remove the cover slip by lifting straight upward and place it on a microscope slide. If done properly, the material under the cover slip should be sufficiently thick.
16. Using the 10× objective, scan the entire slide, counting all parasite eggs.
    - For cattle (for example): 100 eggs counted/ 5 grams of feces equals 20 eggs/gram of feces
    - For horses and swine (for example): 100 eggs counted/2 grams of feces equals 50 eggs/gram of feces

host in the trophozoite form. Trophozoites are one-cell, motile organisms that lack the rigid wall of a cyst, making flotation without distortion or death of the trophozoite impossible. Therefore the direct smear technique, with saline and a stain, is the preferred procedure for examination of a fecal sample for protozoal organisms.

In a direct smear, trophozoites may be recognized by their movement. *Balantidium coli* is bean shaped and covered with tiny hairs, or cilia. It moves in a slow, tumbling fashion. *Giardia* species are tear shaped and have five to eight flagella. They move with a jerky motion. Trichomonads are long, slender organisms with a single flagellum attached to the dorsal surface, forming a sail-like structure that ripples as the organism glides through debris. Amoebas move with a flowing motion, extending a part of the body (pseudopod) and moving the rest of the body after it.

Stains also may be used to recognize certain structural characteristics of trophozoites and cysts. Lugol's iodine and new methylene blue are common stains used with the direct smear procedure. These stains do not preserve the slide but do facilitate examination of the specimen, making identification easier.

If a protozoal parasite cannot be identified on direct smears, fecal smears containing protozoal

PROCEDURE 6-8

Modified Wisconsin Technique

1. Weigh 5 g of feces.
2. Mix the feces thoroughly with 45 ml of water in a small cup.
3. Withdraw 1 ml of suspended mixture and place into a 15-ml centrifuge cup.
4. Fill the tube with sugar solution (specific gravity 1.27) and place a cover slip on the tube.
5. Centrifuge the tube at 1200 rpm for 5 minutes.
6. Remove the cover slip and place on a microscope slide. Scan the slide, counting all parasite eggs or oocysts seen.
7. Multiply the number of eggs or oocysts counted by 10 to determine the eggs per gram of feces.

trophozoites can be dried, stained with Diff-Quik, Wright's, or Giemsa stain, and sent to a diagnostic laboratory. Many other procedures are used for staining and preserving protozoal trophozoites. Most of these procedures are used in diagnostic laboratories and are not explained in this text.

Coccidia

Several coccidian parasites require special staining techniques for identification. Two procedures are discussed.

The acid-fast staining technique is used to identify *Cryptosporidium* species in feces. *Cryptosporidium* is a parasite of the gastrointestinal tract of many animals, including human beings. The oocysts are 2 to 8 μm in diameter and are almost undetectable in flotation solution to the inexperienced eye. Acid-fast staining can help detect the oocysts in a fecal smear.

The second procedure uses Diff-Quik stain for identification of *Isospora* species. *Isospora* species are coccidia found in the gastrointestinal tract (especially the jejunum) of many animals, but

they are of most concern in pigs. This parasite can cause the death of many piglets before any oocysts are found in the feces by conventional flotation methods. Therefore an intestinal mucosal scraping must be stained and examined for other diagnostic stages (schizonts, merozoites) of this parasite. This procedure involves scraping the mucosa of the jejunum and smearing the scrapings onto microscope slides. After the slides are air dried, they are stained with Diff-Quik and examined with the oil-immersion objective.

For accurate results with either of these procedures, several samples should be examined. If such examination is not possible, feces or intestines may be sent to a diagnostic laboratory. Collection and shipping of parasitic specimens are described subsequently.

Antigen Tests

Antigen tests for *Giardia* and *Cryptosporidium* are available and may be used for their detection. See Chapter 8 for more details on antigen testing.

Fecal Culture

Fecal cultures involve rearing infective larvae of strongyles, trichostrongyles, or hookworms for identification. Several techniques are available for this purpose.

The first procedure uses a covered glass jar rinsed with 0.1% sodium carbonate solution. Sodium carbonate solution is used to inhibit mold growth while allowing the parasite eggs to develop. Formed feces are placed in the jar, which is then stored at room temperature in a dark area for 7 to 10 days. The contents of the jar should be kept moist but not soggy. If no water droplets are seen condensing on the inside of the jar, a few drops of water or sodium carbonate are added. Vermiculite or sand should be added to bovine feces or feces that contain a lot of water.

Larvae may be found in the condensation droplets in the culture jar. The veterinary technician may collect the larvae by rinsing the jar with a small amount of water, collecting the rinse, and concentrating the larvae by centrifugation. The larvae found in the sediment after centrifugation are placed on a microscope slide and examined after cover slip application. The slide is then briefly heated with a match to "relax," or straighten, the larvae and curtail their movement.

During examination for larvae, the numbers of larvae do not necessarily correlate with numbers of eggs present in the feces. Development from egg to larva may take longer with some species than with others, and some parasite species may produce more eggs than others. For example, *Haemonchus contortus* and *Strongyloides papillosus* are found in greater numbers and their eggs develop faster than those of *Trichostrongylus* and *Cooperia* species.

Culture of canine feces for *Strongyloides stercoralis* filariform larvae uses the same technique previously described. Most filariform larvae appear within 24 to 48 hours. Rhabditiform larvae may be evident first. If this occurs, the sample should be allowed to stand for no less than 96 hours so that the larvae can mate and produce filariform larvae.

Another method uses a covered Petri dish and filter paper. Feces are placed in the middle of a piece of moistened filter paper, which is then placed in the Petri dish. The Petri dish is covered and placed in a dark area at room temperature for 7 to 10 days. The dish is rinsed and the rinse is collected as previously described. Technicians who want to perform a fecal culture and identify larvae should refer to the chapters on larval identification in the reference by Bowman listed at the end of this chapter.

Sample Collection at Necropsy

Necropsy (postmortem examination) is an important method of diagnosing many diseases, including parasitism. The types of lesions produced by immature parasites, any adult parasites found in the body cavity and tissues, and histopathologic examination of infected tissues are used in diagnosis. Veterinary technicians are responsible for the samples collected, making sure they are properly contained, preserved, labeled, and shipped.

Two methods are used to recover parasites from the digestive tract at necropsy: the decanting

---

BOX 6-1
Decanting Method

- Each section of the digestive tract is opened and the contents poured into a bucket.
- The interior lining of the organ is scraped with a spatula and the scrapings added to the bucket or examined separately.
- An amount of water equal to the contents of each bucket is added and thoroughly mixed
- The bucket is allowed to sit undisturbed for approximately 45 minutes.
- The liquid is poured off, leaving the sediment in the bottom of the bucket.
- An amount of water equal to the volume of the sediment is added and thoroughly mixed
- The process is repeated until the water over the sediment becomes clear.
- The sediment is transferred to a dissecting pan and examined with a dissecting microscope or magnifying glass,
- Any parasites found are gently removed with thumb forceps and preserved.

BOX 6-2
Sieving Method

- The contents (including scrapings of the interior lining) are placed n a bucket and mixed with an equal volume of water
- The mixture is poured through a #18 sieve and then through a #45 sieve.
- The sieves' contents are rinsed with water.
- The solid material in the sieves is examined with a dissecting microscope or magnifying glass,
- Any parasites found are gently removed with thumb forceps and preserved.

---

method and the sieving method (Boxes 6-1 and 6-2). With either method, the veterinary technician must separate the different parts of the digestive tract and work with the contents of each individually.

Parasites recovered from the digestive tract may be preserved in 70% alcohol or 10% neutral buffered formalin for later identification. Occasionally bladderworms or cysticerci may be found attached to the viscera of domestic animals. These should be handled with care because the fluid within the bladder can be allergenic and may also be zoonotic. To identify the parasites recovered, the veterinary technician should consult the references listed at the end of this chapter. If in-hospital diagnosis is not possible, the samples may be preserved as previously described and sent to a diagnostic laboratory for identification.

Shipping Parasitologic Specimens

Any parasitologic specimen shipped to a diagnostic laboratory should be preserved with alcohol or formalin unless otherwise directed by laboratory personnel. Specimens should be packaged in a leak-proof container and sealed with Parafilm (American National Can, Greenwich, CT.) or tape. If specimen containers are found leaking, the shipment will not be delivered. Feces can be sent fresh or mixed at a ratio of 1:3 with 10% formalin. Whole parasites or segments can be preserved in alcohol or formalin and placed in a leak-proof container.

All specimen containers should be labeled with the site from which the specimen was obtained; the owner's name; the animal's species, name, or identification number; and the referring veterinarian (including telephone number and address). The labeled specimen container should be placed in a shock-proof shipping container to prevent breakage during shipping. Styrofoam containers filled with shredded newspaper work well for shipping parasitologic specimens.

A cover letter should be included with the specimen and should contain a brief history of the animal, findings at necropsy, and the reason for submitting the samples to the laboratory (e.g., fecal examination, special staining, species identification). Without this background information, the diagnostic laboratory is unlikely to provide accurate results.

Miscellaneous Procedures for Detection of Endoparasites

Cellophane Tape Technique

The cellophane tape technique is used to detect the equine pinworm *Oxyuris equi* (Procedure 6-9). Pinworms are nematodes found in horses; rodents; rabbits; and primates; including human beings. They live in the colon and, as adults, migrate out the rectum to lay eggs on the skin around the anus. The eggs are contained within a sticky substance and fall off as the substance hardens or as the animal scratches. For this reason, pinworm eggs usually are not seen in a routine fecal examination (see Fig. 6-47).

Baermann Technique

The Baermann technique is used to recover nematode larvae from feces, tissues, or soil. This technique uses warm water to stimulate larvae to move about. As the larvae do so, they sink to the bottom of the funnel for collection and identification (Procedure 6-10). This technique is

PROCEDURE 6-9

Cellophane Tape Technique

Materials

Transparent cellophane tape
Tongue depressor
Microscope slide

Procedure

1. Wrap the cellophane tape in a loop around the tongue depressor with the sticky side out.
2. Press the tape to the skin around the horse's anus. Stand to the side of the horse and not directly behind it.
3. Place a drop of water on the slide. Remove the tape from the tongue depressor and place it, sticky side down, on top of the water.
4. Examine the slide for pinworm eggs (see Fig. 6-47).

PROCEDURE 6-10

Baermann Technique

Materials

Baermann apparatus (Fig. 6-61)
Cheesecloth or gauze square approximately twice the diameter of the funnel
Microscope slides and cover slips

Procedure

1. Spread the cheesecloth out on the support screen in the Baermann apparatus. Take 5 to 15 g of fecal, soil, or tissue sample and place it on the cheesecloth. Fold any excess cheesecloth over the top of the sample. Be sure the sample is covered by the warm water or saline; add more if necessary.
2. Allow the apparatus to remain undisturbed overnight.
3. Hold a microscope slide under the cut-off pipette and open the pinch clamp only long enough to allow a large drop to fall on the slide. Apply a cover slip to the slide and examine it microscopically for larvae. Repeat by examining several slides before concluding the sample is negative.

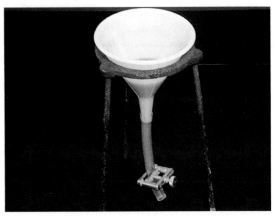

Figure 6-61. Baermann apparatus is used to recover larvae of roundworms from feces, soil, or animal tissues. This apparatus is most useful in recovering larvae of lungworms. (Reprinted from Hendrix CM, Robinson E: *Diagnostic parasitology for veterinary technicians,* ed 3, St Louis, 2006, Mosby.)

Larvae recovered from fresh large animal feces are almost always those of lungworms. Larvae from *Strongyloides stercoralis* can be found in fresh canine feces. If the feces are not fresh, many types of parasitic and nonparasitic larvae and adults may be seen.

DIAGNOSIS OF BLOOD PARASITISM

Dirofilaria immitis, the canine heartworm, is the most important parasite of the vascular system in domestic animals in the United States. For this reason, in-hospital blood examinations are commonly performed to detect heartworms.

The following procedures can be performed by veterinary technicians to identify *D. immitis.* As previously mentioned, a clean environment and proper handling of samples are vital for quality control in any laboratory. Any sample handled improperly may result in inaccurate results.

Collection of Blood Samples

Sterile equipment and alcohol are required for collecting a blood sample from an animal. Blood

performed with a Baermann apparatus. The apparatus consists of a ring stand and ring holder, a glass funnel with a piece of rubber tubing on the end, a clamp, and a wire net or cheesecloth. With the apparatus set up as shown in Figure 6-61, the sample is placed on the wire screen or cheesecloth and warm water is added to barely cover the sample. All air bubbles are allowed to flow from the tube of the funnel by releasing the clamp. The apparatus is allowed to sit undisturbed for 12 to 24 hours.

A drop of fluid from the bottom of the funnel is removed (usually the first drop) and placed on a microscope slide. If any larvae are found swimming on the slide, the slide is heated with a match to render them immobile.

may be collected using by a syringe and needle or a Vacutainer (Becton Dickinson, Rutherford, NJ). All samples should be labeled with the owner's name, animal's name, and date of collection. (See Chapter 2 for more details on blood collection.)

Microfilariae are more numerous in the bloodstream at certain times of the day. To increase the probability of collecting microfilariae, blood should be collected in the afternoon because the microfilariae of *D. immitis* are most numerous in the circulating blood at this time.

Examination of the Blood

General observations of the blood should be noted. For example, a blood sample that appears watery may reflect anemia. Clinical pathology tests on the blood also may aid in diagnosis of parasitism. Heartworm microfilariae may be seen during the differential white blood cell (WBC) count. A high eosinophil count may also indicate parasitism (Procedure 6-11).

Direct Examination

Direct examination of the blood for microfilariae is the simplest procedure to perform (Procedure 6-11). This procedure detects movement of microfilariae and other parasites among the RBCs. As with direct examination of feces, direct examination of blood requires only a small sample. However, unless parasites are present in large numbers, they may be missed. For this reason, the direct smear is not a good technique for detecting microfilariae.

Microfilariae of primary interest are those of *D. immitis,* the canine heartworm, and *Dipetalonema (Acanthocheilonema) reconditum,* a subcutaneous parasite of dogs. Differentiation between the two is extremely important because treatment for heartworms is expensive, somewhat stressful, and often involves use of extremely toxic compounds.

In a direct blood smear, microfilariae of *Dirofilaria* species coil and uncoil, whereas those of *Dipetalonema* species may glide smoothly across the slide. However, this is not always the case. Also, the number of *Dirofilaria* species microfilariae in a sample is greater than that of *Dipetalonema* species. Again, however, this is not always the case. Direct examination of the blood is used to determine only the presence of microfilariae, not the type. For this, a concentration technique that "relaxes" and stains microfilariae is used. These procedures are discussed later.

Trypanosomes are another type of parasite found in the blood. These protozoa occur in tropical areas and occasionally in the United States. Trypanosomes can be seen swimming among the cells of a diluted blood smear (single-cell thickness) but are more easily identified in stained smears.

Microfilariae can also be found in large animals. *Setaria* is a long white nematode found in the serous membranes of cattle and horses. Adults are most often seen during abdominal surgery, and microfilariae are found during differential WBC count.

Thin Blood Smear

The thin blood smear is prepared and stained in exactly the same way as a blood smear for a differential WBC count. The procedure is described in Chapter 2. When doing a differential WBC count on an animal, the veterinary technician should note any parasitic organisms seen. Microfilariae occasionally may be found. Because of their size, microfilariae usually are found along the feathered edge of the blood film. Because differentiation of the microfilariae

---

PROCEDURE 6-11

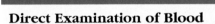

Direct Examination of Blood

Materials
    Blood collection equipment
    Microscope slides and cover slips

Procedure
1. Immediately after collecting the blood sample, place a single drop of blood onto the microscope slide and add a cover slip.
2. Examine the slide with the 10× microscope objective. Watch for localized areas of movement among the RBCs, which may indicate the presence of parasites.

is not possible in a thin blood smear, other procedures must be performed for identification. Trypanosomes, protozoans, and rickettsiae also may be found among or within cells. As with the direct smear procedure, a small blood sample is used and mild parasitic infections may be missed.

Thick Blood Smear

A thick blood smear examines a slightly greater volume of blood than does a thin blood smear. Again, microfilariae may be seen, but they cannot be easily differentiated by this method (Procedure 6-12).

Buffy Coat Method

The buffy coat method is a concentration technique used on a small volume of blood. When blood is placed in a microhematocrit tube and centrifuged for determining the packed cell volume

(PCV), it separates into three layers: plasma, WBC layer (buffy coat), and RBC layer (Fig. 6-62). Microfilariae can be found on the surface of the buffy coat layer (Fig. 6-63). This technique is quick and may be performed in conjunction with a PCV and total protein evaluation. However, differentiation of microfilariae is not possible (Procedure 6-13).

The following concentration techniques may be used for differentiating *D. immitis* from *D. reconditum.*

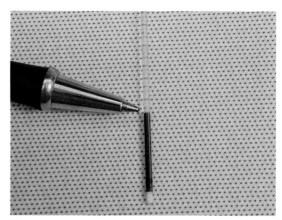

Figure 6-62. Buffy coat in a hematocrit tube. (From Hendrix CM, Robinson E: *Diagnostic parasitology for veterinary technicians,* ed 3, St Louis, 2006, Mosby.)

PROCEDURE 6-12

Thick Blood Smear

Materials

Microscope slides
Distilled water
Methyl alcohol
Giemsa stain, diluted 1:20 with distilled water
Wooden applicator stick

Procedure

1. Place 3 drops of blood on the slide and spread them with a wooden applicator stick to make a 2-cm circle.
2. Allow the slide to air dry.
3. Place the slide in a slanted position, smear side down, in a beaker filled with distilled water. Allow the slide to remain in the water until the smear loses its red color.
4. Remove the slide and allow it to air dry. Immerse the slide in methyl alcohol for 10 minutes. Stain the slide with Giemsa stain for 30 minutes. Rinse off excess stain.

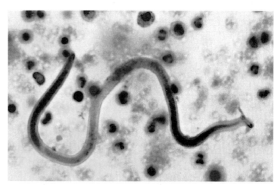

Figure 6-63. Microfilaria in a buffy coat smear from canine blood. (From Hendrix CM, Robinson E: *Diagnostic parasitology for veterinary technicians,* ed 3, St Louis, 2006, Mosby.)

PROCEDURE 6-13

Buffy Coat Method

Materials

Microhematocrit tubes and sealer
Microhematocrit centrifuge
Small file or glass cutter
Microscope slides and cover slips
Saline
Methylene blue stain (diluted 1:1000 with distilled water)

Procedure

1. Fill the microhematocrit tube with blood and seal.
2. Centrifuge for 3 minutes.
3. Read the packed cell volume, if desired, and then find the buffy coat layer between the red blood cells and plasma (see Fig. 6-62).
4. With a file, scratch the tube at the level of the buffy coat. Carefully snap the tube and save the part of the tube containing the buffy coat and plasma. Gently tap the tube onto a slide, ejecting the buffy coat layer with a small amount of plasma. Save the rest of the plasma for a total protein determination if desired.
5. Add a drop of saline and a drop of stain to the buffy coat. Apply a cover slip and examine for microfilariae (see Fig. 6-63).

PROCEDURE 6-14

Modified Knott's Technique

Materials

15-ml centrifuge tube
Centrifuge
2% formalin (2 ml of 40% formalin diluted with 98 ml of distilled water)
Methylene blue stain (diluted 1:1000 with distilled water)
Pasteur pipettes and bulbs

Procedure

1. Mix 1 ml of blood with 9 ml of 2% formalin in a centrifuge tube.
2. Centrifuge the tube at 1300 to 1500 rpm for 5 minutes.
3. Pour off the liquid supernatant, leaving the sediment at the bottom of the tube.
4. Add 2 to 3 drops of stain to the sediment. Using a pipette, mix the sediment with the stain.
5. Place a drop of this mixture onto a glass slide. Apply a cover slip and exami

Modified Knott's Technique

The modified Knott's technique is a simple procedure that allows differentiation of microfilariae (Procedure 6-14). This technique concentrates, relaxes, and stains microfilariae while lysing RBCs to make the microfilariae more visible.

Figures 6-64 and 6-65 and Table 6-1 show the characteristics that may be used when identifying microfilariae. The veterinary technician should always examine as many microfilariae as possible because mixed infections can occur. The most accurate method for differentiation is measuring

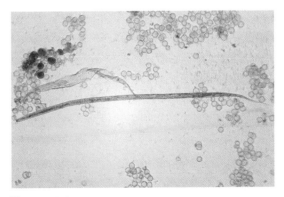

Figure 6-64. Microfilaria of *Dirofilaria immitis*, found by the modified Knott's technique. Note the straight tail and tapering cranial end of the microfilaria. (From Hendrix CM, Robinson E: *Diagnostic parasitology for veterinary technicians*, ed 3, St Louis, 2006, Mosby.)

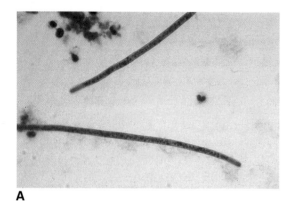

A

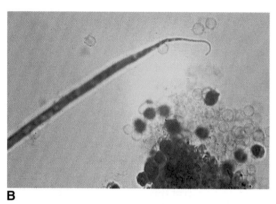

B

Figure 6-65. Cranial **(A)** and caudal **(B)** ends of a *Dipetalonema reconditum* microfilaria. (From Hendrix CM, Robinson E: *Diagnostic parasitology for veterinary technicians,* ed 3, St Louis, 2006, Mosby.)

the length and width of the body. However, with some practice, general characteristics of the microfilariae may be used for identification if a means of measuring microfilariae is not available.

Filter Technique

Filter techniques are a common method used in veterinary practices for detection of microfilariae in the blood. An excellent diagnostic kit, the Di-Fil Test Kit (EVSCO Pharmaceuticals, Buena, NJ), is available for this procedure. This kit comes complete with filters, lysing solution, stain, and directions for use.

Most kits require 1 ml of whole blood to test for heartworms. The blood is mixed with nine parts of lysing solution and passed through a filter. The filter is rinsed, removed, and placed on a slide. A drop of stain is added, a cover slip is applied, and the filter is microscopically examined for microfilariae (Fig. 6-66). Differentiation of microfilariae is possible but difficult with the filter technique. If microfilariae are present, other diagnostic procedures are recommended for identification purposes.

TABLE 6-1

Differentiation of Microfilariae Using the Modified Knott's Technique

	Dirofilaria Immitis	Dipetalonema Reconditum
Body length	310 μm	290 μm
Mid-body width	6 μm	6 μm
Head	Tapered	Blunt
Tail	Straight	Hooked*

*Artifact of formalin fixation.

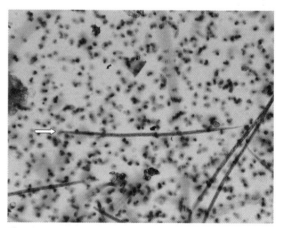

Figure 6-66. Microfilariae of *Dironfuilaria immitis* using the Di-Fil-Test. (From Hendrix CM, Robinson E: *Diagnostic parasitology for veterinary technicians,* ed 3, St Louis, 2006, Mosby.)

Enzyme-Linked Immunosorbent Assay

Enzyme-linked immunosorbent assay (ELISA) kits do not directly detect microfilariae but instead test the host's response to the parasites. These types of tests can be used for differentiating *D. immitis* from *D. reconditum*. They can be used to identify an occult heartworm infection, that is, when microfilariae are not found to be circulating in the peripheral blood. An occult infection can occur in one of several scenarios: when only one adult is present, when only one sex of adult worms is present (all male worms or all female worms), when the adults are unable to reproduce, when the animal's immune system removes microfilariae as they are produced, or when an animal has been treated with drugs that kill circulating microfilariae or render the adults sterile. In all these scenarios, circulating microfilariae would not be found in the peripheral blood.

Some ELISA kits detect the host's antibody response to the adult heartworms, whereas others detect the host's antibody response to the microfilariae (see Chapter 8). A variety of commercially available ELISA tests for the detection of antigens of adult *D. immitis* in both dogs and cats are routinely used in veterinary clinical practice. Test kits that detect circulating antibody are also available although not widely used. The following examples are just a few of the many commercially available heartworm antigen test kits available on the market today: SNAP Heartworm Antigen Test Kit (IDEXX Laboratories, Westbrook, ME), SNAP Feline Heartworm Antigen Test Kit (IDEXX Laboratories), DiroCHEK Canine Heartworm Antigen Test Kit (Synbiotics Corporation, San Diego, CA), and Reference Laboratory Heartworm Test (antigen) (HESKA Veterinary Diagnostic Laboratories, Fort Collins, CO). One of the first actions that the veterinary technician should take is to read the manufacturer's instructions carefully. As with any procedure, ELISA immunodiagnostic tests should be performed exactly according to the manufacturer's directions and in a clean environment to avoid contamination. These ELISA tests are economical and expeditious. Most of the tests rely on a color change in the test kit to determine whether an animal is infected with adults of *D. immitis*. The veterinary technician should rely on caution when using these diagnostic tests because a chance exists for the occurrence of both false-negative and false-positive results in infected and uninfected dogs and cats. In addition, these tests should not be used as a sole means of diagnosis; occasionally a negative result coincides with the finding of microfilariae in the blood, and sometimes such results throw doubt regarding the credibility of these tests. Antigen tests are useful in heartworm diagnosis; however, the veterinary technician should be aware of their limitations as a sole screening test.

Miscellaneous Tests

Another type of heartworm diagnostic test kit (Heartworm Identification Test, ImmunoVet, Tampa, FL) works on the same principle as the Knott's and filter techniques, except the microfilariae remain alive. This test relies on the movement of the microfilariae, which can be unreliable at times.

Other tests use special stains to bring out certain characteristics of the microfilariae. These procedures are too cumbersome to be useful in private practice and usually are performed in diagnostic laboratories.

Recommended Readings

Bowman DD, Lynn RC, Eberhard ML: *Georgi's parasitology for veterinarians,* ed 8, Philadelphia, 2003, WB Saunders.

Hendrix CM, Robinson E: *Diagnostic parasitology for veterinary technicians,* ed 3, St Louis, 2006, Mosby.

Sloss MW, et al: *Veterinary clinical parasitology,* ed 6, Ames, IA, 1994, Iowa State University.

CHAPTER 7

External Parasites

Charles M. Hendrix

KEY POINTS

- Parasites that reside on or outside of the host's body are referred to as ectoparasites.
- Ectoparasites of domestic animals include insects (e.g., fleas, lice, biting flies) and arachnids (e.g., mites, ticks). Leeches (bloodsucking annelids) are also considered to be ectoparasites.
- Infestation by leeches is referred to as hirudiniasis.
- Ectoparasites produce a parasitic infestation or ectoparasitism.
- Immature and/or larval stages of nematodes and some adult stages of nematodes may parasitize an animal's skin or subcutaneous tissues.
- Insects that parasitize domestic animals are primarily members of the Orders Hemiptera (true bugs), Mallophaga (chewing lice), Anoplura (sucking lice), Diptera (two-winged flies), and Siphonaptera (fleas).

- Infestation by chewing or sucking lice is referred to as pediculosis.
- Infestation by larval dipterans is referred to as myiasis.
- Infestation by fleas is referred to as siphonapterosis.
- Infestation by mites or ticks is referred to as acariasis.
- Samples for diagnosis of ectoparasitic infestation may be collected by direct removal and identification of parasite, skin scraping, cellophane tape technique, plucking of individual hairs, or combing the haircoat.

If a parasite resides on the surface of its host, it is termed an ectoparasite. The majority of ectoparasites of domesticated animals are either insects (e.g., fleas, lice, flies) or arachnids (e.g., ticks, mites). However, a few nematodes have been included in this chapter because they demonstrate either immature or adult stages that are found within the animal's skin or subcutaneous tissues.

This chapter is designed to aid the veterinary technician in the diagnosis of ectoparasitism in dogs, cats, cattle, sheep, goats, horses, and swine. To diagnose an ectoparasitic infestation, the technician must be able to collect the ectoparasite or its life cycle stages and then identify the organism involved. This chapter explains procedures most commonly used to collect ectoparasites from the host and describes those parasites so that a correct diagnosis can be made.

Although a complete review of the biology of ectoparasites is beyond the scope of this chapter, a brief review of the life cycles of the major groups of ectoparasites is included.

COLLECTION OF SAMPLES

Skin Scraping

Skin scraping is one of the most common diagnostic procedures used in evaluating animals with dermatologic problems. Equipment needed includes an electric clipper with a #40 blade, a scalpel or spatula, mineral oil in a small dropper bottle, and a compound microscope. Typical lesions or sites most likely to harbor the particular parasite should be scraped (e.g., ear margins for *Sarcoptes scabei* var. *canis*).

The scraping is performed with a #10 scalpel blade, with or without a handle. A 165-mm stainless steel spatula (Sargent-Welsh Scientific, Detroit, MI) is preferred by some clinicians. The scalpel blade should be held between the thumb and forefinger (Fig. 7-1). Before the skin is scraped, the blade is dipped in a drop of mineral oil on the slide, or a drop of mineral oil may be placed on the skin.

During the scraping process, the blade must be held perpendicular to the skin. Holding it at

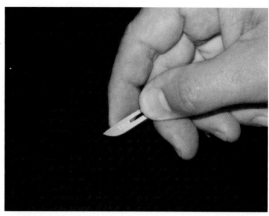

Figure 7-1. A scalpel blade may be held safely between the thumb and forefinger for skin scrapings. (From Hendrix CM, Robinson E: *Diagnostic parasitology for veterinary technicians,* ed 3, St Louis, 2006, Mosby.)

another angle may result in an accidental incision. The average area scraped should be approximately 3 to 4 cm². Multiple sites should be scraped to increase the chances of collecting the parasite.

The depth of the scraping varies with the typical location of the parasite in question. When scraping for mites that live in tunnels (e.g., *Sarcoptes* species) or in hair follicles (e.g., *Demodex* species), the veterinary technician should scrape the skin until a small amount of capillary blood oozes from the scraped area. Clipping the area with a #40 blade before scraping enables better visualization of the lesion and removes excess hair that impedes proper scraping and interferes with collection of epidermal debris. Scraping at the interface between affected and unaffected sites is important. For surface-dwelling mites (e.g., *Cheyletiella, Psoroptes,* or *Chorioptes* species), the skin is scraped superficially to collect any loose scales or crusts. Clipping before scraping is not necessary when infestation with surface-dwelling mites is suspected.

All scraped debris on the forward surface of the blade is then spread in a drop of mineral oil on the glass slide. A glass cover slip is placed on the material, and the slide is ready for microscopic examination using the 4× (scanning) objective.

The slide should be examined systematically in rows so that the entire area under the cover slip is evaluated. Low light intensity and high contrast increase visualization of translucent mites and eggs. If necessary, the slide may be evaluated with the 10× (low power) objective.

Demonstration of the characteristic mite or egg is frequently diagnostic for most diseases. In certain circumstances, however, more than just identification of the parasite is necessary. For example, determination of live/dead ratios and observation of immature larval and nymphal stages of demodectic mites are important in determining a patient's prognosis. A decrease in the number of live mites and eggs during treatment is an excellent prognostic indicator.

Cellophane Tape Preparation

When attempting to demonstrate lice or mites that live primarily on the surface of the skin (e.g., *Cheyletiella, Psoroptes,* or *Chorioptes* species), the veterinary technician may use a cellophane tape preparation instead of a skin scraping. Clear cellophane tape (e.g., Scotch Transparent Tape, 3M, Minneapolis, MN) is applied to the skin to pick up epidermal debris. A ribbon of mineral oil is placed on a glass slide, and the adhesive surface of the tape is then placed on the mineral oil. Additional mineral oil and a cover slip may be placed on the tape to prevent the tape from wrinkling, but this is not necessary. The slide is then examined microscopically for parasites (see Procedure 6-9).

Parasite Identification

When arthropods or helminths cannot be grossly identified, the intact specimen should be collected in a sealed container containing 10% formalin or ethyl alcohol and submitted to an arthropodologist or parasitologist for identification. A complete history should accompany the specimen. The specimen should not be fragmented or squashed, which could distort morphologic features necessary for proper identification. Forensic identification of parasites is difficult.

TERMINOLOGY

Ectoparasites usually live on or in skin surfaces or feed on them. Ectoparasites infest the skin or external surfaces of animals and produce an infestation on the animal. By contrast, internal parasites, or endoparasites, infect the internal organs of domestic animals and produce an infection within that animal. In diagnostic parasitology, these terms always should be used in the proper context.

Life cycle describes the development of a parasite through its various life stages. Every parasite's life cycle has a definitive host and may have one or more intermediate hosts. The definitive host harbors the adult, sexual, or mature stages of a parasite. The intermediate host harbors the juvenile, asexual, or immature stages of a parasite.

Many of the ectoparasites in this chapter belong to the phylum Arthropoda or, more simply, are considered arthropods. All adult arthropods have jointed legs. In addition, a few larval arthropods may be associated with dermal lesions. Later in this chapter is a discussion of ectoparasites that reside within the skin; these ectoparasites are not arthropods but rather belong to the phylum Nematoda, or more simply, the roundworms.

CLASSIFICATION SYSTEM

In beginning biology, students must learn the classification scheme perfected by Linnaeus, an early biologist. Every living organism on this planet may be classified with the following classification scheme: Kingdom, Phylum, Class, Order, Family, Genus, and species. Students often remember this scheme with this simple mnemonic device, "**K**ing **P**hilip **c**ame **o**ver **f**or **g**ood **s**paghetti."

Every living thing is known by a scientific name that is made up of two components: the genus and the specific epithet. The dog's scientific name is *Canis familiaris. Canis* is the Genus and *familiaris* is the specific epithet or species. Similar species are grouped together into the same Genus. Similar Genera (plural of genus) are grouped together into the same Family. Similar Families are grouped together into the same Order. Similar Orders are grouped together into the same Class. Similar Classes are grouped together into the same Phylum. Similar Phyla are grouped together into the same Kingdom. Therefore the dog's classification scheme is as follows:

Kingdom: Animalia
  Phylum: Chordata
    Subphylum: Vertebrata
      Class: Mammalia
        Order: Carnivora
          Family: Canidae
            Genus: *Canis*
              species: *familiaris*

Every living creature on Earth has a distinct classification scheme.

PHYLUM: ARTHROPODA

Class: Insecta

The first part of this chapter discusses the Orders belonging to the Class Insecta and the Families belonging to the Class Acarina and how these ectoparasites are relevant to veterinary practice.

Order: Hymenoptera

Hymenoptera includes ants, bees, and wasps. Fire ants are indigenous to the southeastern United States and can bite and sting almost any domestic animal. "Downer cows" and young newborn animals are particularly susceptible to the bites and stings of fire ants.

Bees, wasps, and hornets can sting domestic animals, particularly curious dogs and cats. When stung, the animals may show an extremely swollen nose or face.

Africanized honeybees, or "killer bees," have now crossed the Mexico/United States border. Almost any domestic animal (or person) could stumble on a hive of these bees, angering the inhabitants. Death often results from thousands of bee stings. Animals are particularly at risk because these bees often nest at or near the surface of the ground.

Diagnosis

If ants, bees, wasps, or hornets are suspected to be causing problems, the intact Hymenopteran should be collected in a sealed container containing 10% formalin or ethyl alcohol and submitted to an entomologist for identification.

Order: Hemiptera

Members of Hemiptera are true bugs. Although some adult Hemipterans are wingless, most adult Hemipterans have two pairs of wings. The posterior pair of wings is membranous in appearance. The anterior pair of wings has a leathery basal portion with a membranous apical portion, which gives the appearance of being a "half wing," hence, the origin of the ordinal name: hemi-, meaning half, and -ptera, meaning wing. Two groups of Hemipterans are of veterinary importance: reduviid bugs ("kissing bugs") and bed bugs. Reduviid bugs are periodic parasites, making frequent visits to the host to obtain a blood meal. These bugs serve as intermediate hosts for *Trypanosoma cruzi*, a protozoan parasite that can produce a rare disease in people and dogs called Chagas disease. This disease also is called South American trypanosomiasis and rarely occurs in dogs and other animals in the United States. Reduviid bugs take blood meals from an infected host and transmit the parasite as they defecate.

Bed bugs are dorsoventrally flattened, wingless Hemipterans that often infest homes. They are periodic parasites, making frequent visits to the host to obtain a blood meal. Although bed bugs are human parasites, they also may be found in rabbit colonies, poultry houses, and pigeon colonies. Bed bugs do not naturally transmit any human or animal pathogen.

Diagnosis

If Reduviid bugs or bed bugs are suspected to be causing problems, the intact Hemipteran should be collected in 10% formalin or ethyl alcohol and submitted to an entomologist for identification.

Orders: Mallophaga and Anoplura

Lice are some of the most prolific ectoparasites of domestic animals. Two orders of lice exist: the

Mallophaga (chewing or biting lice) and the Anoplura (sucking lice). Lice are dorsoventrally flattened, wingless insects. They have three body divisions: the head, with its mouthparts and antennae; the thorax, with its three pairs of legs and its lack of wings; and the abdomen, the portion that bears the reproductive organs. These body divisions and their relations to each other are important in diagnostic veterinary parasitology.

Members of the order Mallophaga, or chewing/biting lice, are smaller than sucking lice. They are usually yellow and have a large, round head. The mouthparts are mandibulate and are adapted for chewing or biting the host. Characteristically, the head of every chewing louse is wider than the widest portion of the thorax. On the thorax are three pairs of legs, which may be adapted for clasping or moving rapidly among feathers or hairs. Chewing/biting lice may parasitize birds, dogs, cats, cattle, sheep, goats, and horses (Fig. 7-2).

Members of the order Anoplura (sucking lice) are larger than members of the order Mallophaga (chewing lice). These lice are red to gray; their color usually depends on the amount of blood ingested from the host. In contrast to the wide head of the Mallophagans, Anoplurans heads are narrower than the widest part of the thorax. Their mouthparts are piercing and are adapted for sucking blood. Their pincerlike claws are adapted for clinging to the host's hairs. Although they are found on many species of domestic animals, sucking lice do not parasitize birds or cats (Fig. 7-3).

Anoplurans and Mallophagans have the same type of life cycle. This life cycle has only three developmental stages: the egg, nymphal, and adult stages.

The egg stage is also called a nit. The nit is tiny, approximately 0.5 to 1.0 mm in length. It is oval, white, and usually found cemented to the hair or feather shaft of the host (Fig. 7-4). Figure 7-5 shows

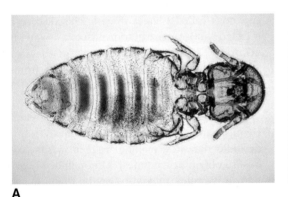

A

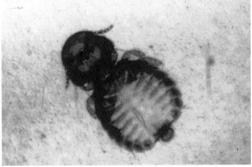

B

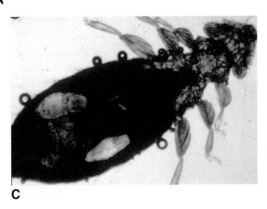

C

Figure 7-2. *Damalinia caprae* **(A)**, *Goniodes dissimilis* **(B)**, and *Goniodes gallinae* **(C)**, assorted chewing lice of goats and fowl. (From Hendrix CM, Robinson E: *Diagnostic parasitology for veterinary technicians,* ed 3, St Louis, 2006, Mosby.)

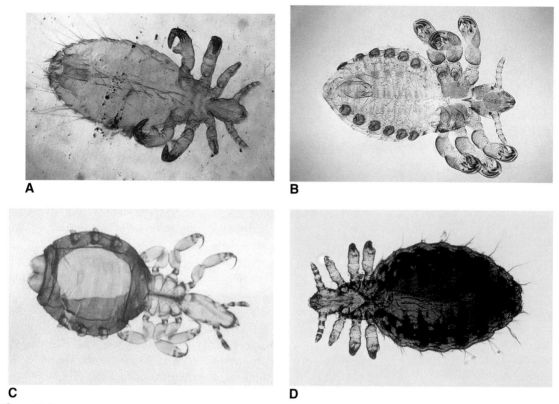

Figure 7-3. *Solenopotes capillatus* (**A**), *Pedicinus obtusus* (**B**), *Pedicinus obtusus* (**C**), and *Linognathus setosus* (**D**), assorted sucking lice of sheep, monkeys, and dogs. (Reprinted from Hendrix CM, Robinson E: *Diagnostic parasitology for veterinary technicians,* ed 3, St Louis, 2006, Mosby.)

a gravid female sucking louse and an associated nit collected from a dog. Nits hatch approximately 5 to 14 days after being laid by the adult female louse.

The nymphal stage is similar in appearance to the adult. However, it is smaller and lacks functioning reproductive organs and genital openings. The three nymphal stages are each progressively larger than its predecessor. The nymphal stage lasts from 2 to 3 weeks.

The adult stage is similar in appearance to the nymphal stage but larger. It has functional reproductive organs. Male and female lice copulate, the female lays eggs, cementing them to the hair or feather, and the life cycle begins again. It takes 3 to 4 weeks to complete the cycle. Nymphal and adult

stages live no longer than 7 days if removed from the host. Eggs hatch within 2 to 3 weeks during warm weather but seldom hatch off the host.

Lice usually are transmitted by direct contact, but all life stages may be transmitted by fomites (inanimate objects such as blankets, brushes, and other grooming equipment). Lice are easily transmitted among young, old, and malnourished animals. Veterinarians often cannot understand why certain animals in a flock or herd are heavily infested, whereas others have only a few lice. Lice are species specific; that is, they will parasitize only their specific hosts. For example, dog lice parasitize dogs. They may temporarily reside on another species of animal, but they will not set up housekeeping on that animal.

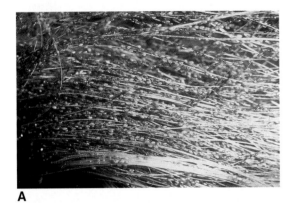

A

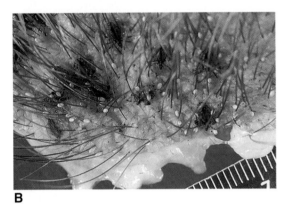

B

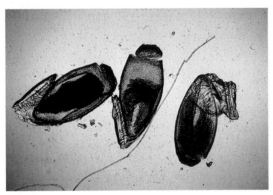

C

Figure 7-4. A, Thousands of nits can be cemented by female lice to the haircoat of domesticated animals. This calf's tail contains thousands of nits. **B,** Pediculosis can be defined as infestation by either chewing or sucking lice, in this case, *Haematopinus suis* infestation in a pig. **C,** Appearance of operculated nits viewed by compound microscope. (From Hendrix CM, Robinson E: *Diagnostic parasitology for veterinary technicians,* ed 3, St Louis, 2006, Mosby.)

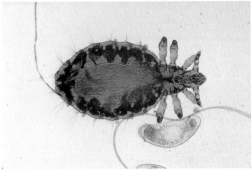

Figure 7-5. *Linognathus setosus,* a gravid female sucking louse, and associated nit collected from a dog. (From Hendrix CM, Robinson E: *Diagnostic parasitology for veterinary technicians,* ed 3, St Louis, 2006, Mosby.)

Infestation by lice (whether Mallophagan or Anopluran) is referred to as pediculosis. Sucking lice can ingest blood to such a degree that they produce severe anemia; fatalities can occur, especially in young animals. The packed cell volume can drop as much as 10% to 20%. Severely infested animals may harbor many thousands of lice. Infested animals become more susceptible to other diseases and parasites and may succumb to stresses not ordinarily pathologic to uninfested animals. When animals are poorly fed and kept in over-crowded conditions, they often become severely infested with lice and quickly become anemic and unthrifty.

Diagnosis

Careful examination of the haircoat or feathers of infested animals easily reveals lice and their accompanying nits. Hair clippings also serve as a good source for lice. Infestation of animals with a thick haircoat may be easily overlooked. A handheld magnifying lens or a binocular headband magnifier may aid observation of adult and nymphal lice crawling through or clinging to hair or feathers or tiny nits cemented to individual hairs.

Any lice and/or their nits observed may be collected with thumb forceps and placed in a drop of mineral oil on a glass microscope slide. A cover slip should be placed over the specimen and the slide examined with the 4× or 10× objective.

Identification of louse to Genus and specific epithet is difficult and best left to a trained specialist. Veterinary technicians should be able to identify the specimen as being Anopluran (sucking) or Mallophagan (chewing or biting) by visual examination of head size in relation to the thorax.

Order: Diptera

Diptera are a large, complex order of insects. As adults, most members have one pair of wings, which is the origin of the ordinal name: di-, meaning two, and -ptera, meaning wing. Its members vary in size, food source preference, and developmental stage that parasitizes the animal or produces lesions.

Dipterans produce two contrasting pathologic scenarios. As adults, they may feed intermittently on vertebrate blood, saliva, tears, or mucus. As larvae, they may develop in the subcutaneous tissues or within internal organs. Adult Dipterans that make frequent visits to the vertebrate host to intermittently feed on blood are referred to as periodic parasites. When Dipteran larvae develop in the tissue or organs of vertebrate hosts, they produce a condition known as myiasis.

As periodic parasites, blood-feeding Dipterans may be classified with regard to which sex feeds on vertebrate blood, as well as food preference. In certain Dipteran groups only the females feed on vertebrate blood; these female flies require vertebrate blood for laying their eggs. In this group are the biting gnats (e.g., *Simulium, Lutzomyia,* and *Culicoides* species), the mosquitoes (e.g., *Anopheles, Aedes,* and *Culex* species), the horse flies (e.g., *Tabanus* species), and the deer flies (e.g., *Chrysops* species).

In the second group of blood-feeding Dipterans, both male and female flies require a vertebrate blood meal. These species include the stable fly *Stomoxys calcitrans,* the horn fly *Haematobia irritans,* and the sheep ked *Melophagus ovinus. Musca autumnalis* (the face fly) feeds on mucus, tears, and saliva of large animals, particularly cattle.

Simulium species

Members of the genus *Simulium* are commonly called "black flies," although their coloration may vary from gray to yellow. They also are called "buffalo gnats" because their thorax is humped over the head, giving the appearance of a buffalo's hump (Fig. 7-6). These are tiny flies, ranging from 1 to 6 mm in length. They have broad, unspotted wings with prominent veins along the cranial margins of the wings. These tiny flies have serrated, scissorlike mouthparts that inflict painful bites.

Because the females lay their eggs in well-aerated water, these flies often are found in the vicinity of swiftly flowing streams. They are swift fliers and move in great swarms, inflicting painful bites and sucking the host's blood. These flies may keep cattle from grazing or cause them to stampede. The animal's ears, neck, head, and abdomen are favorite feeding sites. These flies also feed on poultry and can serve as an intermediate host for the protozoan parasite *Leukocytozoon.*

Diagnosis. Adult black flies are most often collected in the field and are not found on animals presented to a veterinary clinic. They are identified

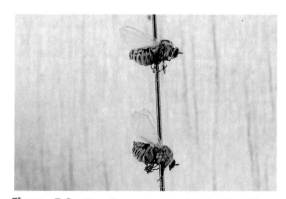

Figure 7-6. *Simulium* species, black flies. These tiny flies range in size from 1 to 6 mm in length. (From Hendrix CM, Robinson E: *Diagnostic parasitology for veterinary technicians,* ed 3, St Louis, 2006, Mosby.)

by their small size, humped back, and strong venation in the cranial region of the wings. Identification of black flies is probably best left to an entomologist.

Lutzomyia (New World Sand Fly)

Members of the genus *Lutzomyia* are commonly referred to as "New World sand flies." They are tiny, mothlike flies, rarely more than 5 mm long. A key feature for identification is that their bodies and wings are covered with fine hairs. They tend to be active only at night and are weak fliers. These tiny flies transmit the protozoan parasite *Leishmania* species.

Diagnosis. Like black flies, adult sand flies most often are collected in the field and are not found on animals presented to a veterinary clinic. They are identified by their small size and hairy wings and body. Identification of sand flies is probably best left to an entomologist.

Culicoides species

Culicoides gnats are also commonly known as "no see-ums," "punkies," or "sand flies." They are tiny gnats (1 to 3 mm in length), similar in appearance to black flies. They inflict painful bites, suck the blood of their hosts, and are active at dusk and dawn, especially during the winter months. These gnats tend to feed on the dorsal or ventral areas of the host; the feeding site depends on the species of biting gnat.

Horses often become allergic to the bites of *Culicoides* gnats, scratching and rubbing bitten areas, causing alopecia, excoriations, and thickening of the skin. This condition has several names, including "Queensland itch," "sweat itch," "sweet itch," and "summer dermatitis" (the latter name because it is often seen during the warmer months of the year). These flies also serve as the intermediate host for *Onchocerca cervicalis*, a nematode whose microfilariae are found in the skin of horses. These flies also transmit the bluetongue virus of sheep.

Diagnosis. In contrast to the clear, heavily veined wings of black flies, the wings of adult *Culicoides* species are mottled. Identification of

Culicoides species is probably best left to an entomologist.

Anopheles, Aedes, and Culex Species (Mosquitoes)

Although they are tiny, fragile Dipterans, mosquitoes are some of the most voracious blood feeders on domestic animals and human beings (Fig. 7-7). Mosquitoes can plague livestock and in swarms have been known to keep cattle from grazing in certain areas or cause them to stampede. The feeding of large numbers of swarming mosquitoes may cause significant anemia in domestic animals. Large numbers of mosquitoes may be produced from eggs laid in relatively small bodies of water. Although they are known for spreading malaria (*Plasmodium* species), yellow fever, and elephantiasis among people, mosquitoes are probably best known in veterinary medicine as the intermediate host for the canine heartworm, *Dirofilaria immitis*.

Diagnosis. Adult mosquitoes have wings and body parts covered by tiny, leaf-shaped scales. Identification of adult and larval *Anopheles*, *Aedes*, and *Culex* species is probably best left to an entomologist.

Hippelates Species (Eye Gnats, "Dog Penis" Gnats)

These tiny, fragile Dipterans are nonbiting gnats with sponging mouthparts that are very similar to the

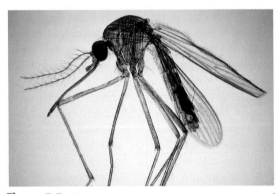

Figure 7-7. *Culex* species, one genus among several genera of mosquitoes. (From Hendrix CM, Robinson E: *Diagnostic parasitology for veterinary technicians,* ed 3, St Louis, 2006, Mosby.)

mouthparts of the common house fly. These tiny gnats are often found around a dog's penis (hence, the nickname "dog penis gnats"). These Dipterans are not capable of biting the host but often feed on liquid secretions from the host. These nonbiting gnats frequently are found around the teats of dairy cattle. They have been know to serve as mechanical vectors of a variety of bacteria.

Diagnosis. Adult *Hippelates* flies possess sponging mouthparts similar to those of the common housefly. Precise identification of adult *Hippelates* species is probably best left to an entomologist.

Chrysops and *Tabanus* Species (Deer Fly, Horse Fly)

Chrysops species (deer flies) and *Tabanus* species (horse flies) are large (up to 3.5 cm long), heavy-bodied, robust Dipterans with powerful wings and large eyes. Horse flies and deer flies are the largest flies in the Diptera group, in which only the females feed on vertebrate blood. Figure 7-8 shows *Tabanus* species, the largest blood-feeding Dipterans. Horse flies are larger than deer flies. Deer flies have a dark band passing from the cranial to the caudal margin of the wings.

Adult flies lay eggs in the vicinity of open water. Larval stages of these flies are found in aquatic

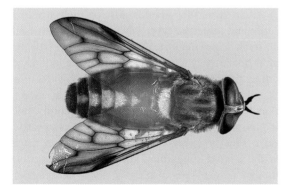

Figure 7-8. *Tabanus* species, the largest blood-feeding Dipteran. This tabanid is approximately 2.5 cm in length. (From Hendrix CM, Robinson E: *Diagnostic parasitology for veterinary technicians,* ed 3, St Louis, 2006, Mosby.)

to semiaquatic environments, often buried deep in mud at the bottom of lakes and ponds. Adults are seen in summer and are fond of sunlight. Female flies feed in the vicinity of open water and have reciprocating, scissorlike mouthparts. They use these sharp, bladelike mouthparts to lacerate tissues and lap up the oozing vertebrate blood. These flies feed primarily on large animals such as cattle and horses. Preferred feeding sites include the underside of the abdomen around the navel, the legs, or the neck and withers.

Horse flies and deer flies feed a number of times at multiple feeding sites before they stop feeding. When disturbed by the animal's swatting tail or by the panniculus reflex (skin twitching), the flies leave the host, but the blood continues to ooze from the open wound. These fly bites are painful. Affected cattle and horses become restless. Because they often feed on multiple hosts, these flies may act as mechanical transmitters of anthrax, anaplasmosis, and the virus of equine infectious anemia.

Diagnosis. These flies are most easily recognized by their large, robust size and lacerating, scissorlike mouthparts. Species identification of intact adult and larval horse and deer flies is probably best left to an entomologist.

In the second group of blood-feeding Dipterans, both male and female adult flies require a vertebrate blood meal. These species include the stable fly *Stomoxys calcitrans,* the horn fly *Haematobia irritans,* the wingless sheep ked *Melophagus ovinus,* and *Lynchia* and *Pseudolynchia* species, the louse flies of raptors and songbirds.

Stomoxys calcitrans (Stable Fly)

The stable fly, *Stomoxys calcitrans,* is often called the "biting housefly." It is approximately the size of *Musca domestica,* the common housefly. Rather than possessing sponging mouthparts, the stable fly has a bayonet-like proboscis that protrudes forward from the head (Fig. 7-9). These flies are found worldwide. In the United States, they are found in the central and southeastern states, where cattle are raised. Both male and female flies are avid blood feeders, feeding on any domestic animal. They usually attack the legs and ventral abdomen and

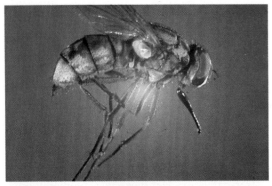

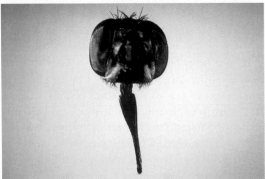

Figure 7-9. *Stomoxys calcitrans,* the stable fly. Note the bayonet-like proboscis that protrudes forward from the head. The stable fly is approximately the same size as a housefly. (From Hendrix CM, Robinson E: *Diagnostic parasitology for veterinary technicians,* ed 3, St Louis, 2006, Mosby.)

may also bite the ears. These flies also feed on the tips of the ears of dogs with pointed ears, especially the German Shepherd. These dogs' ears often demonstrate loss of hair and the presence of dried, crusty blood on the ear tips.

This fly feeds on both horses and cattle, with horses the preferred host. The fly usually lands on the host with its head pointed upward. It is a sedentary fly, not moving on the host. The fly inflicts painful bites that puncture the skin and bleed freely. The stable fly stays on the host for short periods, during which it obtains the blood meals. This is an outdoor fly; however, in the late fall and during rainy weather, it may enter barns.

Stable flies are mechanical vectors of anthrax in cattle and equine infectious anemia. They are the intermediate host for *Habronema muscae,* a nematode found in the stomach of horses. When large numbers of stable flies attack dairy cattle, milk production can fall. Beef cattle may refuse to graze in the daytime when they are attacked by large numbers of flies; as a result, these cattle do not gain the usual amount of weight.

Diagnosis. The veterinary technician can easily identify the stable fly by its size (approximately the same size as a housefly) and its bayonet-like proboscis that protrudes forward from the head.

Haematobia irritans (Horn Fly)

Haematobia irritans is often called the horn fly. This dark-colored fly is approximately 3 to 6 mm in length, half the size of *Stomoxys calcitrans,* the biting housefly. Like the stable fly, the horn fly has a bayonet-like proboscis that protrudes forward from the head. These flies are found almost exclusively on cattle throughout North America.

When the air temperature is less than 70° F, horn flies cluster around the base of the horns; this is the origin of the name horn fly. In warmer climates, thousands of flies often cluster on the hosts' shoulders, backs, and side; these areas are least disturbed by tail switching. On hot, sunny days, horn flies congregate on the ventral abdomen.

Adult horn flies spend most of their lives on cattle and leave the host only to deposit their eggs in fresh cow manure. Using their tiny bayonet mouthparts, they feed frequently, sucking blood and other fluids, and cause considerable irritation. Female flies are more aggressive than males. Harassment by the flies and loss of blood often reduce weight gains and milk production in cattle. Horn flies probably cause greater losses in cattle in the United States than any other blood-sucking fly. Adult horn flies also cause focal midline dermatitis on the ventral abdomen of horses. These flies also serve as the intermediate host for *Stephanofilaria stilesi,* a filarial parasite that produces plaquelike lesions on the ventral abdomen of cattle.

Diagnosis. The veterinary technician can easily identify the horn fly by its dark color and its small size (approximately half the size of a stable fly). Like the stable fly, the horn fly's bayonet-like proboscis protrudes forward from the head.

Melophagus ovinus (Sheep Ked)

Melophagus ovinus is often called the *sheep ked*. Members of the order Diptera usually have one pair of wings (two wings). Keds are an exception to that rule; they are wingless Dipterans. Keds are hairy, leathery, and 4 to 7 mm in length. The head is short and broad, the thorax brown, and the abdomen broad and grayish-brown. The legs are strong and armed with stout claws (Fig. 7-10). Some say that keds have a "louselike" appearance, but they are not related to lice.

Keds are permanent ectoparasites of sheep and goats. Their pupal stages are often found attached to the wool or hair of the host. Keds are avid blood feeders. Heavy infestations can reduce the condition of the host considerably and even cause anemia. Their bites cause pruritus over much of the host's body; infested sheep often bite, scratch, and rub themselves, damaging the wool. Ked feces often stain the wool and do not wash out readily. Keds are most numerous in the cold temperatures of the fall and winter months. Their numbers decline as temperatures warm in the spring and summer months.

Diagnosis. Close inspection of the wool and underlying skin reveals infestation.

Lynchia and *Pseudolynchia* species (Louse Flies)

Lynchia and *Pseudolynchia* species are often called louse flies and, like the keds, they are not related to lice. These Dipterans are closely related to the wingless sheep keds, but they are found to parasitize a wide variety of birds—from songbirds to pigeons to raptors. They are found among the feathers of these birds; however, they enjoy sucking blood from areas of the skin that are sparsely covered with feathers. These winged Dipterans are dark brown in color, hairy, and leathery in appearance. They are from 4 to 6 mm in length with legs armed with stout, fierce claws (Fig. 7-11). They

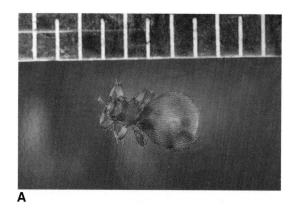

A

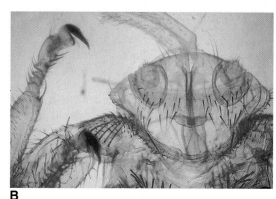

B

Figure 7-10. *Melophagus ovinus,* the sheep ked. Keds are hairy, leathery, and 4 to 7 mm in length. The head is short and broad. The thorax is brown, and the abdomen broad and grayish brown. The legs are strong and armed with stout claws. (From Hendrix CM, Robinson E: *Diagnostic parasitology for veterinary technicians,* ed 3, St Louis, 2006, Mosby.)

are swift fliers and move about quickly—even attempting to get into human hair.

Diagnosis. Close inspection of the feathers and the underlying skin reveals infestation by these winged Dipterans. These insects are swift fliers and often fly from the avian host in an attempt to get into the hair of any human being in the room.

Musca autumnalis (Face Fly)

The final periodic parasite among the Dipteran flies is one that is not a blood feeder but instead feeds on mucus, tears, and saliva of large animals, particularly

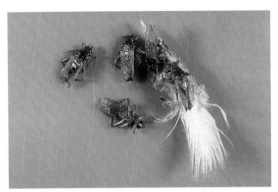

Figure 7-11. Louse flies, *Lynchia* or *Pseudolynchia* species, often parasitize wild birds. (From Hendrix CM, Robinson E: *Diagnostic parasitology for veterinary technicians,* ed 3, St Louis, 2006, Mosby.)

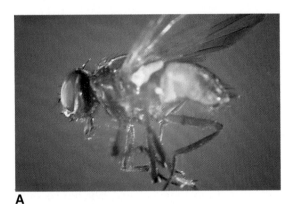

A

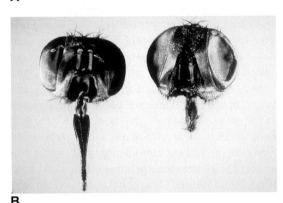

B

Figure 7-12. *Musca autumnalis,* the face fly. Its mouthparts are adapted for sponging saliva, tears, and mucus. (From Hendrix CM, Robinson E: *Diagnostic parasitology for veterinary technicians,* ed 3, St Louis, 2006, Mosby.)

cattle. Face flies, *Musca autumnalis*, are so named because they gather around the eyes and muzzle of livestock, particularly cattle. They also may be found on the withers, neck, brisket, and sides. Face flies feed mostly on liquid media: saliva, tears, and mucus. They usually are not considered blood feeders because their mouthparts are not piercing nor bayonet-like. Instead, their mouthparts are adapted for sponging up saliva, tears, and mucus (Fig. 7-12). They follow blood-feeding flies, disturb them during their feeding process, and then lap up the blood and body fluids that accumulate on the host's skin. Face flies are found on animals outdoors; they usually do not follow animals into barns.

Face flies produce considerable annoyance to the host. The irritation around the host's eyes stimulates the flow of tears, which attracts even more flies. This harassment ultimately interferes with the host's productivity. Face flies may be involved in the transmission of *Moraxella bovis,* a bacterium associated with infectious keratocon-junctivitis or pinkeye in cattle.

Diagnosis. Face flies are morphologically similar to the housefly, *Musca domestica*. These two species may be differentiated by minor differences in eye position and color of the abdomen. The veterinary technician probably should not attempt to speciate this fly; speciation requires the skills of a trained entomologist. If flies are found around the face of cattle or horses, they are probably face flies.

Myiasis-Producing Flies

With regard to their roles as ectoparasites, larval Dipterans may develop in the subcutaneous tissues of many domestic animals. When Dipteran larvae develop in the tissue or organs of vertebrate hosts, they produce a condition known as myiasis. On the basis of the degree of host dependence, the myiases (plural of "myiasis") are divided into two classifications. In facultative myiasis, the fly larvae are usually free living. Under certain circumstances, these normally free-living larvae can adapt to a parasitic dependence on a host. In obligatory myiasis, the fly larvae are completely parasitic; that is, they are completely dependent on the host to develop through the life cycle. In other words, without the host, the obligatory parasites will die.

Facultative Myiasis-Producing Flies

This group of flies includes *Musca domestica* (housefly) and *Calliphora, Phaenicia, Lucilia, Phormia* (blowfly, bottle flies), and *Sarcophaga* (flesh fly) species. The adults of these fly species are colloquially known as "filth flies" because of their propensity to fly from feces to food. Like the face fly, these flies are "vomit drop feeders," disgorging their stomach contents with their associated liquefaction enzymes and then lapping up the resulting liquid food. These adult flies are frequently seen in kennel situations, alighting on feces that have not been removed from dog runs.

Dipteran larvae that produce facultative myiasis include the housefly *M. domestica,* the blowflies or bottle flies *Calliphora, Phaenicia, Lucilia,* and *Phormia* species, and the flesh fly *Sarcophaga* species. Larval stages of these flies usually are associated with skin wounds contaminated with bacteria or with a matted haircoat contaminated with feces or urine.

Under their "normal" living conditions, adult flies of these genera lay their eggs in decaying animal carcasses or in feces. In facultative myiasis, the adult flies are attracted to an animal's moist wound, skin lesion, or soiled haircoat. These sites provide the adult fly with a moist medium on which it feeds. As adult female flies feed in these sites, they lay their eggs. These eggs hatch, producing larvae (maggots) that move independently about the wound surface, ingesting dead cells, exudate, secretions, and debris, but not live tissue. This condition is known as "fly strike" or "strike." These larvae irritate, injure, and kill successive layers of skin and produce exudates.

Maggots can tunnel through the thin epidermal layer into the subcutis. This process produces tissue cavities in the skin that measure up to several cen-timeters in diameter. Unless the process is halted by appropriate therapy, the infested animal may die from shock, intoxication, histolysis, or infection. A peculiar, distinct, pungent odor permeates the infested tissues and the affected animal. Advanced lesions may contain thousands of maggots.

As adults, these flies can be pestiferous flies in a veterinary clinical setting. These flies are "vomit drop" feeders and fly from feces to food, spreading bacteria on their feet and their disgorged stomach contents. A veterinary clinic with outdoor kennels is especially susceptible to the assault of these pestiferous flies.

Diagnosis. A tentative diagnosis of maggot infestation in any domestic animal can easily be made because maggots can be observed in an existing wound or among the soiled, matted haircoat. When facultative myiasis has been diagnosed, the veterinarian must rule out the possibility of obligatory myiasis caused by *Cochliomyia hominivorax.*

Obligatory Myiasis-Producing Flies
Cochilomyia hominivorax (Primary Screwworm)

In obligatory myiasis, the Dipteran larvae must lead a parasitic existence. Only one fly in North America, *Cochliomyia hominivorax,* is a primary invader of fresh, uncontaminated skin wounds of domestic animals. These larvae must not be confused with the larvae of the more common facultative myiasis-producing flies previously described. *C. hominivorax* is often referred to as the screwworm fly. Economically it is the most important fly that may attack livestock in the southwestern and southern United States.

Adult female flies are attracted to fresh skin wounds on any warm-blooded animal, where they lay batches of 15 to 500 eggs in a shinglelike pattern at the edge of wounds. The female lays several thousand cream-colored, elongated eggs during her lifetime. They hatch within 24 hours. Larvae enter the wound, where they feed for 4 to 7 days before developing into third-stage (fully grown) larvae. They may be as long as 1.5 cm in length. At this stage they resemble a wood screw. These larvae also bore down into the tissues, much like a wood screw penetrating a piece of wood. When fully mature, the larvae drop from the host to the ground and pupate for approximately a week, after which the adult flies emerge. The adult male and female fly mate only once during their lifetime, a fact that is used to control these flies biologically, a program known as the sterile male release technique.

Diagnosis. Adult flies are shiny and greenish blue, with a reddish-orange head and eyes, and are 8 to 15 mm long. Larvae often are identified by their wood screw shape and by the deeply pigmented tracheal tubes on the posterior third of the dorsal aspect of the caudal ends. Because of the obligatory nature of the screwworm with regard to breeding in the fresh wounds of any warm-blooded animal, the veterinarian must report any screwworm infestations to both state and federal authorities. *C. hominivorax* has been eradicated from the United States but occasionally surreptitiously enters the country in imported animals (Fig. 7-13).

Cuterebra species (Wolf Warble)

Larvae of the genus *Cuterebra* infest the skin of rabbits, squirrels, mice, rats, chipmunks, and occasionally, dogs and cats. A large discrepancy exists concerning the descriptions of larval *Cuterebra*. Most of the specimens recovered in a veterinary setting are second- or third-stage larvae. Second-stage larvae are grublike, 5 to 10 mm long, and cream to grayish white in color. They are often sparsely covered with tiny, black, toothlike spines. Third-stage larvae are large, robust, black, and heavily spined (Fig. 7-14). Larval stages usually are found in swollen, cystlike subcutaneous sites, with a fistula or pore communicating to the outside environment. The larval *Cuterebra* species breathes through this pore (Fig. 7-15).

Adult flies lay eggs near the entrance to rodent burrows. As a result of this site of egg deposition, the adult flies never annoy the host. Pets usually contract this parasite while investigating or hunting rodent prey. As a result, the most commonly affected sites in dogs and cats are the subcutaneous tissues of the neck and face. Most cases occur during the late summer and early fall. Among the myiasis-producing flies, this Dipteran larva is known for its aberrant or erratic migrations, having been found in a variety of extracutaneous sites, the cranial vault, the eye, and the pharyngeal regions. Clinical signs vary with the site of infection or infestation. Larvae often are discovered in subcutaneous sites during physical examination. The larva usually

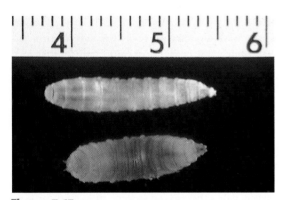

Figure 7-13. Larvae of *Cochliomyia hominivorax* can be identified by wood screw appearance and two deeply pigmented tracheal tubes on the dorsal aspect of the caudal ends of the third larval stage. (From Hendrix CM, Robinson E: *Diagnostic parasitology for veterinary technicians,* ed 3, St Louis, 2006, Mosby.)

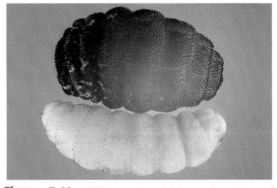

Figure 7-14. Different developmental stages of *Cuterebra* species. Larval *Cuterebra* are either sparsely or thickly covered with tiny black spines. (From Hendrix CM, Robinson E: *Diagnostic parasitology for veterinary technicians,* ed 3, St Louis, 2006, Mosby.)

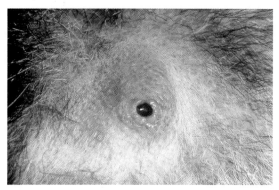

Figure 7-15. Larval *Cuterebra* species are usually found in swollen, cystlike subcutaneous sites, with a fistula (pore, or hole) communicating to the outside environment. (From Hendrix CM, Robinson E: *Diagnostic parasitology for veterinary technicians,* ed 3, St Louis, 2006, Mosby.)

is removed by enlarging the breathing pore and extracting it with thumb forceps. Great care must be taken not to crush the larva during extraction because anaphylaxis might result.

   Diagnosis. Cuterebrosis is diagnosed by observing the characteristic swollen, cystlike subcutaneous lesion, with a fistula or central pore communicating to the outside environment. Second- or third-stage larvae usually are removed from this lesion.

Hypoderma Species (Ox Warble, Cattle Grub)

Two larval stages of *Hypoderma* flies infect cattle: *Hypoderma lineatum* and *Hypoderma bovis*. *H. lineatum* is found in the southern United States; both species are found in the northern United States and Canada. The adult flies are heavy bodied and resemble honeybees; the adults often are called "heel flies."

   The life cycle is almost a year in duration. Adult flies are bothersome to cattle because they approach cattle to lay eggs. Animals often become apprehensive and disturbed and attempt to escape the fly by running away, an action called gadding. The eggs are approximately 1 mm long and attached to hairs on the legs of cattle. *H. lineatum* deposits a row of six or more eggs on an individual

hair shaft, whereas *H. bovis* lays its eggs singly. The larvae hatch in approximately 4 days and crawl down the hair shaft to the skin, which they penetrate. They wander through the subcutaneous connective tissue in the leg, migrating to the esophagus *(H. lineatum)* or the region of the spinal canal and epidural fat *(H. bovis),* until they reach the subcutaneous tissues of the back. Here the larvae create breathing pores in the skin of the dorsum, through which they later exit and fall to the ground to pupate. The adult flies emerge from the pupae.

   Diagnosis. Adults are beelike and covered with yellow to orange hairs. Mature larvae are 25 to 30 mm long, cream to dark brown in color, and covered with small spines (Fig. 7-16). Lesions consist of large, cystlike or boil-like swellings on the back, with a central breathing pore. As with *Cuterebra* species, great care must be taken not to crush the larva during extraction because anaphylaxis might result.

Order: Siphonaptera (Fleas)

Of all the ectoparasites discussed thus far, the flea is perhaps the most economically important insect to the veterinarian; treating and preventing flea

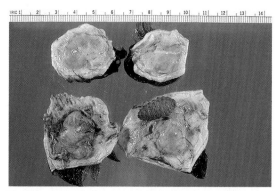

Figure 7-16. Mature larvae of *Hypoderma* species are 25 to 30 mm long, cream to dark brown in color, and covered with small spines. Lesions consist of large, cystlike swellings on the back, with a central breathing pore. (From Hendrix CM, Robinson E: *Diagnostic parasitology for veterinary technicians,* ed 3, St Louis, 2006, Mosby.)

infestations can be a veterinary practice builder. Because of the extreme popularity of dogs and cats and the prolific nature of the flea (it is able to rebound after populations are exterminated on the animal and in the animal's environment), special attention should be paid to detecting the various life cycle stages of fleas both on the pet and in the pet's environment.

Fleas are Siphonapterans, small (4 to 5 mm in length), laterally compressed, wingless insects with powerful hind legs that are used for jumping. Figure 7-17 shows the life stages of *Ctenocephalides felis,* the cat flea. Adult fleas have piercing/sucking (siphonlike) mouthparts that are used to suck the blood of their host. Figure 7-18 shows the morphologic details of the adult female and male *C. felis.* More than 2000 species of fleas have been identified throughout the world. Adult fleas are always parasitic, feeding on both mammals and birds. Dogs and cats are host to comparatively few species of fleas.

C. felis is the most common flea found on dogs and cats. The dog flea, *C. canis,* is uncommon and occurs far less frequently on dogs than does the cat flea.

Echidnophaga gallinacea is also known as the "stick-tight flea" of poultry (Fig. 7-19). A common flea of chickens and guinea fowl, it also feeds on dogs and cats. This flea has unique feeding habits.

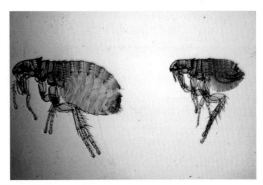

Figure 7-18. Morphologic details of the adult female and male *Ctenocephalides felis,* the cat flea. (From Hendrix CM, Robinson E: *Diagnostic parasitology for veterinary technicians,* ed 3, St Louis, 2006, Mosby.)

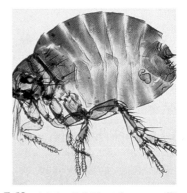

Figure 7-19. Adult *Echidnophaga gallinacea,* the stick-tight flea of poultry. (From Hendrix CM, Robinson E: *Diagnostic parasitology for veterinary technicians,* ed 3, St Louis, 2006, Mosby.)

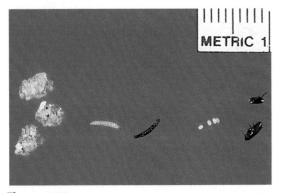

Figure 7-17. Life stages of *Ctenocephalides felis,* the cat flea. *Left to right,* Pupae, larvae, eggs, adult male, and female. (From Hendrix CM, Robinson E: *Diagnostic parasitology for veterinary technicians,* ed 3, St Louis, 2006, Mosby.)

The female flea inserts its mouthparts into the skin of the host and remains attached at that site. These specimens resemble attached ticks; however, they are fleas.

Fleas are not commonly found on horses or ruminants. In barns where feral cats abound and where excessive bedding is used, fleas have been found on calves in large numbers and can produce significant anemia. *Pulex irritans,* the human flea, has been recovered from dogs and cats, especially in the southeastern United States.

Although the adult flea is the stage most commonly encountered, the veterinary technician also may be presented with flea eggs, larval fleas, or flea droppings from the pet's environment. Flea eggs and larvae are commonly found in the owner's bedclothes, the pet's bedding, travel carriers, doghouses, or clinic cages. Flea eggs resemble tiny, smooth pearls; they are nonsticky, 0.5 mm long, white, oval, and rounded at both ends (Fig. 7-20). Flea larvae resemble tiny fly maggots. They are 2 to 5 mm long, white (after feeding they become brown), and sparsely covered with hairs (Fig. 7-21). Flea larvae spin a sticky, silky cocoon that often becomes covered with environmental debris. This is the pupal stage, a stage that is seldom detected in the pet's environment (Fig. 7-22).

Diagnosis

Because adult fleas spend most of their time on the host, flea infestation is usually obvious. However, in animals with flea-allergy dermatitis, fleas may be so few in number on the pet as to make diagnosis of flea infestation difficult.

Definitive diagnosis of flea infestation requires demonstration of the adult fleas and/or their droppings (flea dirt, flea feces, flea frass) (Fig. 7-23). Adult fleas defecate large quantities of partially digested blood, commonly called "flea dirt" or "flea frass." These feces are reddish-black and can appear as fine pepper-like specks, comma-shape columns, or long coils.

Adult fleas usually are encountered on the animal but also may be collected in the pet's environment. When recovered from the pet, the larger fleas with an orange to light brown abdomen are females; the smaller, darker specimens are males.

Flea collection is facilitated by spraying the pet with an insecticide. In a few minutes, dead fleas drop off the animal. Alternatively, fleas may be collected with a fine-tooth flea comb available at any veterinary supply store or pet store.

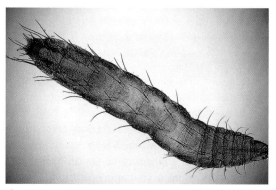

Figure 7-21. Larva of *Ctenocephalides felis,* the cat flea. (From Hendrix CM, Robinson E: *Diagnostic parasitology for veterinary technicians,* ed 3, St Louis, 2006, Mosby.)

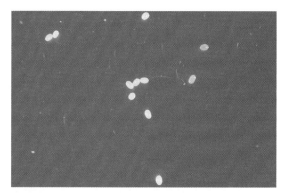

Figure 7-20. Eggs of *Ctenocephalides felis,* the cat flea. (From Hendrix CM, Robinson E: *Diagnostic parasitology for veterinary technicians,* ed 3, St Louis, 2006, Mosby.)

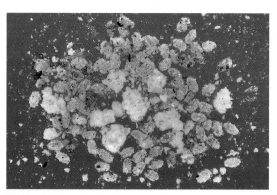

Figure 7-22. Sand-covered pupae of *Ctenocephalides felis,* the cat flea. (From Hendrix CM, Robinson E: *Diagnostic parasitology for veterinary technicians,* ed 3, St Louis, 2006, Mosby.)

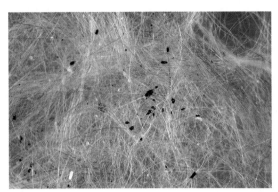

Figure 7-23. Flea dirt, flea feces, or flea frass of *Ctenocephalides felis,* the cat flea. (From Hendrix CM, Robinson E: *Diagnostic parasitology for veterinary technicians,* ed 3, St Louis, 2006, Mosby.)

"Flea dirt" may be used to diagnose current or recent flea infestation. To collect a sample of flea dirt, the pet should be combed with a flea comb and the collected samples of detritus placed on a white paper towel moistened with water. Rubbing the flea dirt with a fingertip causes the flea dirt to dissolve, producing a characteristic blood red or rust-red color.

Control

Flea control is important because fleas cause discomfort and irritation to the pet and serve as intermediate hosts to certain helminth parasites. Fleas serve as intermediate host for *Dipylidium caninum,* the double-pore tapeworm of dogs and cats, and as intermediate host for *Dipetalonema (Acanthocheilonema) reconditum,* a filarial parasite that resides in the subcutaneous tissues of dogs. Some types of fleas also may transmit disease, such as bubonic plague and endemic typhus, to human beings. In many areas throughout the world, flea control on dogs and cats is one of the most economically important scenarios encountered in a small animal veterinary practice.

Class: Acarina (Mites and Ticks)

Mites and ticks of veterinary importance are members of the class Acarina.

Mites of Veterinary Importance

The first group of parasitic mites can be classified together as sarcoptiform mites. Sarcoptiform mites have several common key characteristics or features. These mites may produce severe dermatologic problems in a variety of domestic animals. This dermatitis usually is accompanied by a severe pruritus. Sarcoptiform mites are small, barely visible to the naked eye, and approximately the size of a grain of salt. Their bodies have a round to oval shape. Sarcoptiform mites have legs with pedicels or stalks at the tip. The pedicels may be long or short. If the pedicel is long, it may be straight (unjointed) or jointed. At the tip of each pedicel may be a tiny sucker. Veterinarians and veterinary technicians should use the description of the pedicel (long or short, jointed or unjointed) to identify these sarcoptiform mites.

Sarcoptiform mites are divided into two basic families: *Sarcoptidae,* which burrow or tunnel within the epidermis, and *Psoroptidae,* which reside on the surface of the skin or within the external ear canal. Species of *Sarcoptidae* includes *Sarcoptes, Notoedres,* and *Cnemidocoptes;* species of *Psoroptidae* include *Psoroptes, Chorioptes,* and *Otodectes.*

Family Sarcoptidae

Sarcoptic mites burrow or tunnel within the epidermis of the infested definitive host. The entire four-stage life cycle is spent on the host. Male and female mites breed on the skin surface. Female mites penetrate the keratinized layers of the skin and burrow or tunnel through the epidermis. Over a 10- to 15-day period, the female deposits 40 to 50 eggs within the tunnel. After egg deposition, the female dies. Larvae emerge from the eggs in 3 to 10 days and exit the tunnel to wander on the skin surface. These larvae molt to the nymphal stage within minute pockets in the epidermis. Nymphs become sexually active adults in 12 to 17 days and the life cycle begins again.

Sarcoptes scabei (Scabies Mites)

The disease caused by *Sarcoptes scabei* is called sarcoptic acariasis. This condition is considered extremely pruritic.

Certain varieties of *Sarcoptes* mites infest specific hosts. For example, *S. scabiei* var. *canis* infests only dogs, and *S. scabiei* var. *suis* infests only pigs. Almost every domestic species has its own distinct variety of this mite.

Scabies in dogs is caused by *S. scabiei* var. *canis,* which produces an erythematous, papular rash. Scaling, crusting, and excoriation are common. The ears, lateral elbows, and ventral abdomen are most likely to harbor mites. The host's entire body, however, may be infested. These mites are spread by direct contact and can affect all dogs in a household or kennel. Scabies is extremely contagious. Also, the dog owner can become infested with this mite, but the infestation in people is self-limiting. The mites burrow into human skin, producing a papulelike lesion, but they do not establish a full-blown infestation in people. This mite is considered to be zoonotic, that is, able to transmit disease from animals to human beings. Some dogs may be asymptomatic carriers of this mite. *S. scabiei* var. *felis,* which causes scabies in cats, is an extremely rare mite.

Among large animals, pigs most commonly are affected by scabies. Lesions caused by *S. scabiei* variety *suis* include small, red papules; alopecia; and crusts, most commonly on the trunk and ears. The mite is rare in cattle (*S. scabiei* var. *bovis*). The main infested areas are the head, neck, and shoulders. *S. scabiei* var. *equi* of horses is even rarer. The main infested area is the neck. *S. scabiei* var. *ovis* infests the face and muzzle of sheep and goats instead of the fleece.

Diagnosis. Areas with an erythematous, papular rash and crust should be scraped, especially the areas most associated with sarcoptic infestation (ears, lateral elbows, and ventral abdomen of dogs). Repeated scrapings (as many as six scrapings) may be necessary to detect mites. Adult sarcoptic mites are oval and 200 to 400 µm in diameter and have eight legs. The key morphologic feature used to identify this species is the long, unjointed pedicel with a sucker on the end of some of the legs (Fig. 7-24). The anus is located on the caudal end of the body. The eggs of *Sarcoptes* mites are oval (Fig. 7-25).

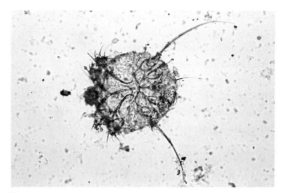

Figure 7-24. Adult *Sarcoptes scabiei* mite. Note the long, unjointed pedicels (stalks), with suckers on the ends. (From Hendrix CM, Robinson E: *Diagnostic parasitology for veterinary technicians,* ed 3, St Louis, 2006, Mosby.)

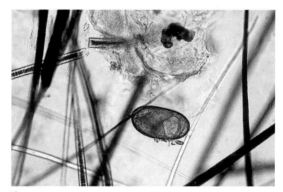

Figure 7-25. Oval eggs of Sarcoptes scabiei. (From Hendrix CM, Robinson E: *Diagnostic parasitology for veterinary technicians,* ed 3, St Louis, 2006, Mosby.)

Notoedres cati (Feline Scabies Mite)

Notoedres cati infests mainly cats but on occasion parasitizes rabbits. This sarcoptiform mite is found chiefly on the ears, back of the neck, face, feet, and in extreme cases, on the entire body. The life cycle is like that of *S. scabiei,* with the mite burrowing or tunneling in the superficial layers of the epidermis. The characteristic lesion of notoedric acariasis is a yellowing crust in the region of the ears, face, or neck.

Diagnosis. Notoedric mites are easier to demonstrate in cats than are sarcoptic mites in dogs. Likely infestation sites should be scraped. Like *Sarcoptes* species, *Notoedres* mites have a long, unjointed pedicel with sucker on the end of some of the legs. Adult notoedric mites are similar to sarcoptic mites but are smaller, with a dorsal anus. The eggs of notoedric mites are oval.

Cnemidocoptes pilae (Scaly Leg Mite of Budgerigars)

Cnemidocoptes pilae causes scaly leg in budgerigars, or parakeets. This mite tunnels in the superficial layers of the epidermis of the pads and shanks of the feet. In severe cases the beak and cere also may be affected. The mite characteristically produces a yellow to gray-white mass that resembles a honeycomb. This condition may be disfiguring to the parakeet. The parasites pierce the skin underlying the scales, causing an inflammation with exudate that hardens on the surface and displaces the scales superficially. This process causes the thickened, scaly nature of the skin. A related species, *Cnemidocoptes mutans,* produces "scaly leg" in chickens and turkeys.

Diagnosis. Infested sites should be scraped. Great care should be taken in handling infested birds because parakeets are fragile. The eight-legged, globular mites are approximately 500 μm in diameter. Adult female mites have very short legs and no suckers on the end of their legs (Fig. 7-26). Adult males have longer legs and a long, unjointed pedicel with suckers on the end of some of the legs.

Family: Psoroptidae

Members of the family Psoroptidae reside on the surface of the skin or within the external ear canal. The entire five-stage life cycle (egg, larva, protonymph, deutonymph or pubescent female, and adult egg-laying female) is spent on the host. Adult male and female mites breed on the skin surface. The female produces 14 to 24 elliptic, opaque, shiny white eggs that hatch within 1 to 3 days. The six-legged nymphs are small, oval, soft, and grayish brown. The eight-legged nymphs are slightly larger than larvae. Larval and nymphal stages may last 7 to

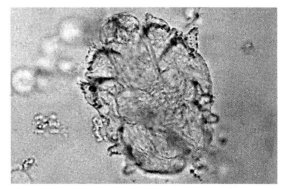

Figure 7-26. Adult female *Cnemidocoptes pilae* mite. The adult male has longer legs and a long, unjointed pedicel with suckers on the end of some of the legs. (From Hendrix CM, Robinson E: *Diagnostic parasitology for veterinary technicians,* ed 3, St Louis, 2006, Mosby.)

10 days. The life cycle is completed in 10 to 18 days. Under favorable conditions, psoroptic mites can live off the host for 2 to 3 weeks or longer. Under optimal conditions, mite eggs may remain viable for 2 to 4 weeks.

Psoroptes cuniculi (Ear Canker Mite of Rabbits)

Psoroptes cuniculi occurs most commonly in the external ear canal of rabbits but also has been found in horses, goats, and sheep. These mites live on the surface of the skin and feed on the rabbit host by puncturing the epidermis to obtain tissue fluids. Within the external ear canal of the infested host are the characteristic dried crusts of coagulated serum. The rabbit's ears appear to be packed with dried corn flakes. Affected animals shake the head and scratch their ears. Lesions sometimes occur on the head and legs. Severely infested animals may become debilitated. Loss of equilibrium may occur, with head tilt.

Diagnosis. The mites within the crusty debris inside the ear can be easily isolated. The brownish-white female is large, up to 750 μm long. The mites exhibit characteristic long, jointed pedicels with suckers on the ends of some of the legs (Figs. 7-27 and 7-28). The anus is in a terminal slit.

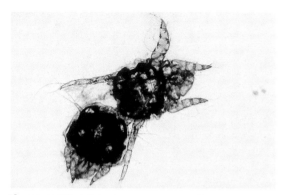

Figure 7-27. Adult Psoroptes cuniculi mites. (From Hendrix CM, Robinson E: *Diagnostic parasitology for veterinary technicians,* ed 3, St Louis, 2006, Mosby.)

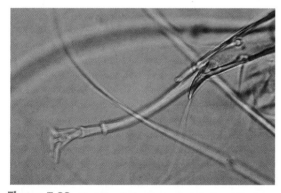

Figure 7-28. Detail of the long, jointed pedicel on the leg of *Psoroptes cuniculi.* (From Hendrix CM, Robinson E: *Diagnostic parasitology for veterinary technicians,* ed 3, St Louis, 2006, Mosby.)

Psoroptes species (Scab Mite of Large Animals)

Psoroptes ovis, Psoroptes bovis, and *Psoroptes equi* are the scab mites of large animals, residing on sheep, cattle, and horses, respectively. These mites are host specific and reside within the thick hair or long wool areas of the animal. They are surface dwellers and feed by puncturing the epidermis to feed on lymphatic fluid. Serum exudes through the puncture site. After the serum coagulates and forms a crust, wool is lost. The feeding site is extremely pruritic and the animal excoriates itself, producing

further wool loss. The mites then migrate to adjacent undamaged skin. As the mites proliferate, tags of wool are pulled out and the fleece becomes matted. Finally, patches of skin are exposed and the skin becomes parchmentlike, thickened, and cracked. The skin may bleed easily. Infested sheep constantly rub against fences, posts, farm equipment, and anything else that might serve as a scratching post. The disease is spread by direct contact or infested premises.

P. bovis in cattle produces lesions on the withers, neck, and rump. These consist of papules; crusts; and wrinkled, thickened skin. *P. equi* in horses is rare and affects the base of the mane and the tail.

Because of the intense pruritus and the highly contagious nature of the infestation, the occurrence of *Psoroptes* species in large animals should be reported to state and federal authorities and the United States Department of Agriculture.

Diagnosis. These mites are host specific. Adults are up to 600 μm long. Psoroptic mites exhibit characteristic long, jointed pedicels with suckers on the ends of some of the legs.

Chorioptes species (Foot and Tail Mite, Itchy Leg Mite)

Chorioptes equi, Chorioptes bovis, Chorioptes caprae, and *Chorioptes ovis* are the foot and tail mites of large animals, residing on horses, cattle, goats, and sheep, respectively. These mites are found on the skin surface on the distal (lower) part of the hind legs but may spread to the flank and shoulder area. On cattle, they are frequently found in the tail region, especially in the area of the escutcheon. These mites do not spread rapidly or extensively. They puncture the skin, causing serum to exude. Thin crusts of coagulated serum form on the skin surface. The skin eventually wrinkles and thickens although pruritus is not severe.

Infested horses stamp, bite, and kick, especially at night. Mites typically infest the pasterns, especially those of the hind legs.

Diagnosis. The characteristic mites can be identified from skin scrapings of infested areas. Chorioptic mites have short, unjointed pedicels, with suckers on the ends of some of the legs

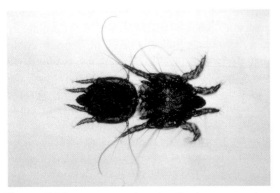

Figure 7-29. Female and male Chorioptes species. Note this mite's short, unjointed pedicels. (From Hendrix CM, Robinson E: *Diagnostic parasitology for veterinary technicians,* ed 3, St Louis, 2006, Mosby.)

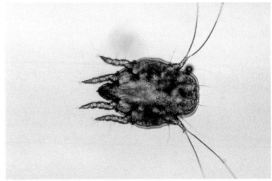

Figure 7-30. Adult female *Otodectes cynotis* mite. (From Hendrix CM, Robinson E: *Diagnostic parasitology for veterinary technicians,* ed 3, St Louis, 2006, Mosby.)

(Fig. 7-29). The female mites are approximately 400 μm long.

Otodectes cynotis (Ear Mite)

Ear mites, *Otodectes cynotis,* are a common cause of otitis externa in dogs, cats, and ferrets. Although they occur primarily in the external ear canal, ear mites may be found on any area of the body. A common infestation site is the tail and head region. As dogs and cats curl up to sleep, their head (and ears) are often in close proximity to the base of the tail. These mites are spread by direct contact and are highly transmissible both among and between the canine and feline species.

Ear mites are found within the external ear canal, where they feed on epidermal debris and produce intense irritation. Infection is usually bilateral. The host responds to the mite infestation by shaking its head and scratching its ears. Severe infestations may cause otitis media, with head tilt, circling, and convulsions. Auricular hematomas may develop.

Diagnosis. Mites usually are identified by an otoscope; through an otoscope the mites appear as white, motile objects. The brown exudate collected by swabbing the ear may be placed in mineral oil on a glass slide and the mites observed with a low power microscopic objective. These mites are

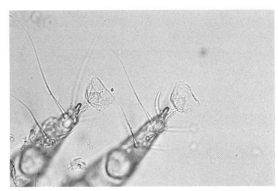

Figure 7-31. Detail of the leg of *Otodectes,* with a short, unjointed pedicel. (From Hendrix CM, Robinson E: *Diagnostic parasitology for veterinary technicians,* ed 3, St Louis, 2006, Mosby.)

fairly large, approximately 400 μm; they also may be easily seen with a magnifying glass or even the unaided eye. The mites exhibit characteristic short, unjointed pedicels, with suckers on the ends of some of the legs (Figs. 7-30 and 7-31). The anus is terminal.

Miscellaneous Mites

Other parasitic mites can be grouped together because they are not sarcoptiform mites. They can, however, produce severe dermatologic problems in a variety of domestic animals. These mites lack pedicels or stalks on their legs that identify sarcoptiform mites.

Demodex species

Mites of the genus *Demodex* reside in the hair follicles and sebaceous glands of most domesticated animals and human beings. In many species they are considered normal, nonpathogenic fauna of the skin. These mites are host specific and are not transmissible from one host species to another. The clinical disease, caused by an increased number of these mites, is called demodicosis.

Demodex mites resemble eight-legged alligators. They are elongated mites with short, stubby legs on the anterior half of the body. Adult and nymphal stages have eight legs, whereas the larvae have six. Adult *Demodex* mites are approximately 250 μm long (Fig. 7-32). The eggs are spindle shaped or tapered at each end (Fig. 7-33).

The life cycle of *Demodex* species has five stages: egg, larva, protonymph, deutonymph, and adult. The developmental periods of these various life cycle stages are not well known.

Of all the domestic animals infested with *Demodex* species, the dog is the most commonly and most seriously infested. Small numbers of these mites are considered part of the normal skin flora of all dogs. In dogs with immunodeficiencies, however, these mites proliferate and cause skin disease.

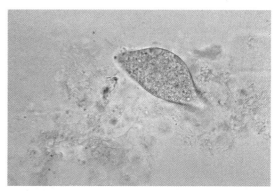

Figure 7-33. Egg of Demodex canis. (From Hendrix CM, Robinson E: *Diagnostic parasitology for veterinary technicians,* ed 3, St Louis, 2006, Mosby.)

Demodicosis occurs in two forms in dogs: localized demodicosis and generalized demodicosis. The predominant clinical sign of the localized form is patchy alopecia, especially of the muzzle, face, and forelimbs. The mites presumably are acquired during intimate contact when the puppy nurses the dam. As a result of that close contact, localized demodicosis often develops in the region of the face. Generalized demodicosis is characterized by diffuse alopecia, erythema, and secondary bacterial contamination over the entire body surface of the dog. An inherited defect in the dog's immune system is thought to be an important factor in the development of generalized demodicosis.

Cats are infested by two species of demodectic mites: *Demodex cati* and an unnamed species. *D. cati* is an elongated mite similar to *D. canis*. The unnamed species has a broad, blunted abdomen compared with the elongated one of *D. cati*. The presence of either species on the skin of cats is rare. Localized feline demodicosis is characterized by patchy areas of alopecia and erythema and occasionally crusting on the head (especially around the eyes), ears, and neck. In generalized feline demodicosis, the alopecia, erythema, and crusting usually involve the entire body. Demodicosis also has been associated with ceruminous otitis externa.

Demodectic mites reside in the hair follicles of other species of domestic animals but rarely produce clinical disease. Cattle and goats are most commonly infested but only rarely.

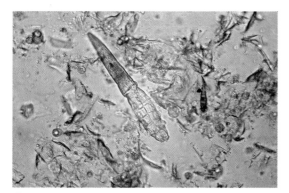

Figure 7-32. Adult *Demodex canis* mite. (From Hendrix CM, Robinson E: *Diagnostic parasitology for veterinary technicians,* ed 3, St Louis, 2006, Mosby.)

In cattle, *D. bovis* causes large nodules (abscesses) on the shoulders, trunk, and lateral aspects of the neck. In goats, *D. caprae* occurs in small papular or nodular lesions on the shoulders, trunk, and lateral aspect of the neck. In sheep, *D. ovis* rarely causes pustules and crusting around the coronet, nose, ear tips, and periorbital areas. In pigs, *D. phylloides* rarely produces pustules and nodules on the face, abdomen, and ventral neck. In horses, *D. equi* occurs around the face and eyes and rarely produces clinical disease.

Diagnosis. Skin areas with altered pigmentation, obstructed hair follicles, erythema, or alopecia should always be scraped. In localized demodicosis, the areas most commonly affected are the forelegs, perioral region, and periorbital regions. In generalized demodicosis, the entire body may be affected; however, the face and feet usually are the most severely involved. In dogs, areas of apparently normal skin also should be scraped to determine if the disease is generalized. The areas should be clipped and a fold of skin gently squeezed just before scraping. Gentle scraping of affected areas should be continued until capillary blood oozing is observed because these mites live deep in the hair follicles and sebaceous glands (Fig. 7-34).

Nodular lesions in large animals should be incised with a scalpel and the caseous material within smeared on a slide with mineral oil, covered with a cover slip, and examined microscopically for mites.

The mites on the slide should be counted and the live/dead ratio determined. The presence of any larval or nymphal stages or eggs should be noted. During therapy for *Demodex* species, a decrease in the number of eggs and live mites is a good prognostic indicator.

Cheyletiella species (Walking Dandruff)

Mites of the genus *Cheyletiella* are surface dwelling (nonburrowing), residing in the keratin layer of the skin and in the haircoat of the definitive host, which may be a dog, cat, or rabbit. These mites ingest keratin debris and tissue fluids. *Cheyletiella* mites are sometimes referred to as "walking dandruff" because the mites resemble large, mobile flakes of dandruff. Cheylettid mites have distinct key morphologic features. They are large (386 μm by 266 μm) and visible to the unaided eye. With the compound microscope, their most characteristic key morphologic feature may easily be seen: their enormous hooklike accessory mouthparts (palpi). These palpi assist the mite in attaching to the host as it feeds on tissue fluids. The mite also has comblike structures at the tip of each leg. Members of the genus also are known for their characteristic body shape resembling a shield, a bell pepper, an acorn, or a western horse saddle when viewed from above (Fig. 7-35). Eggs are 235 to 245 μm long and 115 to 135 μm wide (smaller than louse nits) and are supported by cocoonlike structures bound to the host's hair shaft by strands of fibers. Two or three eggs may be bound together on one hair shaft.

Diagnosis. The key feature of *Cheyletiella* species infestation is often the moving white "dandruff" flakes along the dorsal midline and head of the host. A handheld magnifying lens or binocular headband magnifier (e.g., OptiVISOR, Donegan Optical Company Inc., Lenexa, KS) often are used to view questionable dandruff flakes or hairs; these are perhaps the quickest methods of diagnosing cheyletiellosis. A fine-tooth flea comb may be used to collect mites; combing dandrufflike debris onto black paper often facilitates visualization of these highly mobile mites. The use of clear cellophane

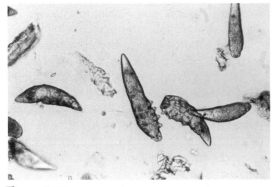

Figure 7-34. A deep skin scraping produces numerous mites of *Demodex canis*. (From Hendrix CM, Robinson E: *Diagnostic parasitology for veterinary technicians,* ed 3, St Louis, 2006, Mosby.)

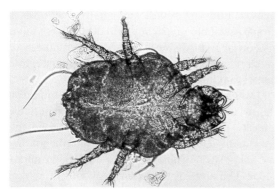

Figure 7-35. Adult *Cheyletiella* mite. (From Hendrix CM, Robinson E: *Diagnostic parasitology for veterinary technicians,* ed 3, St Louis, 2006, Mosby.)

tape to entrap mites collected from the haircoat often simplifies viewing with the compound microscope.

Lynxacarus radovskyi (Feline Fur Mite)

Lynxacarus radovskyi, the feline fur mite, is found attached to the shafts of individual hairs on the back, neck, thorax, and hind limbs of cats residing in tropical or warm areas of the United States, such as Florida, Puerto Rico, and Hawaii. These fur mites are laterally compressed. The adults are approximately 500 μm long (Fig. 7-36). Pruritus is not always associated with infestations of *L. radovskyi* in cats. This mite also may affect human

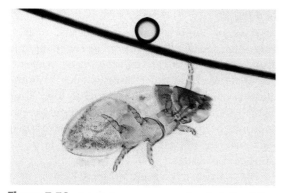

Figure 7-36. Adult *Lynxacarus radovskyi,* the feline fur mite, attaches to the hair shafts on the back, neck, thorax, and hind limbs of cats. (From Hendrix CM, Robinson E: *Diagnostic parasitology for veterinary technicians,* ed 3, St Louis, 2006, Mosby.)

beings who handle infested cats, producing a papular dermatitis.

Diagnosis. These mites are diagnosed by observation of the mites attached to individual hair shafts and by examination of the dander and other debris after combing.

Trombicula species (Chigger)

The chigger (*Trombicula* species) is yellow to red, has six legs, and is 200 to 400 μm in diameter. The larval stage is the only developmental stage that parasitizes human beings, domestic animals, and wild animals. The larvae are most common in the late summer and early fall and are transmitted by direct contact with the ground or with foliage in fields or heavy underbrush. Nymphal and adult chiggers are nonparasitic and are free living in nature.

Chigger larvae do not burrow into the skin as commonly believed, and they do not feed primarily on host blood. Their food consists of the serous components of tissues. Chiggers attach firmly to the host and inject a digestive fluid that liquefies host cells. The host's skin becomes hardened and a tube called a stylostome forms at the chigger's attachment site. Chiggers suck the liquefied host tissues. When the mite has finished feeding, it loosens its grip and falls to the ground. The injected digestive fluid causes the attachment site to itch intensely. Cutaneous lesions tend to be restricted to areas of the body that come in contact with the ground, such as the limbs, interdigital areas, and ventrum, in addition to the head and ears.

The most common chigger mite affecting animals and people is *Trombicula alfreddugesi* (the North American chigger). Lesions consist of an erythematous, often pruritic papular rash on the ventrum, face, feet, and legs.

Diagnosis. Chigger infestation (trombiculosis) is diagnosed by an orange, crusting dermatosis; a history of exposure (roaming the outdoors); and identification of the typical six-legged larvae in skin scrapings or on collection from the host. The larvae remain attached to the skin only for several hours. Consequently, trombiculosis may be difficult to diagnose because the pruritus persists after the larvae have dropped.

Pneumonyssoides (Pneumonyssus) caninum (Nasal Mite of Dogs)

Pneumonyssoides (Pneumonyssus) caninum is a rare mite that lives in the nasal passages and associated sinuses of dogs. Nasal mites are generally considered to be nonpathogenic; however, reddening of the nasal mucosa, sneezing, head shaking, and rubbing of the nose often accompany infestation. Fainting, labored breathing, asthmalike attacks, and orbital disease have been associated with this mite. Sinusitis caused by these mites may lead to disorders of the central nervous system. Owners may observe these mites exiting the animal's nostrils.

The life cycle is unknown, but it apparently takes place entirely on the host. Adult males, adult females, and larvae have been identified, but no nymphal stages have been observed. Transmission probably occurs by direct contact with an infested animal.

Diagnosis. The mites are oval and pale yellow. They measure 1 to 1.5 mm by 0.6 to 0.9 mm. They have a smooth cuticle, with few hairs. The larvae have six legs and the adults have eight legs. All legs are located on the cranial half of the body.

Ornithonyssus sylviarum (Northern Mite of Poultry) and *Dermanyssus gallinae* (Red Mite of Poultry)

These two mites parasitize poultry, but they differ in the sites they tend to infest. *Ornithonyssus sylviarum* is a 1-mm, elongated to oval mite usually found on birds but also in their nests or houses. They feed intermittently on the birds, producing irritation, weight loss, decreased egg production, anemia, and even death. These mites have been known to bite human beings.

Dermanyssus gallinae is a 1-mm, elongated to oval, whitish, grayish, or black mite that feeds on birds. This mite has a distinct red color when it has recently fed on its host's blood. *D. gallinae* lays its eggs in cracks and crevices in the walls of poultry houses. Nymphs and adults are periodic parasites, hiding in the crevices of the poultry houses and making frequent visits to the host to feed. Because of their blood-feeding activity, they may produce significant anemia and much irritation to the host.

Infested birds are listless and egg production may drop. Loss of blood may result in death. These mites also occur in birds' nests in the eaves of houses or in air conditioners. The mites can migrate into homes and infest human beings.

Diagnosis. *O. sylviarum* usually is found on the avian host, whereas *D. gallinae* is a periodic parasite, usually found in the host's environment. Specimens should be cleared in lactophenol and the anal plates examined with a compound microscope. The anus of *O. sylviarum* is on the cranial half of the anal plate, whereas the anus of *D. gallinae* is on the caudal half.

Ticks of Veterinary Importance

Ticks are small- to medium-sized acarines with dorsoventrally compressed, leathery bodies. The tick's head, the capitulum, serves as an organ of cutting and attachment. It is made of a penetrating, anchorlike sucking organ, the hypostome; and four accessory appendages, two cutting chelicerae and two pedipalps, which act as sensors and supports when the tick fastens to the host's body. The tick's body may be partially or entirely covered by a hard, chitinous plate, the scutum. Mouthparts may be concealed under the tick's body or may extend from the cranial border. Most ticks are inornate; that is, they are reddish or mahogany, without markings. Some species are ornate and have distinctive white patterns on the dark scutum background. Adult ticks have eight legs, with claws on the ends of the legs.

Ticks are important parasites because of their voracious blood-feeding activity. They are important also because they can transmit many parasitic, bacterial, viral, and other diseases, such as borreliosis (Lyme disease), among animals and from animals to human beings. These pathogenic organisms may be passively transmitted, or the tick may serve as an obligatory intermediate host for protozoan parasites.

The salivary secretions of some female ticks are toxic and can produce a syndrome known as "tick paralysis" in human beings and animals. Tick species commonly associated with tick paralysis are *Dermacentor andersoni* (the Rocky Mountain spotted fever tick), *Dermacentor occidentalis* (the Pacific Coast tick), *Ixodes holocyclus* (the Australian paralysis tick), and *Dermacentor variabilis* (the wood tick).

Ticks of veterinary importance are divided into two families: the Argasid, or soft ticks and the Ixodid, or hard ticks. Argasid ticks lack a scutum, or hard, chitinous plate. The mouthparts of the adults cannot be seen when viewed from the dorsal aspect. Ixodid ticks have a hard, chitinous scutum that covers all the male tick's dorsum and approximately one third or less of the female's dorsum. Depending on the degree of engorgement, male ticks are much smaller than female ticks.

Two species of Argasid ticks are important: *Otobius megnini* (the spinose ear tick) and *Argas persicus* (the fowl tick). Thirteen economically important tick species are in the Ixodid family. These include *Rhipicephalus sanguineus, Ixodes scapularis, Dermacentor* species, and *Amblyomma* species. Of these species, only *R. sanguineus* infests buildings; the remaining ticks attack their hosts outdoors.

Specific identification of ticks is difficult and should be performed by a veterinary parasitologist or a trained arthropodologist. Ticks usually are identified by the shape and length of the capitulum, the shape and color of the body, and the shape and markings on the scutum. Male and unengorged female ticks are easier to identify than engorged females. Determining the species of larval or nymphal ticks is difficult. Common species may be identified by their size, shape, color, body markings, host, and location on the host.

Four major stages exist in the life cycle of ticks: egg, larva, nymph, and adult. After engorgement on the host, female ticks drop off the host and seek protected places, such as within cracks and crevices or under leaves and branches to lay their eggs (Fig. 7-37). The six-legged larvae, or seed ticks, hatch from the eggs and feed on a host (Fig. 7-38). The larva molts to the eight-legged nymphal stage, which resembles the adult stage but lacks the functioning reproductive organs of the adult stage. After one or two blood meals, the nymph matures and molts to the adult stage. During the larval,

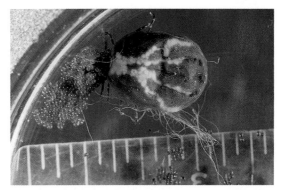

Figure 7-37. Adult female *Dermacentor variabilis* tick laying hundreds of eggs. (From Hendrix CM, Robinson E: *Diagnostic parasitology for veterinary technicians,* ed 3, St Louis, 2006, Mosby.)

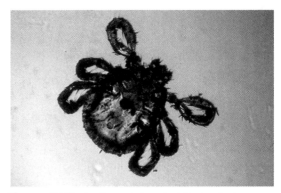

Figure 7-38. Six-legged larval *Rhipicephalus sanguineus.* (From Hendrix CM, Robinson E: *Diagnostic parasitology for veterinary technicians,* ed 3, St Louis, 2006, Mosby.)

nymphal, and adult stages, ticks may infest one to three or even many different host species. This ability to feed on several hosts during the life cycle plays an important role in the transmission of disease pathogens among hosts. Any infestation of domestic animals by mites or ticks is referred to as acariasis.

Most ticks do not tolerate direct sunlight, dryness, or excessive rainfall. They can survive as long as 2 to 3 years without a blood meal, but females require blood before egg fertilization and deposition. Tick activity is restricted during the cold winter months.

Argasid (Soft) Ticks
Otobius megnini (Spinose Ear Tick)

Otobius megnini, the spinose ear tick, is an unusual soft tick in that only the larval and nymphal stages are parasitic. The adult stages are not parasitic but are free living, found in the environment of the definitive host, usually in dry, protected places, in cracks and crevices, under logs, and on fence posts. The larval and nymphal stages feed on horses, cattle, sheep, goats, and dogs. These ticks usually are associated with the semiarid or arid areas of the southwestern United States. With widespread interstate movement of animals, this soft tick may occur throughout North America. As with most soft ticks, the mouthparts may not be visible when viewed from the dorsal aspect (Fig. 7-39). The nymphal stage is widest in the middle, almost violin shape. It is covered with tiny, backward-projecting spines, which is the origin of the name spinose. Larvae and nymphs usually are found within the ears of the definitive host.

Spinose ear ticks are extremely irritating to the definitive host. They often occur in large numbers, deep within the external ear canal. These ticks imbibe large amounts of host blood; however,

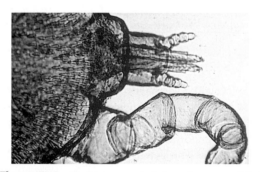

Figure 7-39. *Otobius megnini,* the spinose ear tick, is an unusual soft tick in that only the larval and nymphal stages are parasitic. The mouthparts may not be visible when viewed from the dorsal aspect. (From Hendrix CM, Robinson E: *Diagnostic parasitology for veterinary technicians,* ed 3, St Louis, 2006, Mosby.)

because they are soft ticks, they do not enlarge with feeding. Large numbers may produce ulceration deep within the ear. The ears become highly sensitive and the animals may shake their heads. The pinnae may become excoriated by the animal's shaking and rubbing its head.

Diagnosis. The ticks may be visualized in the ear with an otoscope. Any waxy exudate should be examined for larval and nymphal spinose ear ticks.

Argas persicus (Fowl Tick)

Argas persicus, the fowl tick, is a soft tick of chickens, turkeys, and wild birds. These ticks are periodic parasites, hiding in cracks and crevices during the day and becoming active during the night, when they feed intermittently on the avian host. The adults are 7 mm long and 5 mm wide. In the unengorged state, they are reddish brown. After engorgement, they are slate blue. These ticks are flat and leathery, and the tegument is covered with tiny bumps. As soft ticks, they lack a scutum. The mouthparts are not visible when the adult tick is viewed from the dorsal aspect.

Heavily infested birds may develop anemia. These ticks are worrisome to birds, particularly at night. Egg production by hens may decrease or cease.

Diagnosis. All stages of this tick may be collected from birds, but they usually are found in cracks, crevices, and contaminated bedding in poultry houses.

Ixodid (Hard) Ticks
Rhipicephalus sanguineus (Brown Dog Tick)

Rhipicephalus sanguineus, the brown dog tick, is an unusual hard tick; it may invade both kennel and household environments. This tick is distributed throughout North America. It has an inornate, uniformly reddish-brown scutum, and it feeds almost exclusively on dogs. *R. sanguineus* also has a distinguishing morphologic feature. Its basis capitulum has prominent lateral extensions that give this structure a decidedly hexagonal appearance (Fig. 7-40). The engorged female is often slate gray. In southern climates, the tick is found

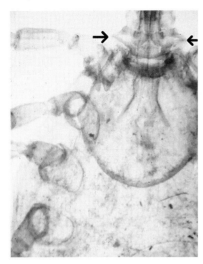

Figure 7-40. Lateral expansion of the basis capitulum (base of the head) *(arrows)* of an adult *Rhipicephalus sanguineus.* This key morphologic feature is used to identify this parasite, which can breed in the host's environment. (From Hendrix CM, Robinson E: *Diagnostic parasitology for veterinary technicians,* ed 3, St Louis, 2006, Mosby.)

outdoors but in northern climates it becomes a serious household pest, breeding indoors.

The bites of this tick can irritate dogs. Severe infestations may cause heavy blood loss. This tick is also an intermediate host for *Babesia canis,* the agent that causes piroplasmosis in dogs.

Diagnosis. This tick may be identified by its inornate brown color and characteristic lateral projections of the basis capitulum. These ticks are unique; they may be found in indoor or kennel environments.

Dermacentor variabilis (American Dog Tick, Wood Tick)

Dermacentor variabilis, the American dog tick or wood tick, is found primarily in the eastern two thirds of the United States; however, with increased mobility of American households, the tick may occur throughout the country. Unlike *R. sanguineus,* this tick inhabits only grassy, scrub brush areas, especially roadsides and pathways. This three-host tick initially feeds on small mammals and

rodents; however, dogs (and human beings) can serve as hosts for this ubiquitous tick. This tick is a seasonal annoyance to human beings and domestic animals. It can serve as a vector of Rocky Mountain spotted fever, tularemia, and other diseases and may also produce tick paralysis in animals and human beings. This tick has a dark-brown, ornate scutum with white striping. Unfed adults are approximately 6 mm long, whereas adult engorged females are about 12 mm long and blue-gray (Fig. 7-41).

Diagnosis. This tick may be identified by its morphologic features. It has a rectangular base of the capitulum and characteristic white markings on the dorsal shield.

Amblyomma americanum (Lone Star Tick)

Amblyomma americanum, the "lone star" tick, gets its common name from a characteristic white spot on the apex of its scutum. The spot is more conspicuous on male ticks than on female ticks. This tick is distributed throughout the southern United States but also is found in the Midwest and on the Atlantic coast.

This three-host tick is found most often in the spring and summer months, parasitizing the head, belly, and flanks of wild and domestic animal hosts. It also feeds on human beings and is said to have a

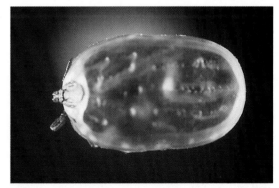

Figure 7-41. Adult female *Dermacentor variabilis.* Unfed adults are approximately 6 mm long, whereas engorged adult females are about 12 mm long and a blue-gray color. (From Hendrix CM, Robinson E: *Diagnostic parasitology for veterinary technicians,* ed 3, St Louis, 2006, Mosby.)

painful bite. It can produce anemia and has been incriminated as a vector of tularemia and Rocky Mountain spotted fever.

Diagnosis. *A. americanum* is easily identified by a characteristic white spot on the apex of the scutum.

Amblyomma maculatum (Gulf Coast Tick)

Amblyomma maculatum, the Gulf Coast tick, is a three-host tick found in the ears of cattle, horses, sheep, dogs, and human beings. It occurs in areas of high humidity on the Atlantic and Gulf coasts. It produces severe bites and painful swellings and is associated with tick paralysis. This tick has silvery markings on its scutum. Larval and nymphal stages occur on ground birds throughout the year. The number of adult ticks on cattle decreases during the winter and spring and increases in the summer and fall. When the ear canals of cattle and horses are infested, the pinna may droop and become deformed.

Diagnosis. *A. maculatum* is easily identified by the silvery markings on its scutum (Fig. 7-42).

Boophilus annulatus (Texas Cattle Fever Tick)

Boophilus annulatus is often called the Texas cattle fever tick or the North American tick. This one-host tick has historic significance in that it is the first arthropod shown to serve as an inter-mediate host for a protozoan parasite, *Babesia bigemina* of cattle, a milestone in veterinary parasitology. This tick has been completely eradicated from the United States; however, any *Boophilus* species infestation should be reported to the proper regulatory agencies. The tick should be identified by a specialist and control methods applied. *B. annulatus* frequently enters the United States from Mexico.

The engorged female is 10 to 12 mm long and the male 3 to 4 mm. The mouthparts are short and no festoons are on the caudal aspect of the abdomen.

Because this is a one-host tick, larvae, nymphs, and adult ticks may be found on the same animal. They do not have to leave the host to complete the life cycle. Animals with heavy infestations are restless and irritated. In an attempt to rid themselves of ticks, they rub, lick, bite, and scratch themselves. Irritated areas may become raw and secondarily infected. Heavily infested cattle may become anemic.

Diagnosis. Suspect ticks from an enzootic area or from animals originating from the Texas-Mexico border should be submitted to a laboratory recommended by regulatory agencies.

PHYLUM: NEMATODA (ROUNDWORMS)

Class: Secernentea

The next part of this chapter discusses the super-families belonging to the class Secernentea and how these skin-dwelling parasites are relevant to veterinary practice.

Superfamily: Rhabditoidea

Pelodera strongyloides (Free-Living Saprophytic Nematode)

Pelodera strongyloides is a free-living saprophytic nematode that normally lives in moist soil. These are facultative parasites. They are normally free living; however, under certain circumstances they can invade mammalian skin and develop to a parasitic existence. Male and female adult *P. strongyloides* nematodes are found in soil mixed

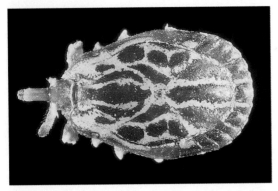

Figure 7-42. Ornate adult male *Amblyomma maculatum.* (From Hendrix CM, Robinson E: *Diagnostic parasitology for veterinary technicians,* ed 3, St Louis, 2006, Mosby.)

with moist organic debris, such as straw. The females produce eggs that hatch into first-stage larvae. These larvae invade the superficial layers of damaged or scarified skin, producing mild dermatitis. The skin may become reddened, denuded, and covered with a crusty material. Occasionally a pustular dermatitis develops. Because dogs become infested by lying on contaminated soil, these lesions usually are observed on the ventrum or medial (inner) surface of the limbs. Larvae of *P. strongyloides* also may be recovered from the skin of cattle recumbent on soil containing these larvae.

Diagnosis. These larvae (and possibly adults) can be identified in superficial skin scrapings. Larvae of *P. strongyloides* are 596 to 600 μm long. These larvae must be differentiated from the microfilariae of the canine heartworm, *D. immitis;* the microfilariae of *D. reconditum;* and the first-stage larvae of *Dracunculus insignis.*

Superfamily: Spiruroidea (Spirurid Nematodes)
Habronema and *Draschia* species

Adult *Habronema* nematodes are found on the stomach mucosa of horses under a thick layer of mucus. Adult *Draschia* species produce large, fibrous nodules in the equine stomach wall; the nematodes reside within the nodules. The adults do not parasitize the skin (see Chapter 6). However, the larval stages of these stomach parasites can be deposited by flies *(Musca domestica, Stomoxys calcitrans)* into skin wounds on horses. Here the larvae produce a condition known as "cutaneous habronemiasis," "cutaneous draschiasis," or "summer sores."

The lesions vary in size and have an uneven surface consisting of a soft, reddish-brown material covering a mass of firmer granulations. These lesions are seen on body parts most susceptible to trauma, such as the legs, withers, male genitalia, and medial canthus of the eye. Infested wounds tend to increase in size and do not respond to ordinary treatment until the following winter, when they spontaneously heal.

Diagnosis. Diagnosis of cutaneous habronemiasis is made on the basis of clinical signs and skin biopsies, which may reveal cross or longitudinal

sections of these aberrant *Habronema* or *Draschia* larvae.

Superfamily: Filarioidea (Filarial Nematodes)
Onchocerca cervicalis

Microfilariae of *Onchocerca cervicalis,* the filarial parasite of horses, produce recurrent dermatitis and periodic ophthalmia. The adults live in the ligamentum nuchae. Females produce microfilariae that migrate to the dermis by way of connective tissue. This parasite is spread by the biting midge *Culicoides* species. The midge feeds on a horse's blood and ingests the microfilariae, which develop to the infective third stage within the fly. When the fly bites another horse, larvae are injected into the connective tissue and develop to adults during migration to the ligamentum nuchae. The characteristic signs of cutaneous onchocerciasis include patchy alopecia; scaling on the head, neck, shoulders, and ventral midline; and sometimes, intense pruritus.

Many infected horses are asymptomatic. Microfilariae of *Onchocerca* species concentrate in certain areas, with the ventral midline the most common area of concentration. Because more than 90% of normal hosts are probably infected with *O. cervicalis,* detection of microfilariae in the skin of the ventral midline is not diagnostic for cutaneous onchocerciasis. However, the presence of microfilariae in diseased skin is highly indicative, though not diagnostic, of cutaneous onchocerciasis.

Diagnosis. *Onchocerca* microfilariae may be demonstrated by the following procedure. After clipping the skin site and performing a surgical scrub, a 6-mm punch biopsy is used to obtain a skin sample (see Chapter 9). With a single-edge razor blade or scalpel blade, half of the tissue is minced in a small amount of preservative-free physiologic saline on a glass slide and allowed to stand for 5 to 10 minutes. Drying of the specimen is prevented by placing the slide in a covered chamber with a small amount of saline. The slide is then examined with the low power (10×) objective. Because the translucent microfilariae are difficult to observe, low-intensity light and high contrast (achieved by lowering the condenser) are essential. Live microfilariae are identified by their vigorous swimming activity at the edge of the tissue. *O. cervicalis* microfilariae are slender and 207 to 240 μm long. The other half of the biopsy should be submitted for routine histopathologic examination.

Stephanofilaria stilesi

Stephanofilaria stilesi is a small filarial nematode found in the skin of ruminants such as cattle, goats, and buffalo and of wild mammals. It commonly causes dermatitis along the ventral midline of cattle in the United States. The infective larvae are transmitted by the bites of horn flies, *Haematobia irritans*. The skin lesions are thought to be caused by both adult and microfilarial stages.

The lesions caused by *S. stilesi* are located near the umbilicus and initially consist of small red papules. Later the lesions develop into large pruritic areas (up to 25 cm) of alopecia, with thick, moist crusts.

Diagnosis. The adults (less than 6 mm long) and microfilariae may be found in deep skin scrapings after the crusts have been removed from the lesions.

Dipetalonema (Acanthocheilonema) reconditum (Subcutaneous Filarial Parasite of Dogs)

Adult *Dipetalonema (Acanthocheilonema) reconditum* is a nonpathogenic parasite that resides in the subcutaneous tissues of the dog. It also may be found within a body cavity. Occasional subcutaneous abscesses and ulcerated areas have been associated with this parasite. The intermediate host for this parasite is the flea, *C. felis*. Because this parasite is found in enzootic areas where *D. immitis* is present, differentiation of the microfilariae of these two filarial parasites is necessary (see Chapter 6).

Diagnosis. Adults of *D. (Acanthocheilonema) reconditum* rarely are recovered from their subcutaneous sites. Microfilariae may be recovered rarely in deep skin scrapings that draw blood. When subjected to the modified Knott's procedure, the microfilariae of *D. reconditum* average approximately 285 μm long, with a button-hook tail and a blunt (broom handle–shaped) cranial end. They must be differentiated from microfilariae of *D.*

immitis, first-stage larvae of *Pelodera strongyloides*, and first-stage larvae of *Dracunculus insignis*.

Dirofilaria immitis (Canine Heartworm)

Dirofilaria immitis, the canine heartworm, normally resides in the right ventricle and pulmonary arteries of its definitive host, the dog. Adult heartworms also may occur aberrantly and may be found in a variety of extravascular sites, including cystic spaces in the subcutaneous sites (Fig. 7-43). When adult heartworms are found aberrantly, they are usually single, immature, isolated worms. Any female heartworms found within the cyst have not been fertilized by a male heartworm. Therefore such females are not gravid and do not produce microfilariae.

Adult female heartworms in the right ventricle and pulmonary arteries may produce microfilariae after mating with adult males. These microfilariae may be recovered occasionally in deep skin scrapings that draw blood.

Diagnosis. Aberrant adult *D. immitis* heartworms within cystic spaces in the skin can be surgically removed. When subjected to the modified Knott's procedure, the microfilariae of *D. immitis* are 310 to 320 μm long, with a straight tail and tapering cranial end. They must be differentiated from the microfilariae of *D. (Acanthocheilonema) reconditum*, first-stage larvae of *Pelodera strongy-*

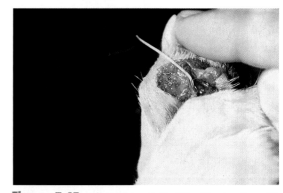

Figure 7-43. Aberrant adult *Dirofilaria immitis* heartworm in a subcutaneous interdigital cyst in a dog. (From Hendrix CM, Robinson E: *Diagnostic parasitology for veterinary technicians*, ed 3, St Louis, 2006, Mosby.)

loides, and first-stage larvae of *Dracunculus insignis.*

Superfamily: Dracunculoidea
Dracunculus insignis (Guinea Worm)

Dracunculus insignis, the Guinea worm, is a nematode found in the skin of dogs. The adult female nematode resides subcutaneously and produces a draining, ulcerous lesion in the skin, usually on the dog's limb. The cranial end of the female worm extends from this ulcer. When the female worm within the lesion comes in contact with water, its uterus prolapses through the worm's cranial end and ruptures, releasing a mass of first-stage larvae into the water. These larvae are 500 to 750 μm long and have a unique, long tail (Fig. 7-44). The larvae are ingested by tiny crustaceans in the water; within the crustaceans, the larvae develop to the infective third stage. Dogs become infected with *D. insignis* by drinking water containing the infected crustaceans.

Diagnosis. If *D. insignis* infection is suspected, the ulcer with its associated worm should be dipped in cool water. The cool water is a stimulus for the female worm to expel her larvae. The water containing expelled larvae should be centrifuged and the sediment examined for the characteristic first-stage larvae. Larvae of *D. insignis*

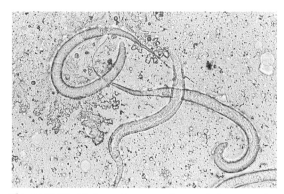

Figure 7-44. Unique first-stage larva of *Dracunculus insignis.* These larvae are 500 to 750 μm long and have a characteristic long tail. (From Hendrix CM, Robinson E: *Diagnostic parasitology for veterinary technicians,* ed 3, St Louis, 2006, Mosby.)

must be differentiated from the microfilariae of *D. immitis,* microfilariae of *D. reconditum,* and first-stage larvae of *P. strongyloides.* Once identified, the adult female worm may be surgically removed.

PHYLUM: ANNELIDA (SEGMENTED WORMS)

Class: Hirudinea (Leeches)

Order: Gnathobdellida
Hirudo medicinalis (Medicinal Leech)

Leeches are annelids; they are not considered true helminths but are often described as parasitic worms. As ectoparasites of human beings, domestic animals, and wild animals, leeches are members of the phylum Annelida and the class Hirudinea. Leeches may have a pathologic or beneficial role in veterinary medicine.

The term hirudiniasis is derived from the classic Linnaean nomenclature and is defined as invasion of the nose, mouth, pharynx, or larynx by leeches, or the attachment of leeches to the skin. Leeches are voracious blood feeders; depending on the number that attach to the host, the host may become anemic and die from blood loss. Leeches have recently gained favor as postsurgical tools in reconstructive and microvascular surgery. *H. medicinalis,* the medicinal leech, has been used in reconstructive and microvascular surgery in human beings; such use in veterinary medicine is forthcoming.

Diagnosis. Leeches are segmented worms with slender, leaf-shaped bodies devoid of bristles. A typical leech has two suckers, a large and adhesive caudal sucker and a smaller cranial one that surrounds the mouth. Most leeches are found in fresh water and a few in salt water; some are terrestrial varieties.

Recommended Reading

Bowman DD, Lynn RC, Eberhard ML: *Georgi's parasitology for veterinarians,* ed 8, Philadelphia, 2003, WB Saunders.
Hendrix CM, Robinson E: *Diagnostic parasitology for veterinary technicians,* ed 3, St Louis, 2006, Mosby.
Zajac AM, Conboy GA: *Veterinary clinical parasitology,* ed 7, Ames, IA, 2006, Blackwell Publishing.

CHAPTER 8

Immunology, Serology, and Molecular Diagnostics

Eloyes Hill

KEY POINTS

- Vertebrate species have two major internal defense systems: the innate, or nonspecific, immune system and the adaptive, or specific, immune system.
- Cytokines are chemical messengers produced by a variety of cells that interact with components of the immune system.
- Five classes of immunoglobulins are produced by B lymphocytes. Each class has a specific role in immunity.
- The complement system is a series of chemicals that interact with the cells of the immune system.
- Immune system disorders include hypersensitivity reactions and autoimmune disease.
- Serologic tests are designed to identify the presence or absence of an antigen or specific antibody.
- Most commercially available tests for measuring the immune response use enzyme-linked immunosorbent technology.
- Transfusion of foreign cells can result in antibody production and transfusion reaction.
- Typing or cross matching of donor and recipient blood is essential to minimize the possibility of transfusion reaction.
- Molecular diagnostic testing, such as the polymerase chain reaction, uses DNA or RNA analysis to identify pathogens, classify cancers, detect genetic defects, verify animal pedigrees, and determine bacterial contaminants in food science applications.

This chapter reviews basic principles of the immune system; some of its disorders; the practical applications of immunology, including vaccinations and serology tests; and molecular diagnostic tests.

THE IMMUNE RESPONSE

Vertebrate species have two major internal defense systems: the innate, or nonspecific, immune system and the adaptive, or specific, immune system (also called acquired immunity).

Innate Immune System

Foreign bodies, such as bacteria, viruses, and fungi, first encounter barriers of the innate immune system. These barriers include the skin; physical and biochemical components in the nasopharynx, gut, lungs, and genitourinary tract; and populations of commensal bacteria that compete with invading pathogens and the body's inflammatory response. The inflammatory response is a response to infection or tissue injury. Alerted by chemicals released from the infected site, blood vessels dilate and allow neutrophils to pass into tissue where they phagocytize infectious agents and kill the pathogens with chemicals stored in their cytoplasm. The classic signs of inflammation are pain, heat, redness, swelling, and loss of function. Each of these is related to physiologic mechanisms taking place in the inflammatory process. Inflammation is a protective mechanism of the innate immune system, but it can overreact and actually cause tissue damage itself.

Monocytes also follow neutrophils to inflammatory sites. Here, like neutrophils, they ingest and destroy inert particles, viruses, bacteria, and cellular debris by phagocytosis. In the blood they are called monocytes, but when they migrate to various tissues and organs they become macrophages and are given specialized names. They locate in connective tissue, liver, brain, lung, spleen, bone marrow, and lymph nodes and together make up the mononuclear phagocytic system.

In addition to the phagocytic cells, natural killer (NK) cells, interferons, and the complement system are important components of the innate immune system. NK cells are not T or B lymphocytes, but rather a small subset of lymphocytes found in the blood and peripheral lymphoid organs. NK cells recognize and destroy host cells that are infected with microbes, such as viruses. They also activate phagocytes by releasing interferon-γ. Interferons are cytokines (soluble proteins secreted by cells to mediate immune responses) that elicit other cellular reactions, such as prevention of viral replication, and influence the actions of NK cells. They are also active in the adaptive immune response.

The complement system consists of a group of proteins found in the blood. Collectively they are referred to as complement and are integral in both the innate and adaptive systems. When activated, a series of chemical reactions, known as the complement cascade, occurs. The system can be activated through one of three pathways, but the later steps are the same for all pathways. The components of the complement system are numbered C1 through C9, with some having several subunits designated by letters.

The classical pathway, a mechanism of the adaptive immune system, is activated when C1 is bound to an antigen-antibody complex. The other pathways of complement activation are part of the innate immune system and are triggered by microbial surfaces and plasma lectins that bind to microbes. All three initial pathways catalyze a series of reactions of other complement molecules that have numerous physiologic effects. These include opsonization of the microbes to promote phagocytosis, the stimulation of inflammation and cell lysis by the formation of a membrane attack complex on the surface of the antigen.

Adaptive Immune System

If foreign bodies evade the innate immune system, they then encounter the adaptive immune system, which is more sophisticated. The adaptive immune system is divided into two components: the humoral immune system and the cell-mediated immune system. The adaptive immune system has the ability to respond specifically to foreign substances. These substances, or antigens, may be bacterial, viral, fungal, or altered endogenous cells of the host's body. Their presence initiates humoral and cellular responses that neutralize, detoxify, and eliminate these foreign materials from the host.

Lymphocytes and their progeny are the cell types largely responsible for the adaptive immune system. This line of defense is not, however, divorced from the innate immune system. Macrophages process antigens and present them to antigen-committed lymphocytes. That is, they act as antigen-presenting cells.

Lymphoid stem cells develop first in the yolk sac and then in the fetal liver. The bone marrow assumes this responsibility near parturition and serves as the source of these cells throughout postnatal life. The lymphoid stem cells are destined to further mature in one of two places: the bone marrow or the thymus. B lymphocytes mature in the bone marrow, whereas T lymphocytes mature in the thymus (Fig. 8-1).

Humoral Immune System

Lymphocytes that mature in the bone marrow (B cells) are concerned chiefly with production and secretion of immunoglobulin (Ig) molecules, which are also known as antibodies. This is referred to as humoral immunity because the antibodies are secreted into the body's fluids or "humors". Their maturation process consists of three stages: the lymphoblast, the prolymphocyte, and the mature lymphocyte. The mature cells leave the bone marrow to seed secondary lymphoid organs, chiefly the spleen and lymph nodes, where they encounter antigens. The humoral immune system can recognize billions of different antigens because as B cells mature, each B cell develops a specific receptor molecule to a specific antigen. When an

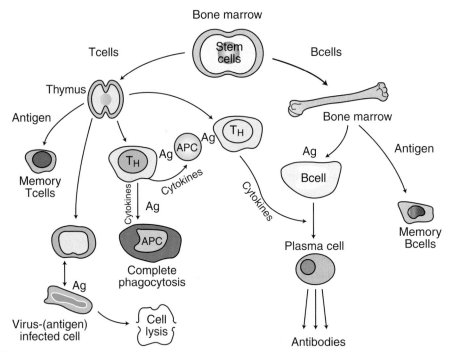

Figure 8-1. Pathways of lymphoid cells in the immune response. Stem cells in the bone marrow give rise to T and B lymphocytes. Lymphocytes mature in the thymus and bone marrow. Exposure to antigens causes lymphocytes to differentiate and proliferate into memory and effector cells. *Ag,* Antigen; *TH,* T-helper lymphocytes; *TC,* T-cytotoxic lymphocyte.

antigen enters the body, a mature B cell that is committed to that particular antigen will react with it. Stimulation of that B cell to produce antibodies is a complex process, requiring the help of specialized T lymphocytes called helper T cells. Helper T cells produce cytokines that activate the B cells. The antigen-stimulated B cell then quickly divides and differentiates, producing a clone of identical B cells that all produce the same type of antigen-specific antibody. These antibody-secreting B cells are now called plasma cells, a type of effector cell. An effector cell is a cell of the immune system that performs specific functions to destroy foreign antigen. Some of the antigen-stimulated B cells differentiate into memory B cells, which respond faster to a second exposure of that antigen (see Fig. 8-1).

Antibodies (immunoglobulins) are protein molecules consisting of two pairs of polypeptide chains configured in a Y shape (Fig. 8-2). Each immunoglobulin (Ig) molecule contains two variable regions and one constant region. The variable regions (Fab) bind to the antigen, and the constant region (Fc) is responsible for the unique functions of the different antibody classes.

Five distinct classes of immunoglobulins are produced: IgM, IgG, IgE, IgA, and IgD. The first antibody type produced in response to an antigen is IgM. IgM is a pentameric molecule (i.e., contains five monomers) and comprises approximately 5% of circulating immunoglobulin. IgM is relatively large and is therefore unable to enter tissue spaces. The most abundant circulating immunoglobulin is IgG. It comprises approximately 75% of circulating immunoglobulin and remains in circulation longest. IgG is a relatively small monomer that is capable of entering tissue spaces and is usually produced during a secondary immune response. IgE is usually present in very small amounts and is similar in structure to IgG. IgA comprises approximately 20% of circulating antibody, and IgD is a monomer that, when present, is in very low abundance.

The following are the functions of the different classes:

IgG: neutralization of microbes and toxins; opsonization of microbes for phagocytosis by

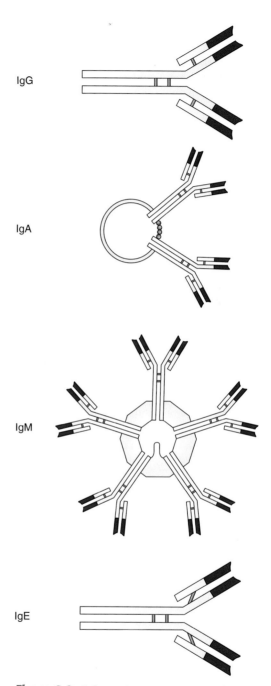

Figure 8-2. Schematic representation of IgM (pentamer), IgG and IgE (monomers), and IgA (dimer). (From Gershwin L, et al: *Immunology and immunopathology of domestic animals,* ed 2, St Louis, 1995, Mosby.)

macrophages and neutrophils; activation of complement; fetal and neonatal immunity by passive transfer across placenta and in colostrums

IgM: activation of complement

IgE: immediate hypersensitivity reactions, such as allergies and anaphylactic shock; coating of helminth parasites for destruction by eosinophils

IgA: mucosal immunity; protection of respiratory, intestinal, and urogenital tracts

IgD: B-lymphocyte surface antigen receptor in some species

Antibodies interact with antigens in different ways to prevent antigenic attachment or invasion of body cells. A neutralization antibody reaction occurs when antibody binds directly with the antigen. For example, if a foreign microbe or microbial toxin is bound by antibody, it cannot infect or damage body cells. This essentially neutralizes the potential effect of the antigen. Sometimes antibodies coat microbes. The Fab region of the antibody attaches to receptors on the microbial surface. The Fc region of the antibody then binds to macrophages or neutrophils and the microbe is phagocytized. If the antigenic material is a helminth parasite, IgE antibodies opsonize the worms; but instead of phagocytosis, which would be ineffectual against the large worms, eosinophils bind to and destroy the parasites. When complement is activated by some antibodies the end result is antigenic cell lysis.

Precipitation reactions occur when antigens bind with antibodies and form an insoluble complex. This precipitate forms on surfaces and the precipitant itself may cause pathology. For example, precipitation of bacterial fragments in the glomerular membrane can result in glomerular nephritis, described later as a type III hypersensitivity reaction.

Cell-Mediated Immune System

Lymphoid stem cells that mature in the thymus develop into T-cell lymphocytes. Like that of B cells, their maturation process consists of three morphologically distinct stages: lymphoblast, pro-lymphocyte, and lymphocyte. As these cells mature, they also develop receptors to specific antigens and become immunocompetent or antigen-committed T lymphocytes. Some references refer to T and B cells at this stage as naive lymphocytes. Then, after contact with their specific antigens, these cells proliferate and differentiate into either clones of memory cells or clones of effector cells against those antigens.

Memory cells recognize antigens to which they have previously been exposed. On a subsequent encounter, they elicit a more rapid immune response.

Different types of T-effector cells exist, such as helper T cells (CD4+) and cytolytic T cells (CD8+). CD4+ and CD8+ refer to surface molecules, or markers, found on helper T and cytolytic T lymphocytes, respectively. Cytolytic T lymphocytes are also called cytotoxic T lymphocytes. HIV (human immunodeficiency virus), the AIDS virus, has a special affinity for the helper T lymphocytes.

Helper T lymphocytes recognize antigen that has been phagocytized by an antigen-presenting cell (APC), such as a macrophage. The APC displays a portion of the antigen on its surface and presents it to the helper T lymphocyte. This stimulates the helper lymphocyte to release cytokines. These cytokines then in turn are the chemical signal that helps the APC to further phagocytize the ingested microbe. T helpers, when stimulated, also release cytokines that help B cells differentiate into antibody-producing cells.

Cytolytic T lymphocytes recognize antigen particles that are on the surface of infected body cells and are able to lyse and kill the infected cells. Microbe infected cells, tumor cells, and cells of foreign tissue graft all may be eliminated in this manner (see Fig. 8-1).

Immunologic Tolerance

One of the most important features of an animal's immune system is that it does not destroy its own cells. This may seem obvious, but it can actually happen. Maturing lymphocytes develop antigen receptors for foreign antigens but also for the animal's antigens on its own cells. Therefore these self-reactive lymphocytes could attack the self-antigens. However, in the healthy animal, mechanisms normally are in place that prevent this self-destruction. The immune system can discriminate between self and non-self, which results in immunologic tolerance.

Invading microbes typically are immunogenic; that is, they will interact with their specific naive lymphocytes, which then proliferate and differentiate into effector cells that destroy the foreign microbes. However, to tolerate self-antigens, the animal relies on mechanisms such as antigenic tolerance and ignorance. Self-antigens are normally tolerogenic; the lymphocytes are either unable to respond when they encounter self-antigens (anergy) or they die when they encounter self-antigens (apoptosis). Self-antigens may also be ignored by the naive lymphocytes, in which case the self-antigens are called nonimmunogenic.

These mechanisms are elaborate. When naive lymphocytes are destroyed by apoptosis, the immune system is in effect selecting for the beneficial lymphocytes that have receptors for foreign antigens and eliminating the self-lymphocytes that would cause self-destruction. This is called negative selection and takes place in the bone marrow, thymus, and peripheral lymphoid tissues.

Another mechanism of immunologic tolerance is through the activity of regulatory lymphocytes. Some T lymphocytes, formerly called "suppressor T cells," become regulatory lymphocytes. Regulatory T cells prevent self-reactive lymphocytes from differentiating into effector cells. They are unable to destroy self-antigens.

This is an oversimplification of the intricacies involved in how immunologic tolerance is maintained. When these mechanisms fail, autoimmune disease results and the animal's immune system is directed against itself.

DISORDERS OF THE IMMUNE SYSTEM

Some immune responses have an adverse effect on the host animal. The immune responses are uncontrolled, or hypersensitive, and cause tissue injury. Four types of hypersensitivity diseases have been categorized. Type I hypersensitivity is an immediate hypersensitivity that occurs when chemical mediators from mast cells are released. Allergies (atopy) and anaphylactic shock, a severe reaction that may occur within seconds after an antigen enters the circulation, are type I hypersensitivity diseases.

Autoimmune hemolytic anemia, a condition causing destruction of red blood cells (RBCs) by the host itself, is a type II hypersensitivity. These are antibody-mediated diseases in which the antibodies are directed against the animal's own cells.

Immune complex disease, or type III hypersensitivity, occurs when antibodies and antigens form complexes that deposit in various blood vessels. Glomerulonephritis, caused by deposition of antibody-antigen complexes in the kidney, is an example of type III hypersensitivity.

Type IV hypersensitivity is T cell–mediated disease caused by the reaction of T lymphocytes against self-antigens in tissues. Contact hypersensitivity reactions, such as those that may occur in dogs from contact with plastic in food dishes and collars or in human beings from contact with poison ivy, cause tissue injury in a delayed response. The chemicals from these substances react with skin proteins, and the immune system recognizes this chemical-protein complex as foreign, resulting in dermatitis.

In addition to hypersensitivity reactions, the immune system also may show deficiencies. A deficiency may exist in phagocytes or in immunoglobulins. A condition called combined immunodeficiency affects animals in early life, after serum levels of maternally derived antibodies have declined. Arabian foals with this disease often die from opportunistic infection resulting from an absence or deficiency of immunoglobulins.

Lymphoma, a type of tumor characterized by uncontrolled proliferation of lymphocytes, is another abnormality of the immune system. The immune system normally recognizes and destroys cancer cells before they become established in the body, but sometimes the cancer seems to become resistant and escapes the immune defense mechanisms.

Passive Immunity

Animals become passively resistant to disease by receiving maternal antibodies in the colostrum or by receiving preformed antibodies by injection. These antibodies have been produced in a donor animal. A donor animal is vaccinated with a pathogen. When its serum antibodies reach a high concentration, the animal is bled and the globulin portion containing the antibodies is separated and purified. The protection that an animal receives from an injection of this immunoglobulin is short-lived but immediate.

Immunization

Animals become actively resistant to disease by having the disease and developing antibodies, or by being vaccinated or immunized, in which case they also develop their own antibodies. Immunization is accomplished by injecting a suspension of microorganisms into an animal for the purpose of eliciting an antibody response but not causing the disease. The microorganisms may be either attenuated (weakened but still alive) or inactivated (killed). Attenuated vaccines normally cause a longer-lasting, more potent immune response. Inactivated vaccines are generally safer and have less ability to cause disease, although vaccine-associated sarcomas in cats have been an issue. An adjuvant may be added to the vaccine to enhance the normal immune response. Some adjuvants do this by simply slowing the rate of antigen elimination from the body so that the antigen is present longer to stimulate antibody production. Killed vaccines require more adjuvant; the increased adjuvant is thought to cause the sarcomas.

Effective DNA vaccines are now being developed by using molecular genetics. They are expected to be safer than traditional vaccines and can be made more quickly. Once the technology is in place, more DNA vaccines should be developed quickly.

Vaccines may be given subcutaneously or intramuscularly depending on the vaccine. Other vaccines are aerosolized and given intranasally. Some vaccines are put in the feed or drinking water. Veterinary technicians working at fish hatcheries may vaccinate fish by putting the vaccine in their water.

TESTS OF HUMORAL IMMUNITY

The science of detection and measurement of antibodies or antigens is called serology. Detection depends on the binding of antibodies and antigens. Unfortunately, this binding phenomenon is ordinarily invisible. Visualization, and thus detection, of the antigen-antibody reaction depends on secondary events by which the union is easily detected and therefore of diagnostic use in the veterinary practice.

Commercial production of monoclonal antibodies to many different antigens has resulted in a variety of test kits for use in the veterinary laboratory. These specific antibodies to many different antigens can be produced and used in the laboratory for rapid identification of disease-producing organisms.

Immunization with viruses, bacteria, or other entities stimulates antibody production in an animal. The antibody-secreting, transformed lymphocytes (plasma cells) may be isolated from the animal and chemically fused with a type of "immortal" cell that propagates indefinitely, such as mouse myeloma cells. The antibodies these hybrid cells produce, called monoclonal antibodies, are collected. Because each monoclonal antibody attaches to only one specific part of one type of molecule (antigen), use of these antibodies in diagnostic kits makes the tests specific and greatly reduces interpretation problems of the result. For example, the feline leukemia virus antigen reacts with only the feline leukemia virus antibody. A specific reaction is diagnostically significant for this complicated disease. In addition to their specificity, these procedures allow rapid identification of the pathogen.

Many serologic tests use monoclonal antibodies. Enzyme immunoassay, latex agglutination, immunodiffusion, and rapid immunomigration are methods used in veterinary laboratories. Other methods, such as complement fixation, immunofluorescence, immunoelectron microscopy, virus neutralization, and polymerase chain reaction (PCR) DNA amplification are used in veterinary reference laboratories and research facilities and are not included in this discussion, except for a brief explanation of PCR. Many of the principles are the same, however, and understanding a few procedures gives readers a good basis for understanding others.

Reference laboratories offer myriad serologic tests specifically developed for veterinary samples. Tests for blood types, allergies, bovine leukemia virus, reproductive hormones, Lyme disease, and brucellosis are a few of the diagnostic tests available (Table 8-1).

Enzyme-Linked Immunosorbent Assay

The enzyme-linked immunosorbent assay (ELISA) has been adapted to many agents commonly tested for in the veterinary laboratory (Figs. 8-3 to 8-7). With monoclonal antibodies, the specificity of ELISA is high; that is, little cross-reactivity occurs with other agents. This phenomenon makes ELISA an accurate way to detect specific antigens such as viruses, bacteria, parasites, or hormones in serum. ELISA also may be used to test for an antibody in the serum, in which case the test kit contains the specific antigen. Some of the available ELISA kits detect heartworms, feline leukemia virus, feline immunodeficiency virus, canine parvovirus, and progesterone. For the ELISA antigen detection system, monoclonal antibody is bound to the walls of wells in a test tray, to a membrane, or to a plastic wand (Boxes 8-1 to 8-3). Antigen, if present in the sample, binds to this antibody and to a second enzyme-labeled antibody that is added to aid in detection of the antigen. This is followed by rinsing. When a chromogenic (color-producing) substrate is added to the mixture, it reacts with the enzyme to develop a specific color, indicating the presence of antigen in the sample. If the sample contained no antigen, the entire enzyme-labeled antibody was washed away in the rinsing process and no color reaction develops.

A similar procedure is used for ELISA antibody detection. In this procedure, antigen is bound to the wells, membrane, or wand, and the patient sample is assayed for the presence of a specific antibody.

Competitive Enzyme-Linked Immunosorbent Assay

The competitive ELISA (CELISA), when used to test for patient antigen, uses an enzyme-labeled antigen, as well as monoclonal antibodies. Patient antigen, if present, competes with enzyme-labeled antigens for the antibodies coating the test wells. Color developer reacts with the enzyme to produce a color. The intensity of the color produced varies with the concentration of the patient antigen (Box 8-4). Equine infectious anemia antibodies may be detected in horse serum with a CELISA test.

Latex Agglutination

The latex agglutination test uses small, spherical latex particles coated with antigen suspended in water. If serum containing the corresponding antibody is added to the mixture, formation of antibody-antigen complexes causes agglutination (clumping). Agglutination changes the appearance of the latex suspension from smooth and milky to clumpy because the latex particles have clustered together. If no antibody is present in the sample, the mixture of latex and serum remains evenly dispersed. Bovine serum may be tested for brucellosis antibodies with this method (Fig. 8-8 and Box 8-5; also see Table 8-1).

Rapid Immunomigration

Rapid immunomigration (RIM) is a technology that historically has been called immunochromatography or lateral flow immunoassay. The signal-generating component of this test is colloidal gold. Its counterparts in other technologies are enzymes and color reagent or agglutinated latex particles. All three types of components create a positive result.

In this type of procedure colloidal gold is conjugated to antibodies specific for the antigen

TABLE 8-1

Commercially Available Immunologic Test Kits

Disease/Condition	Product Name	Manufacturer	Type of Test	Use
Allergies	Allercept	Heska	ELISA	Determination of allergen-specific IgE antibodies in dogs and cats
Bile acids test	SNAP Reader	IDEXX	ELISA	Measurement of serum bile acids
Blood group test	RapidVet-H	DMS Laboratories	Monoclonal antibody agglutination test	To classify dogs as DEA 1.1 or cats types A, B, or AB
Borreliosis, heartworm, and *Ehrlichia canis*	SNAP 3 Dx Test	IDEXX	ELISA	Detection of *Borrelia burgdorferi* antibodies, heartworm antigens, and *Ehrlichia* antibodies in dogs
Bovine leukemia virus (BLV) infection	Herdchek: Anti-BLV	IDEXX	Enzyme immunoassay antibody test kit	Detection of antibodies to bovine leukemia virus in cattle
Brucellosis	Herdchek: Anti-*B. abortus* test	IDEXX	ELISA	Detection of antibodies to *Brucella abortus* in cattle
Equine infectious anemia	Lab-EZ/EIA	Synbiotics	Agar gel immunodiffusion	Detection of infectious anemia antibodies in horses
Equine infectious anemia	Diasystems EIA	IDEXX	CELISA antibody test kit	Detection of infectious anemia antibodies in horses
Failure of passive transfer	SNAP Foal IgG Test Kit	IDEXX	ELISA	Semiquantitative measurement of IgG levels in equine serum or whole blood
Feline infectious peritonitis	Virachek/CV	Synbiotics	ELISA	Detection of antibodies to feline infectious peritonitis virus in cats
Feline leukemia virus	Assure/FeLV	Synbiotics	ELISA	Detection of feline leukemia virus antigens in cats
	SNAP FeLV antigen test kit	IDEXX	ELISA	Detection of feline leukemia virus antigens in cats
	Virachek/FeLV	Synbiotics	ELISA	Detection of feline leukemia virus antigens in cats
	WITNESS FeLV	Synbiotics	RIM	Detection of feline leukemia virus antigens in cats
Feline leukemia virus and Immunodeficiency virus	SNAP Combo	IDEXX	ELISA	Detection of feline leukemia virus antigens and FIV antibodies in cats

TABLE 8-1

Commercially Available Immunologic Test Kits—cont'd

Disease/Condition	Product Name	Manufacturer	Type of Test	Use
Heartworm infection	Petchek	IDEXX	ELISA	Detection of heartworm antigens in dogs
	Dirochek	Synbiotics	ELISA	Detection of heartworm antigens in dogs and cats
	Heska Solo Step FH & CH	Heska	Lateral flow immunoassay	Detection of heartworm antibodies in cats and antigens in dogs
	SNAP Heartworm Ag Test	IDEXX	ELISA	Detection of heartworm antigens in dogs
	Witness HW	Synbiotics	ELISA	Detection of heartworm antigens in dogs
Paratuberculosis (Johne's disease)	Herdchek Mycobacterium	IDEXX	ELISA	Detection of antibody to *M. paratuberculosis* in bovine serum or plasma
	rjt(™)	ImmuCell	Agarose gel immunodiffusion	Detection of antibodies to *M. paratuberculosis* in bovine serum
Mycoplasma species	Mycoplasma Plate Antigens	Intervet	Plate agglutination test	Detection of *Mycoplasma* antibodies in poultry; screening method
Neospora caninum	Herdchek Neospora	IDEXX	ELISA	Detection of antibodies to *Neospora caninum* in bovine serum
Newcastle disease	Flockchek: Newcastle disease virus antibody test	IDEXX	ELISA	Detection of antibodies to Newcastle disease virus in chicken serum
Ovulation timing	ICG Status-LH	Synbiotics	Immunochromatographic assay	Semiquantitative measurement of luteinizing hormone levels in dogs and cats
Parvovirus infection	SNAP canine parvovirus antigen test kit	IDEXX	ELISA	Detection of parvovirus antigens in canine feces
Pregnancy, canine	Relaxin	Synbiotics	RIM	Detection of pregnancy by measurement of relaxin
Progesterone	Ovuchek Premate	Synbiotics	ELISA	The determination of progesterone in canine serum
Pseudorabies	Herdchek pseudorabies virus antibody test kit	IDEXX	ELISA	Detection of pseudorabies virus antibodies in pig serum

Continued

TABLE 8-1

Commercially Available Immunologic Test Kits—cont'd

Disease/Condition	Product Name	Manufacturer	Type of Test	Use
Rheumatoid arthritis	Synbiotics CRF (canine rheumatoid factor)	Synbiotics	Latex agglutination	Detection of rheumatoid arthritis factor in canine serum
Salmonellosis	Flockchek SE test kit	IDEXX	ELISA	Detection of antibodies to *Salmonella enteritidis* in chicken serum or egg yolk
Tuberculosis	Tuberculin PPD	Synbiotics	Intradermal test	Intradermal testing of cattle for bovine tuberculosis
Von Willebrand factor	vWF ZYMTEC	DMS Laboratories	ELISA	Determination of von Willebrand factor in multiple species

DMS Laboratories, Inc., 2 Darts Mill Road, Flemington, NJ 08822.
Synbiotics Corporation, 11011 Via Frontera, San Diego, CA 92127.
IDEXX Laboratories, One Idexx Drive, Westbrook, ME 04092.
Heska Corporation, 3760 Rocky Mountain Ave., Loveland, CO 80538.
ImmuCell Corporation, 56 Evergreen Drive, Portland, ME 04103.
Intervet Inc., 405 State Street, P.O. Box 318, Millsboro, DE 19966.

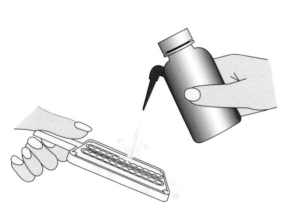

Figure 8-3. A critical step in the Microwell enzyme immunoassay is washing away the unbound enzyme-labeled antibodies. (Pet Check Heartworm PF Antigen Test Kit, courtesy IDEXX Laboratories, Westbrook, ME.)

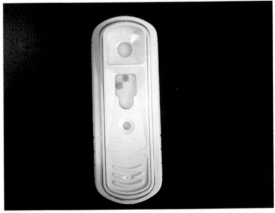

Figure 8-4. A positive test result indicated on the ELISA membrane format (SNAP Test for *Ehrlichia* antibodies, IDEXX). A positive control spot is also seen. (Courtesy IDEXX Laboratories, Westbrook, ME.)

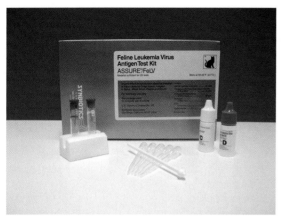

Figure 8-5. Kit to detect feline leukemia antigens in cat serum (Assure/FeLV, Synbiotics) based on the ELISA wand format. (Courtesy Synbiotics Corporation, San Diego, CA.)

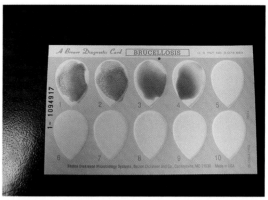

Figure 8-7. Clumped latex particles representing antigen-antibody complexes. Samples 1 and 2 indicate a positive reaction. Samples 3 and 4, showing no clumping, indicate a negative reaction.

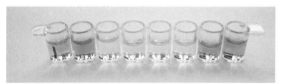

Figure 8-6. With the ELISA wells format for the determination of progesterone in canine serum (Ovuchek Premate, Synbiotics), a positive reaction is indicated by color development. (Courtesy Synbiotics Corporation, San Diego, CA.)

being tested. These conjugated antibodies are present in the membrane of the test cassette where the patient sample is applied. If antigens are present in the patient sample, they bind to the conjugated antibodies and the antibody-antigen complexes migrate along the membrane to another area of the cassette, where the results are read. Buffer may be added to aid the migrational flow of the antibody-antigen complexes. In the reading area a second antibody is present in the membrane. If antigen is in the sample it is captured, along with the first antibody and the colloidal gold, by the second antibody. The accumulation of colloidal gold in that area causes a color change. To ensure quality results, control antigen is present in another area of

BOX 8-1
Microwell ELISA Methodology

- Plastic wells are supplied precoated with antibodies specific for the antigen being tested (primary antibody).
- Patient serum samples (which may contain antigen) are added to the wells.
- If the suspected antigen is present, it binds to the antibodies on the wells.
- A second antibody, labeled with an enzyme, is added to the wells.
- If antigen was present, the second antibody binds to the antigens that are themselves bound to the primary antibody on the well surface.
- The wells are washed to remove any unbound secondary antibodies.
- A chromogenic substrate is added that reacts with the enzyme on the secondary antibody causing a color to develop.
- Development of a color indicates the presence of the antigen in the sample.
- If no antigen was present, no color change will occur since the secondary antibody would have been washed away and no binding of the chromogenic substrate could occur.

BOX 8-2
Membrane ELISA Methodology

- The test system incorporates a membrane that is precoated with antibodies specific for the antigen being tested (primary antibody).
- The patient serum sample (which may contain antigen) is added to the test system.
- If the suspected antigen is present, it binds to the antibodies on the membrane.
- Typically, positive-control spots containing the antigen also have been precoated on the membrane.
- A second enzyme-labeled antibody is added to the membrane. If the patient sample contained the specific antigen, this antibody binds to the captured patient antigen and the control antigen. The antigen is now "sandwiched" between two antibodies.
- Unbound enzyme-labeled antibodies are washed away.
- A chromogen is added to the membrane, which reacts with the enzyme on the second antibody to produce a color.
- Color appears where the positive control and patient antigens are present on the membrane.

BOX 8-3
Wand ELISA Methodology

- The bulbous ends of plastic wands are supplied precoated with antibodies specific for the antigen being tested (primary antibody).
- The wand is placed in a tube along with the patient sample.
- If the suspected antigen is present in the patient sample, it binds to the antibodies on the wand.
- A second antibody, labeled with an enzyme, is added to the wells.
- If antigen was present, the second antibody binds to the antigens that are themselves bound to the primary antibody surface of the wand.
- Unbound enzyme-labeled antibody is washed away and a chromogenic reagent is added.
- The reagent reacts with the enzyme-labeled antibodies that are bound to the antigens, producing a color reaction.

BOX 8-4
CELISA Methodology

- Test wells are supplied precoated with monoclonal antibodies.
- Patient samples (that may contain antigen) are added to test wells.
- Enzyme-labeled antigens are then added to the same test wells.
- The two antigens compete for antibodies on the test wells. The antigen in higher concentration binds more antibodies on the wells.
- After incubation, the wells are rinsed to wash away excess enzyme-labeled antigens.
- Color developer is added, which reacts with the enzyme on the enzyme-labeled antigen.
- If the sample contains low levels of patient antigen, most of the antigen bound to the antibodies on the test wells is enzyme-labeled antigen and a deep color develops.
- If the sample contains high levels of patient antigen, most of the antigen bound to the antibodies on the test wells is antigen from the patient and little color develops.

BOX 8-5
Latex Agglutination Methodology

- A dark glass slide or coated card is used to make the reactions more visible.
- Positive and negative reference sera (positive contains antibodies being tested) and patient sera (with possible antibodies) are placed in separate areas on the slide.
- A suspension of latex particles that have been coated with antigens is added
- If the patient sample contained the specific antibody, visible agglutination will be evident.

the membrane strip. The conjugated first antibody binds to the antigen in the control area. Its accumulation also causes a color change and occurs whether or not antigen is present in the patient sample. A positive patient result shows two areas of color change, one for the patient and one for the quality control antigen. If the control antigen area does not change color, the test is considered invalid regardless of color change in the patient area. Feline leukemia test kits (e.g., WITNESS FeLV, Merial UK, Essex, England; Synbiotics, Lyons, France) that use rapid immunomigration are available (Fig. 8-8 and Box 8-6; also see Table 8-1).

Immunodiffusion

In immunodiffusion, patient serum samples (possibly containing antibodies) and the antigen to this antibody (supplied in the test kit) are placed in separate wells in an agar gel plate. Both components diffuse into the agar and form a visible band of precipitation when they combine. If no band forms, no antibody exists in the patient's serum sample or the patient's antibody levels are insufficient to cause precipitation in the gel. Diseases that may be detected by immunodiffusion are equine infectious anemia and Johne's disease (Fig. 8-9 and Box 8-7; also see Table 8-1).

Radioimmunoassay

A competitive form of radioimmunoassay has primarily been used in research and diagnostic laboratories for many years. The test principle is similar to the CELISA technique except that a radioisotope is used in place of the enzyme. The

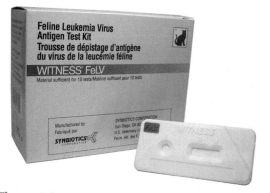

Figure 8-8. WITNESS FeLV uses rapid immunomigration, a reliable one-way flow of sample and reagent, giving accurate answers in minutes. (Courtesy Synbiotics Corporation, San Diego, Calif.)

BOX 8-6
RIM Methodology

- The test system incorporates a membrane that contains colloidal gold conjugated with antibodies to the test antigen.
- Patient sample is applied to the membrane.
- If antigen is present in the patient sample, it binds to the conjugated antibodies and flows along the membrane to a reading area.
- The reading area of the membrane contains capture antibodies to the test antigen.
- If the patient sample contains antigen, it will be captured along with the bound conjugated antibody, by the second antibody in the reading area.
- The accumulation of colloidal gold (now complexed with the first antibody, the antigen and the capture antibody) causes a color change.

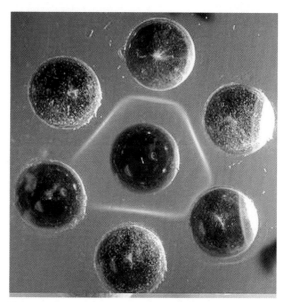

Figure 8-9. Agar plate showing lines of precipitation. No lines of precipitation are evident near negative patient wells. (LAB-EZ/EIA immunodiffusion, courtesy Synbiotics Corporation, San Diego, CA.)

assay typically consists of an antigen labeled with a radioisotope and an antibody. When combined with patient serum that contains the same antigen, both antigens compete for the antibody. With

BOX 8-7
Immunodiffusion Methodology

- An agar plate is prepared with one central well and multiple surrounding wells.
- Antigens from the test kit are placed in the center well.
- Patient serum samples (with possible antibodies) and positive controls (with antibodies) are placed in alternating surrounding wells.
- Antigen from the center well and antibodies from the surrounding wells diffuse through the agar toward each other.
- A line of visible precipitation forms where the diffusing antigens and antibodies meet.
- A line of precipitate in front of a patient well indicates antibodies present in the patient serum.

increasing amounts of patient antigen, more labeled antigen is displaced from the antibody. The remaining amount of radioactivity is measured and compared with a standard curve to determine the concentration of antigen in the patient's serum.

Fluorescent Antibody Testing

Although not commonly performed in veterinary practices, fluorescent testing is available at most veterinary reference laboratories. These test procedures are frequently used to verify a tentative diagnosis made by the veterinarian. Two methods are available—direct and indirect antibody testing—both of which detect the presence of specific antibody in a sample (see Fig. 8-10). In the direct procedure, patient sample is added to a test slide

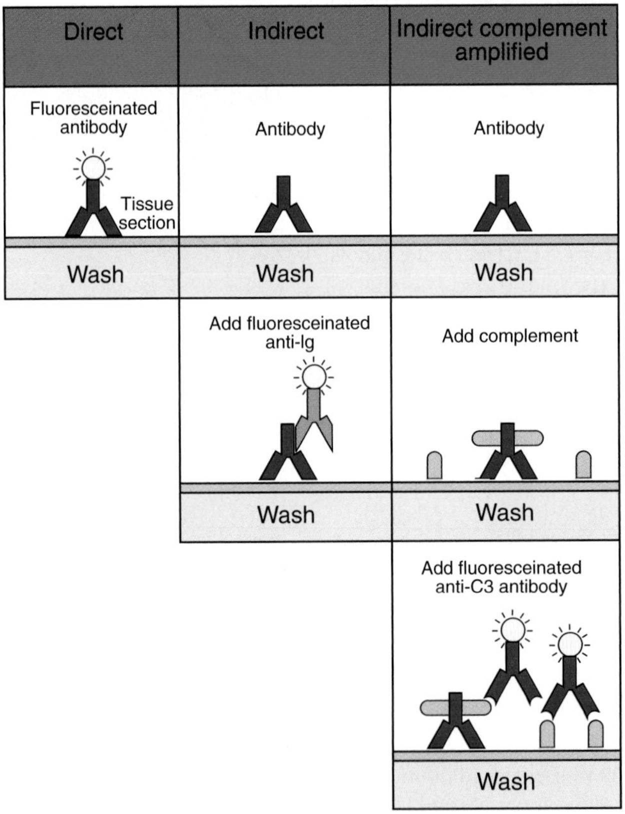

Figure 8-10. Flourescent antibody technique. (Redrawn from Roitt I, Brostoff J, Male D: *Immunology,* ed. 3, London, 1993, Mosby–Year Book Europe.)

that has been precoated with a fluorescent dye-conjugated antigen. The dye combines with a specific antibody if present in the patient sample. The slide is then examined with a special microscope designed for fluorescent microscopy. For cellular antigens, the cell will appear outlined with fluorescent material.

With an indirect fluorescent antibody (IFA) technique, the patient sample is incubated on a slide that contains the specific test antigen. The slide is then washed to remove any unbound antibody. Fluorescent-labeled antiantibody is added to the system. The slide is then microscopically examined. Any fluorescence indicates a positive test result. Fluorescent techniques exist for antigen detection as well.

Coombs Testing

The presence of inappropriate antibodies (i.e., antibodies against the body's own tissues) are detected with the Coombs test (see Fig. 8-11). The direct Coombs reaction is used to detect antibody that has attacked the body's own erythrocytes.

A positive direct Coombs test provides evidence of immune-mediated hemolytic disease. The

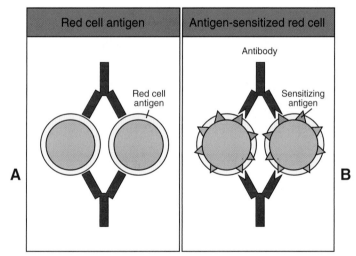

Fig. 8-11. Principles of the Coombs reaction. **(A)** direct Coombs test; **(B)** indirect Coombs test. (Redrawn from Roitt I, Brostoff J, Male D: *Immunology,* ed. 3, London, 1993, Mosby–Year Book Europe.)

procedure involves incubating the suspect sample with antisera, which reacts with the species' immunoglobulins. If the erythrocytes in the sample are coated with immunoglobulin (self-antibody), the antisera and immunoglobulin on the erythrocytes will react and result in visible agglutination of the erythrocytes.

Indirect Coombs testing detects circulating antibody. A positive indirect Coombs test result indicates the presence of circulating antibodies against the body's own tissues. To visualize the reaction, patient serum is incubated with erythrocytes from a normal animal of the same species. If antibody is present in the patient serum, it will bind to these erythrocytes just like it would to its own. Subsequent addition of an anti–gamma globulin for the species being tested results in hemagglutination.

Intradermal Tests

Skin tests are used to diagnose various allergies to allergens in the environment. Allergies are mediated by IgE antibody molecules and can be detected by using allergenic extracts of grasses, trees, weed pollens, molds, dust, insects, and other possibly offending antigens. The extracts are injected intradermally, and the injection sites are monitored for allergic reactions. A positive reaction appears as a raised welt, meaning that the animal is allergic to that antigen.

Antibody Titers

Although not routinely performed in the veterinary practice laboratory, antibody titer tests may be needed by the clinician to distinguish between active infection and prior exposure to certain antigens. This is particularly important when no reliable antigen test is available. Titer refers to the greatest dilution at which a patient sample no longer yields a positive result for the presence of a specific antibody.

The test requires making serial dilutions of a sample. Each dilution is then examined for the presence of the antibody. The reciprocal of the greatest dilution that still elicits a positive test result is the titer. A high titer often indicates active infection. Low titers usually indicate previous exposure to the specific antigen.

BLOOD GROUPS AND IMMUNITY

Red cell antigens are structures on the surface of RBCs from one animal that may react with antibodies in the plasma of another animal. The specific surface markers present in an individual animal are genetically determined and are referred to as blood group antigens. The number of blood groups varies among species. Antigen-antibody reactions can occur with blood transfusions as a result of variation in blood group antigens between the recipient and donor. This usually results in clumping or agglutination of RBCs. However, in some species the antigen-antibody reaction is more likely to result in RBC lysis.

Although erythrocytes of common domestic animals possess antigens, naturally occurring antibodies (alloantibodies) present in human beings are less common in animals. However, they do occur in cats, cattle, sheep, and pigs. Once a transfusion has been given to an animal, antibodies against the RBC antigen (immune antibodies) are formed. Breeding females, especially mares, should always be given properly matched blood to avoid sensitization that results in destruction of the foal's RBCs.

Blood Types

Dogs

More than a dozen different canine blood groups have been identified. Nomenclature for the blood group systems is designated by the letters DEA (for dog erythrocyte antigen) followed by a number. For DEA systems other than DEA 1, the erythrocytes are designated as positive or negative for that specific antigen. The DEA 1 group has three subgroups designated as DEA 1.1 (A1), DEA 1.2 (A2), and DEA 1.2 (A3). Canine erythrocytes may be positive or negative for each of the DEA 1 subgroups. DEA-3 (B), DEA-4 (C), DEA-5 (D), and DEA-7 (Tr) also designate major blood groups. The only groups considered to be clinically significant are DEA-1.1 and DEA-7. The DEA1.1 subgroup elicits the greatest antigen response and causes the most serious transfusion reactions. Approximately 50% of all dogs are positive for the DEA 1.1 antigen. Transfusion reactions to the other blood groups are not known to cause clinical signs. Because naturally occurring anti-A antibodies do not exist, the first transfusion of A-positive blood into an A-negative recipient may not result in an immediate reaction. However, antibodies can develop and result in a delayed transfusion reaction in as little as a week after the original mismatched transfusion. If a previously immunized A-negative dog receives A-positive blood, severe reactions occur in less than 1 hour.

Cats

One blood group system has been identified in the cat, designated the AB system. Blood groups of cats include A, B, and AB. Few cats have group AB. The majority of cats have group A, which probably explains the low incidence of transfusion reactions in cats. Type B occurs in certain purebred breeds and certain geographic areas. Unlike dogs, cats do possess naturally occurring antibodies to the erythrocyte antigen they are lacking. Type B cats have strong anti-A antibodies, whereas type A cats have weak anti-B antibodies. Transfusing type B cats with type A blood may result in serious transfusion reactions and death. Thus blood for transfusion of purebred cats should be selected by typing or crossmatching.

Neonatal isoerythrolysis has been documented in type A and type AB kittens born of type B queens with naturally occurring anti-A antibodies.

Cattle

Eleven blood groups have been described in cattle, designated A, B, C, F, J, L, M, R, S, T, and Z. Group B is polymorphic, with more than 60 different antigens. Anti-J antibodies are the only common natural antibodies in cattle. J-negative donors may be used to minimize transfusion reactions.

Sheep and Goats

Seven blood group systems have been identified in sheep, designated A, B, C, D, M, R, and X. Similar to cattle, the B system is highly polymorphic. Naturally

occurring R antibodies may be present. Neonatal isoerythrolysis may occur in lambs administered bovine colostrum. This is caused by the presence of antibodies to sheep erythrocytes in bovine colostrum. Five major systems have been identified in goats, designated A, B, C, M, and J. Naturally occurring J antibodies may be present.

Horses

More than 30 blood groups have been described in eight major blood group systems in horses, designated A, C, D, K, P, Q, T, and U. Naturally occurring antibodies do exist, but antibodies may be present as a result of vaccinations containing equine tissue or transplacental immunization. Crossmatching should be done before the first transfusion in a horse. Transfusion reactions in horses are commonly fatal.

The mare-foal incompatibility test is a crossmatch procedure that detects the presence of antibodies in mare serum (or colostrum) to foal erythrocytes to confirm or prevent neonatal isoerythrolysis.

Typing and crossmatching of blood

Methods for identification of some canine and feline blood groups are available for use in the veterinary practice (Fig. 8-12). Detailed determination of blood type requires the use of antisera, which consist of antibodies specific for each possible blood type of a given species. Commercial antisera for canine and feline group testing are available. The procedure requires a whole blood sample collected with ethylenediamine tetraacetic acid (EDTA), heparin, or acid-citrate-dextrose (ACD) anticoagulant. The blood is centrifuged at 1000g for 10 minutes. After removal of the plasma and buffy coat, the erythrocytes are washed three times in a saline solution and resuspended. The red cell suspension is distributed among as many tubes as required for the number of blood type antisera being tested. A small amount (usually 0.1 ml) of the antisera in question is added to the appropriately labeled tube. The tubes are incubated for 15 minutes at room temperature and then recentrifuged for 15 seconds at 1000g. Each tube

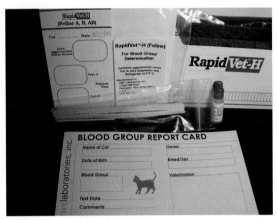

Figure 8-12. Methods for identification of some canine and feline blood groups are available for use in the veterinary practice.

is examined for evidence of hemolysis or agglutination, both macroscopically and microscopically. Weak positive results may require additional testing.

Blood typing of large animals is impractical for routine analysis before transfusion. Literally thousands of different antisera would be required because of the large number of different blood groups in the sheep, cow, and horse.

In the absence of commercial antisera, crossmatching of a blood donor and recipient animal reduces the possibility of a transfusion reaction. The procedure for crossmatching requires both a serum and a whole blood sample and is divided into two parts. Red cell suspensions, collected as for the blood typing procedure, are prepared. The major crossmatch procedure involves the addition of a few drops of serum from the recipient animal to a few drops of washed cells from the donor. The mixture is incubated and then centrifuged. The presence of hemolysis or agglutination, either macroscopically or microscopically, indicates a blood type mismatch. The minor crossmatch procedure is similar except that donor serum and recipient cells are used.

Both procedures should be performed on all animals with unknown blood types that require transfusion. Two controls are used for the test, which consists of running the procedure using donor cells together with donor serum and recipient cells together with recipient serum.

TESTS OF CELL-MEDIATED IMMUNITY

Tests of humoral immunity involve detection of circulating antibodies; evaluation of cell-mediated immunity is much more difficult.

Tuberculin Skin Test

The tuberculin skin test correlates with a specific cell-mediated immune reaction. Animals infected with *Mycobacterium tuberculosis, M. bovis,* and *M. avium* bacteria develop characteristic delayed hypersensitivity reactions when exposed to purified derivatives of the organism called tuberculin. In the tuberculin skin test, tuberculin is injected intradermally at a site in the cervical region or in a skin fold at the base of the tail in large animals (see Table 8-1). A delayed local inflammatory reaction is observed if the animal has been exposed to *Mycobacteria.* The reaction to injection is delayed because a day or more passes before the T lymphocytes migrate to the foreign antigen injected into the dermis.

COLLECTING SAMPLES FOR SEROLOGIC TESTING

Nearly all serologic tests require serum or plasma as the sample. Whole blood should not be sent to the diagnostic laboratory when serum or plasma is specified. The most practical method of collection is the Vacutainer System (Becton Dickinson, Franklin Lakes, NJ), commonly available from many veterinary and medical supply companies. A red-topped vacuum tube is used when serum is required and a lavender-topped tube is used to collect plasma unless heparinized plasma (green-topped tube) is specifically requested.

Reference laboratories have strict requirements concerning specimen type, quality, and handling. If any uncertainty exists, the laboratory should be contacted for specific details. For each test, the requirements should be read carefully and exactly what is requested should be submitted. If a blood sample is to be collected in a syringe, a 5-ml syringe and 20-gauge needle combination should be used because it causes the least hemolysis.

Handling Serologic Samples

When serum is to be submitted, the blood sample is allowed to clot for 20 to 30 minutes at room temperature and then is centrifuged for 10 minutes at a speed no faster than 1500 rpm. If little serum has separated after centrifuging, "rimming" the tube with a wooden applicator stick to loosen the clot may help; however, this also may cause hemolysis. If plasma is desired, the sample may be centrifuged immediately after collection.

After centrifugation, a small pipette is used to aspirate the serum or plasma (upper layer) off the packed erythrocytes. The aspirate is placed into a transfer tube or other sealable test tube and clearly labeled. The serum or plasma may be tested immediately or frozen or refrigerated for later use. See Chapter 3 for more details on collection of serum samples..

Samples for most serologic tests need not be frozen but should be shipped cold, especially during hot weather. The major problem with shipping tubes is breakage. The tubes must be packed firmly in place with packing material so they do not move around when the package is jarred. Each sample must be clearly and correctly labeled and the pertinent paperwork enclosed to facilitate proper reporting of the results from the laboratory.

MOLECULAR DIAGNOSTICS

Leptospira spp., slow-growing bacteria on a culture plate, are one of many bacteria that can now be identified by using molecular diagnostic testing. Its DNA molecule, which contains its genetic information, is the molecule of interest in the test. Molecular diagnostics is based on analyzing DNA or RNA. Although too sophisticated for use in veterinary practices, veterinarians can send samples out to be tested in a short amount of time. Many of the state veterinary diagnostic laboratories now offer several molecular tests. The obvious use for the veterinarian is to identify the presence of pathogens such as viruses, fungi, or bacteria, but there are many other uses for this technology (Tables 8-2 and 8-3).

The branches of medicine and science that use these types of DNA tests include microbiology, genetics, immunology, pharmacology, forensics, biology, food science, agriculture, archaeology, and ecology. DNA tests are available to classify cancers, detect genetic defects, verify animal pedigrees, and

TABLE 8-2

Molecular Diagnostic Tests for Veterinary Pathogens

Organism	Suggested Samples
Bacillus anthracis	Blood
BVD1, BVD2	Lymph nodes, spleen, serum
Chlamydia spp.	Placenta, liver
Clostridium perfringens	Isolated colony from bacterial culture
Escherichia coli virulence typing panel	Isolated colony from bacterial culture
Leptospira spp.	Urine, liver, kidney
Mycobacterium paratuberculosis	Intestinal mucosa, mesenteric lymph nodes
PPRS virus	Serum, spleen, lung
Salmonella spp.	Intestinal mucosa, feces, other tissues
West Nile virus	Kidney, heart, brain, liver, spleen

BVD, Bovine viral diarrhea virus
PRRS, Porcine reproductive and respiratory syndrome

TABLE 8-3

Selected Veterinary DNA Tests

Animal	Test	Test Sample
Avian	Bird sexing	Blood or freshly plucked feathers
Canine	DNA banking and profiling	Buccal swab (for animal identification)
Canine	Inherited disease screening	Buccal swab
Canine	Parentage verification	Buccal swab
Equine	DNA banking (for animal identification)	15-20 hairs pulled from mane, including hair root bulbs
Equine	Hyperkalemic periodic paralysis screening	15-20 hairs pulled from mane, including hair root bulbs
Feline	DNA banking and profiling	Buccal swab (for animal identification)
Feline	Parentage verification	Buccal swab
Feline	Polycystic kidney disease	Buccal swab

determine bacterial contaminants in food science applications, to name a few uses.

The advantages of these kinds of tests are increased sensitivity (degree to which a test can detect and consistently measure small amounts of sample) and increased specificity (ability of a test to detect and measure only the desired sample and not cross-react with other substances). The amount of specimen needed for the test can be exceedingly small, the tests are safe, and many factors that influence other procedures—such as age and condition of sample, fastidious growth requirements, and viability of the organism—are not as crucial with molecular diagnostic tests. The newer techniques also have faster turnaround times. Whereas traditional identification of a bacterium may take 2 to 3 days or more, molecular diagnostic testing can be accomplished in a matter of hours depending upon the test.

Disadvantages have been contamination leading to false-positive results, a high level of technical expertise needed to run the tests, the need for more than one room in which to perform the tests, and high costs. Many of these problems are being solved, and commercial kits and automated instruments are making these tests available to clinical diagnostic laboratories.

Many varieties of molecular diagnostic tests are available, but perhaps the most familiar, if not most widely used, is the polymerase chain reaction (PCR). This test detects the DNA segment of interest in the specimen submitted and amplifies its amount (Box 8-8).

Reverse Transcriptase Polymerase Chain Reaction

Sometimes RNA is the nucleic acid used for the molecular test, such as when testing for RNA viruses. The process used is called reverse

---

BOX 8-8
Interesting PCR Facts

In the 1960s bacteriologist Thomas Brock from the University of Wisconsin was studying bacteria in a hot stream at Yellowstone National Park. As he approached the hot spring that fed the stream, he was still finding bacteria—bacteria that were living in water that nearly reached boiling temperatures, 100° C. He named one of these bacteria *Thermus aquaticus*. It was later discovered that *T. aquaticus* produces an enzyme that can catalyze chemical reactions at high temperatures, just what was needed for the PCR.

In the 1980s Kary Mullis, a biochemist for Cetus Corporation, was driving along a highway in northern California one night when he had a sudden flash of insight. It was while driving on this mountain road that he conceived the concept that became the basis for the PCR. Mullis won the Nobel Prize in chemistry for PCR in 1993.

transcriptase PCR (RT-PCR). It is similar to PCR, but the single-stranded RNA must first be converted to double-stranded DNA before the PCR process can continue.

Real-Time Polymerase Chain Reaction

Another significant test is real-time PCR. Compared with PCR, this method decreases the risk of contamination, is more easily automated, and is generally faster and easier to run. A fluorescent probe is added to the sample mix; it attaches to the DNA segments and, as the quantity of segments is amplified, fluorescence increases. At a set amount of fluorescence, the sample is considered positive.

Polymerase Chain Reaction

Polymerase chain reaction is called an amplification assay because a small amount of a DNA segment detected in the sample is amplified to run the test better and determine the results. That is, a PCR test produces many copies of a small, select region of the DNA molecule. Before performing the test, the nucleotide sequence of this section of DNA must be known so that the proper reagents are used. The region of the DNA that will identify the virus or bacterium is predetermined.

The amplification process consists of three basic steps: denaturation, annealing, and extension (Fig. 8-13). After amplification, the DNA segments are separated on an electrophoretic gel for identification. The sample mixture contains the specimen with the original DNA in question (if present), primers, nucleotides, and Taq DNA polymerase (the enzyme that can read the DNA code and assemble the complimentary nucleotide bases).

Denaturation
The sample is heated to break apart the double-stranded DNA molecule into two separate strands. Each strand serves as a template on which new nucleotides will attach.

Annealing
The temperature is lowered to cause the primers to bind (anneal) to the separated strands. Primers mark the beginning and the end of the section of DNA to be copied. This will happen only if DNA is present in the sample that is complementary to the primers.

Extension
Once more the temperature is raised and Taq DNA polymerase causes new complementary DNA

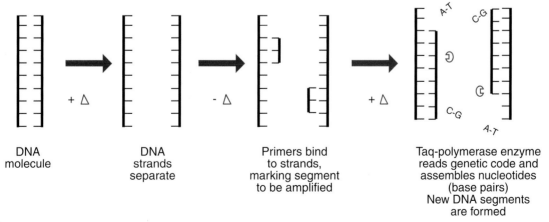

DNA
molecule

+ Δ

DNA
strands
separate

- Δ

Primers bind
to strands,
marking segment
to be amplified

+ Δ

Taq-polymerase enzyme
reads genetic code and
assembles nucleotides
(base pairs)
New DNA segments
are formed

Figure 8-13. PCR showing denaturation of DNA into two strands, annealing of primers to single strands, and extension of DNA molecule with nucleotides by enzymatic action of Taq polymerase.

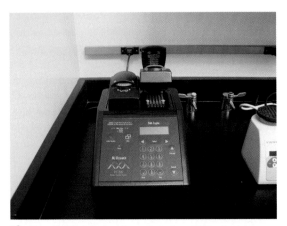

Figure 8-14. Thermal cycler for PCR. Instrument automatically controls the temperature and timing. (Courtesy Bio-Rad Laboratories, Inc., Hercules, CA.)

segments to be produced (extended). Portions of two DNA molecules have been obtained, each with two strands. They are not the complete DNA molecule but do contain the desired segment.

This process is repeated 25 to 30 times in an automated thermal cycler (Fig. 8-14). The timing, temperature, and number of cycles are regulated by the instrument. The amount of DNA segments produced is far greater than the original amount of DNA in the specimen. This is why PCR is useful for detecting minute quantities of the unknown in a mixed specimen.

Finally, to see if the DNA segment was present in the specimen, agarose gel electrophoresis is used. The DNA segments are negatively charged particles and will move along the gel toward the positive electrode when a current is applied. The segments separate according to size, appearing as separate bands on the gel. Controls are run at the same time as the test samples. By knowing the identity of the control bands, the test bands can be compared and identified.

Interpretation of PCR tests must be done carefully. A microbe may be present in the sample, but may not cause disease. As with any laboratory test, the results must be evaluated along with all the information from the clinical case.

Recommended Reading

Birchard SJ, Sherding RG, editors: *Saunders manual of small animal practice,* ed 3, St Louis, 2006, Elsevier.

Sirois M: Clinical chemistry and serology. In *Principles and practice of veterinary technology,* St Louis, 2004, Mosby.

Tizard IR, Schubot RM: *Veterinary immunology: an introduction,* St Louis, 2004, Elsevier.

CHAPTER 9

Cytology

Elaine Anthony, Margi Sirois

KEY POINTS

- The primary purpose of the cytology evaluation is to differentiate inflammation and neoplasia.
- Cytology samples from solid masses on an animal's body or obtained from a surgical procedure can be collected by the swab, scrape, or imprint technique.
- Fine needle biopsy can also be used for some solid samples as well as fluid samples
- Centesis refers to fluid samples collected from body cavities.
- Fine needle biopsy can be performed by either an aspiration or a nonaspiration method.
- Fluid samples must be evaluated for volume, color, turbidity, cell types present, nucleated cell count, and total protein.
- Commonly performed methods for preparing solid samples for cytologic evaluation include the compression smear, starfish smear, and combination methods.
- Fluid samples can be prepared with the compression smear or line smear.

- A systematic approach to slide examination is vital to ensuring quality diagnostic results.
- Samples that appear inflammatory can be categorized as suppurative (purulent), granulomatous, pyogranulomatous, or eosinophilic on the basis of the relative numbers of the various cell types present.
- Neoplastic specimens normally contain homogeneous populations of a single cell type.
- Benign neoplasia is described as hyperplasia with no criteria of malignancy present in the nucleus of the cells.
- Nuclear criteria of malignancy can include anisokaryosis; pleomorphism; high or variable nucleus/cytoplasm ratio; increased mitotic figures; coarse chromatin pattern; nuclear molding; multinucleation; and nucleoli that vary in size, shape, and number.

Exfoliative cytology is the study of cells shed from body surfaces. It refers to examination of cells present in body fluids (such as cerebrospinal, peritoneal, pleural, and synovial fluids), on mucosal surfaces (such as the trachea or vagina), or in secretions (such as semen, prostatic fluid, and milk). The primary purpose of the cytology evaluation is to differentiate inflammation and neoplasia. The types and numbers of cells present in a properly collected and prepared cytology specimen can provide rapid diagnostic information to the clinician. Samples for cytology evaluation can be collected quickly and do not generally require specialized materials or equipment for proper evaluation. With careful attention to quality control, including the use of appropriate collection, preparation, and staining techniques, a high-quality cytology sample can be obtained. Such samples yield valuable results for the clinician and often preclude the need for more invasive procedures to determine diagnosis, treatment, and prognosis for a patient.

Several different preparations are usually made from each sample. This allows for additional diagnostic testing without additional collection. Samples may be processed by a variety of techniques, including impression smears, compression or modified compression preparations, line smears, starfish smears, or wedge smears. The exact type of preparation depends on the characteristics of the sample. Some samples may also require concentration by centrifugation. Fluid samples may require anticoagulant and/or preservatives. A variety of staining techniques are also available for cytology specimens. Some samples require processing with more than one staining procedure.

Cytology provides somewhat different information than a histopathologic evaluation. Histopathology observes cells in relation to their neighboring cells. The histopathologist evaluates the cellular architecture. The preparation of a sample for histopathology involves several complex steps and some specialized equipment. To prepare a sample for histopathology, the tissue is first immersed in fixative. Several steps are involved in dehydrating the tissue before it is imbedded in paraffin. The paraffin block is then sliced and the

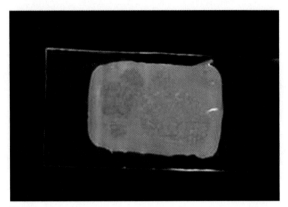

Figure 9-1. A prepared tissue slide for histopathologic evaluation.

slice mounted on a glass slide before staining (Fig. 9-1). Cytologic evaluations observe the cells individually or in small groups. The cells in a cytologic preparation are randomly distributed with no evidence of their *in vivo* relationship to each other.

SAMPLE COLLECTION

Cytology samples from solid masses on an animal's body or obtained from a surgical procedure can be collected by the swab, scrape, or imprint technique. Fine needle biopsy can also be used for some solid samples as well as fluid samples. Centesis refers to fluid samples collected from body cavities.

Swabs

Swabs generally are collected only when imprints, scrapings, and aspirates cannot be made, such as with fistulous tracts and vaginal collections. The area is swabbed with a moist, sterile cotton or rayon swab (Procedure 9-1 and Fig. 9-2). Sterile isotonic fluid, such as 0.9% saline, should be used to moisten the swab. Moistening the swab helps minimize cell damage during sample collection and smear preparation. For collection of vaginal swabs, restrain the animal in a standing position with the tail elevated. Clean and rinse the vulva, then insert a lubricated speculum or smooth plastic tube to a point just cranial to the urethral orifice in the

PROCEDURE 9-1

Collecting Swab Samples

1. Premoisten a swab with saline.
   a. May need rayon swab, rather than cotton.
   b. May need sterile swab.
2. Place the premoistened swab into the cavity.
3. Roll the swab in a single stroke in layers down the length of a clean slide.
4. Make two or three rows.
5. Air dry the slide before staining by gently waving it in the air.

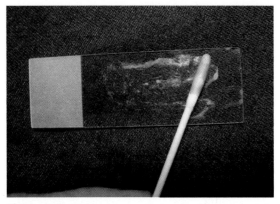

Figure 9-3. The swab is rolled on a clean glass slide to make the smear.

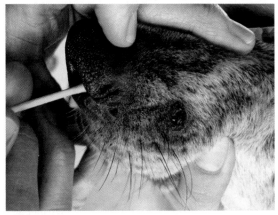

Figure 9-2. A moist cotton swab can be used to collect some cytology samples.

vagina. The cells collected are those exfoliated, or shed, from the vaginal wall (epithelial cells and neutrophils) and those passing through the vagina from the uterus, especially erythrocytes in proestrus and estrus in the bitch. If collecting a sample from a moist lesion, the swab need not be moistened. After sample collection, the swab is gently rolled along the flat surface of a clean glass microscope slide (Fig. 9-3). The swab should not be rubbed across the slide surface because this causes excessive cell damage.

Ear swab samples may contain excess amounts of wax. This may interfere with the evaluation of the sample. To minimize this effect, gentle heating of the slide may be necessary. Passing the slide briefly through a flame or gentle heat from a warm hair dryer may be used to dissolve the wax. Excess heat must be avoided because it will destroy the cellular components of the sample. Aside from the Gram stain procedure, this is the only circumstance under which cytology samples might require heat application.

Scrapings

Smears of scrapings may be prepared from tissues collected during necropsy or surgery or from external lesions on the living animal. Scraping has the advantage of collecting many cells from the tissue and therefore is advantageous when the lesion is firm and yields few cells. The major disadvantages of scrapings are that they are more difficult to collect and they collect only superficial samples. As a result, scrapings from superficial lesions often reflect only a secondary bacterial infection and/or inflammation-induced tissue dysplasia, which markedly hinders their use in diagnosis of neoplasia.

Veterinary technicians may prepare a scraping by holding a scalpel blade perpendicular to the lesion's cleaned and blotted surface and pulling the blade toward themselves several times

PROCEDURE 9-2

Collecting a Scraping Sample

1. For biopsy specimens, use a scalpel blade to expose a fresh edge of the tissue.
2. Blot the sample until it is nearly dry.
3. Hold the blade at a 90-degree angle and scrape across the tissue.
4. Spread the sample onto a clean slide.
   a. Use a motion similar to spreading peanut butter.
   b. If the sample appears thick on the slide, make a compression smear from it.
5. Air dry the slide before staining by gently waving it in the air.

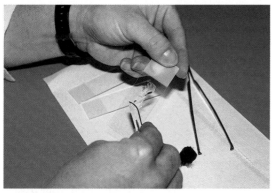

Figure 9-4. A scalpel blade can be used to collect cells from solid masses. (From Raskin RE, Meyer DJ: *Atlas of canine and feline cytology,* St Louis, 2001, Saunders.)

(Procedure 9-2 and Fig. 9-4). The material collected on the blade is transferred to the middle of a glass microscope slide and spread by one or more of the techniques described in the following sections for preparation of smears from aspirates of solid masses.

Imprints

Imprints for cytologic evaluation may be prepared from external lesions on the living animal or from tissues removed during surgery or necropsy. They are easy to collect and require minimal restraint, but they collect fewer cells than scrapings and usually contain a greater amount of contamination (bacterial and cellular) than fine needle biopsies (FNBs). As a result, imprints from superficial lesions often reflect only a local secondary bacterial infection and/or inflammation-induced tissue dysplasia. In many instances the bacteria and tissue dysplasia markedly hinder making an accurate diagnosis of neoplasia.

The Tzanch preparation is a type of imprint collection that can be used on external lesions (Procedure 9-3). To perform this procedure, prepare four to six clean glass slides. The lesion is imprinted before it is cleaned and that first slide designated as number one. The lesion should then be cleaned with a saline-moistened surgical sponge and reimprinted with the slide marked as imprint number two. The lesion is then debrided and reimprinted with the slide, marked as imprint number three. If a scab is present, the underside of the scab should be imprinted and the slide

PROCEDURE 9-3

Collecting a Tzanch Sample

1. Assemble four clean slides, and number them.
2. Touch the slide to the lesion on the patient as follows:
   - Slide 1 – Touch the slide to the unprepped lesion
     - May first lightly wipe the lesion with saline
   - Slide 2 – Prep, gently debride, and lightly clean the lesion and touch the slide to the lesion.
   - Slide 3 – Fully debride the lesion, removing any scabs, etc and imprint the exposed area.
   - Slide 4 – Imprint the bottom of the scab if present
3. Air dry all slides before staining by gently waving in the air.

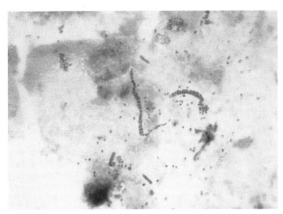

Figure 9-5. This sample was prepared with an imprint of the underside of a scab. Squamous epithelial cells and chains of coccoid organisms *(Dermatophilus congolensis)* are present. (Reprinted from Cowell RL, Tyler RD, Meinkoth JH: *Diagnostic cytology and hematology of the dog and cat,* ed 2, St Louis, 1999, Mosby.)

marked as imprint number four (Fig. 9-5). Imprints from the tissue exposed from the scab removal and scrapings or swabs from that exposed tissue can both be collected.

To collect imprints from tissues collected during surgery or necropsy, blood and tissue fluid first should be removed from the surface of the lesion being imprinted by blotting with a clean, absorbent material (Procedure 9-4 and Fig. 9-6). Excessive blood and tissue fluids inhibit tissue cells from

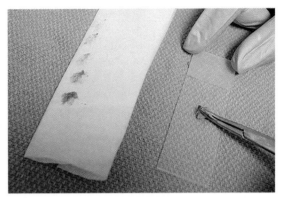

Figure 9-6. The tissue must be thoroughly blotted to remove blood and tissue fluid before preparing the imprint slide.

adhering to the glass slide, producing a poorly cellular preparation. Also, excessive fluid inhibits cells from spreading and assuming the size and shape they usually have on air-dried smears. If a delay occurs from the time of sample collection until the imprint is taken, a scalpel blade should be used to expose a fresh surface before blotting and sampling the surface. The middle of a clean glass microscope slide is then touched against the blotted surface of the tissue to be imprinted. Multiple imprints generally are made on each slide (Fig. 9-7). Several slides may be imprinted so that slides are available for special stains if necessary.

PROCEDURE 9-4

Collecting an Imprint Sample

1. Expose a fresh edge on a small piece of tissue.
2. Blot the sample until it is nearly dry.
3. Touch the tissue repeatedly in rows in single file on a clean slide.
   - Repeat blotting as needed
4. Air dry the slide before staining by gently waving it in the air.

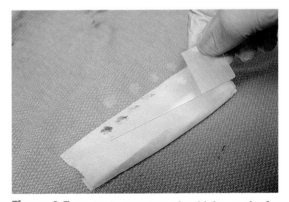

Figure 9-7. Multiple imprints should be made for each tissue. Blot the sample again if tissue fluid and blood remain on the imprint slide.

Fine Needle Biopsy

Fine needle biopsies may be collected from masses, including lymph nodes, nodular lesions, and internal organs. For cutaneous lesions, they provide an advantage over other methods by avoiding superficial contamination (bacterial and cellular). However, fewer cells are usually collected than with other methods, such as scrapings. Fine needle biopsy can be performed by either an aspiration or a nonaspiration method.

Preparation of the Site for Fine Needle Biopsy

If microbiologic tests are to be performed on a portion of the sample collected or a body cavity (such as peritoneal and thoracic cavities and joints) is to be penetrated, the area of aspiration is surgically prepared. Otherwise preparation is essentially that required for a vaccination or venipuncture. An alcohol swab may be used to clean the area.

Selection of Syringe and Needle

For the aspiration method of fine needle biopsy, use a 21- to 25-gauge needle and a 3- to 20-ml syringe. The softer the aspirated tissue is, the smaller the needle and syringe used. The use of a needle larger than 21 gauge for aspiration is seldom advantageous, even for firm tissues such as fibromas. When larger needles are used, tissue cores tend to be aspirated, resulting in a poor yield of free cells suitable for cytologic preparation. Also, larger needles tend to cause greater blood contamination.

The size of the syringe used is influenced by the consistency of the tissue being aspirated. Softer tissues, such as lymph nodes, often may be aspirated successfully with a 3-ml syringe. Firm tissues, such as fibromas and squamous cell carcinomas, require a larger syringe to maintain adequate suction for sufficient collection of cells. Because the ideal size of the syringe is not known for many masses before aspiration, a 12-ml syringe is a useful size.

Aspiration Procedure

The mass to be aspirated is held firmly to aid penetration of the skin and mass and to control the direction of the needle (Procedure 9-5). The needle, with syringe attached, is introduced into the center of the mass and strong negative pressure is applied by withdrawing the plunger to approximately three fourths the volume of the syringe (Fig. 9-8). Several areas of the mass should be sampled, but aspiration of the sample into the barrel of the syringe and contamination of the sample by aspiration of tissue surrounding the mass must be avoided. To accomplish this, when the mass is large enough to allow the needle to be redirected

PROCEDURE 9-5

Fine Needle Biopsy Aspiration

1. Stabilize mass.
2. Insert needle.
3. Retract plunger to create negative pressure.
4. Redirect the needle several times.
   a. Do not exit the mass.
   b. Maintain negative pressure.
5. Remove needle from mass.
6. Remove syringe from needle.
7. Fill syringe with air.
8. Reattach needle.
9. Gently force sample from needle onto clean slide.
10. Air dry the slide before staining by gently waving it in the air.

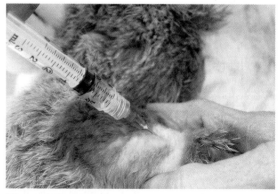

Figure 9-8. Collection of sample by the fine needle biopsy aspiration technique.

and moved to several areas in the mass without danger of the needle's leaving the mass, negative pressure is maintained during redirection and movement of the needle. However, when the mass is not large enough for the needle to be redirected and moved without danger of the needle leaving the mass, negative pressure is relieved during redirection and movement of the needle. In this situation, negative pressure is applied only when the needle is static. Often high-quality collections do not have aspirate material visible in the syringe and sometimes not even in the hub of the needle.

When material is observed in the hub of the needle or after several areas are sampled, the negative pressure is relieved from the syringe and the needle is withdrawn from the mass and skin. Next the needle is removed from the syringe and air is drawn into the syringe. Then the needle is replaced onto the syringe and some of the tissue in the barrel and hub of the needle is expelled onto the middle of a glass microscope slide by rapidly depressing the plunger. When possible, several preparations should be made as described in the following sections.

Nonaspirate Procedure (Capillary Technique, Stab Technique)

This technique is easier to perform than aspiration because it does not involve directing the syringe and needle and pulling the plunger with the same hand (Procedure 9-6). The mass to be sampled is held firmly to aid penetration of the skin and mass and to help direct the needle. A 22-guage needle is introduced into the mass. The needle is moved rapidly back and forth through the mass five to six times along the same tract. The cells are collected by shearing and capillary action. The needle is removed from the mass and attached to a 10-ml syringe prefilled with air. The material is expelled onto a clean glass microscope slide by rapidly depressing the plunger. The expelled material should be smeared using one of the techniques described for preparation of smears. A variation of this procedure involves attachment of the needle to an empty air-filled syringe without the plunger. The syringe can then be held by the barrel and the sample collected as described previously (Fig. 9-9).

PROCEDURE 9-6

Fine Needle Biopsy Nonaspirate Technique

1. Stabilize mass.
2. Insert needle (may have a syringe barrel attached without the plunger.
3. Redirect the needle several times.
   a. Do not exit the mass.
   b. Maintain negative pressure.
4. Remove needle from mass.
   a. Remove syringe barrel (if used) from needle.
5. Fill syringe with air.
6. Reattach needle.
7. Gently force sample from needle onto clean slide.
8. Air dry the slide before staining by gently waving it in the air.

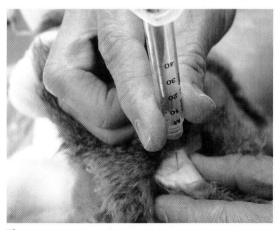

Figure 9-9. Collection of sample by the fine needle biopsy nonaspiration technique. Note that the syringe plunger has been removed.

Generally, enough material is collected to make only one smear. Therefore the procedure should be repeated two or three times in different sites of the mass to have adequate slide numbers and areas of the mass to evaluate.

Tissue Biopsy

Tissue biopsy is the sampling of a piece of tissue for cytologic and/or histopathologic examination. Many organs or tissues, including kidney, liver, lung, lymph node, prostate, skin, spleen, and thyroid, or masses (tumors) may be biopsied. Biopsy techniques include gentle abrasion with a blade, needle aspiration, and excision, including punch biopsy and endoscope-guided biopsy. The technique used varies with the tissue to be biopsied. Considerations include its location, accessibility, and nature. Prospective skin biopsy sites are clipped of hair, being careful to avoid skin irritation and inducement of an inflammatory artifact. Cleansing of the site is neither recommended nor necessary. The lesion must not be scrubbed nor any scales, crusts, or surface debris disturbed because they may offer valuable diagnostic clues.

Tissue samples for histopathologic examination often are fixed in 10% neutral phosphate-buffered formalin. To ensure adequate fixation, slabs of tissue no more than 1 cm wide should be placed in fluid-tight jars containing formalin at approximately 10 times the specimen's volume. With large tissues, the sample can be removed to a smaller jar with less formalin once it has been fixed for 24 hours.

Wedge Biopsy

Elliptic wedge biopsy specimens are commonly obtained with a scalpel. The wedge biopsy offers the advantages of a large, variably sized specimen that is easily oriented by the pathology technician. Solitary lesions are often best removed with this technique. When a wedge biopsy specimen is taken, a sharp scalpel blade is used to excise the entire lesion, or the wedge is taken from an area of the lesion, through a transition zone, to normal tissue. The pathology technician then can trim the specimen on its long axis to provide the pathologist with a slide showing abnormal tissue, a transition zone, and normal tissue.

Punch Biopsy

The punch biopsy technique has a number of advantages over wedge biopsy, particularly the ease and speed of the procedure (Procedure 9-7). Keyes cutaneous biopsy punches (4-, 6-, and 8-mm disposable skin biopsy punches) are most commonly used (Fig. 9-10). Used punches may be placed in the sterilization tray and reused until dull. Most disposable punches may be reused at least three or four times.

With the biopsy punch, 4-mm specimens require no sutures and 6- or 8-mm biopsy specimens require only one or two sutures. Ideally, two or three punch biopsy specimens of various lesions should be collected. The punch is gently rotated in one direction until the punch blade has sectioned the tissue. The punch is rotated in only one direc-

PROCEDURE 9-7

Punch Biopsy Sample Collection

1. Gently rotate the biopsy punch in one direction until the punch blade has sectioned the tissue.
2. Grasp the margin of the tissue with a pair of fine forceps or flush the tissue onto a small piece of wooden tongue depressor.
3. Allow the tissue to dry onto the tongue depressor
4. Place the tissue with the attached tongue depressor "splint" into a formalin jar, specimen-side down.

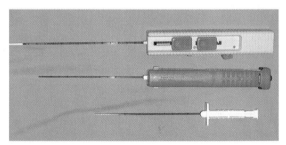

Figure 9-10. Examples of punch biopsy instruments. (From Busch SJ: *Small animal surgical nursing: skills and concepts,* St Louis, 2006, Mosby.)

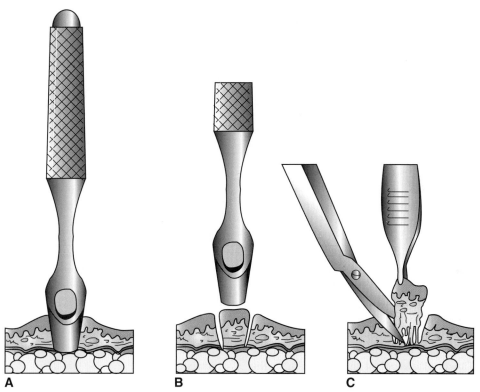

Figure 9-11. Technique for collecting a specimen with a biopsy punch. (From Busch SJ: *Small animal surgical nursing: skills and concepts,* St Louis, 2006, Mosby.)

tion because back-and-forth rotation increases the likelihood of specimen damage from shearing forces (Fig. 9-11).

Once the specimen has been collected, by either the wedge or the punch method, the specimen should be gently removed by grasping the margin of the tissue with a pair of fine forceps. Fresh, unfixed tissue is extremely fragile. Specimens collected by endoscopy can be gently flushed from the tip of the endoscope with sterile saline (Fig. 9-12). The specimen then is blotted gently on a paper towel to remove excess blood and is placed on a small piece of wooden tongue depressor or cardboard (Fig. 9-13). Skin specimens should be placed with the subcutaneous side down. Gently

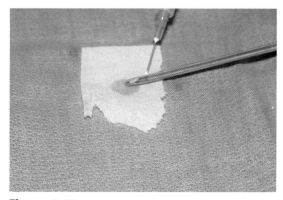

Figure 9-12. Specimens collected by endoscopy should be gently flushed from the tip of the endoscope.

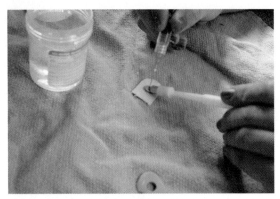

Figure 9-13. A sterile needle can be used to remove a punch biopsy specimen onto a splint.

pressing the biopsy specimen flat facilitates adherence and allows proper anatomic orientation of the specimen in the laboratory. Allow the tissue to dry onto the "splint."

Specimens with the attached "splint" are then immersed or floated specimen side down in the fixative. Timely placement of the specimen in the fixative is critical because artifactual changes may begin to occur within 1 minute after the biopsy specimen is obtained. Adequate specimen fixation requires at least 24 hours before processing. Formalin freezes at $-11°$ C ($-24°$ F), and this freezing may cause substantial artifactual damage in unfixed specimens. Therefore, to ensure proper fixation without freezing artifact, specimens should remain at room temperature for at least 6 hours before exposure to possible extreme cold.

Centesis

Centesis refers to the introduction of a needle into any body cavity or organ for the purpose of removing fluid. Collection of fluid from the peritoneal cavity (abdominocentesis or paracentesis) and thoracic cavity (thoracocentesis) are commonly performed in small animal practice. Cystocentesis (percutaneous aspiration of urine from the urinary bladder) is discussed in Chapter 5. Fluid samples for cytologic evaluation may also be collected from around the spinal column, from within joints (arthrocentesis), and from the eye. General anes-

thesia is required for collection of cerebrospinal fluid, synovial fluid, and aqueous and vitreous humor.

Before collection of peritoneal or pleural fluid, the site should be aseptically prepared and all equipment and supplies gathered. Preparing several smears from the fluid as soon as it is collected is helpful, so a plentiful supply of glass slides should be ready. A portion of the fluid should be collected in an ethylenediamine tetraacetic acid (EDTA) tube. A 21-gauge needle is most commonly used and should be attached to a 60-ml syringe. For small animal patients, thoracocentesis is usually performed with the animal in a standing position and the needle inserted in the seventh or eighth intercostal space along the cranial aspect of the rib. Abdominocentesis may be performed in a standing animal or with the patient in lateral recumbency (Fig. 9-14). The needle is introduced into the ventral abdomen to the right of the midline approximately 1 to 2 cm caudal to the umbilicus. The procedure is slightly different for exotic and farm animals.

Ease of collection may reflect the volume of fluid present and/or the pressure within that body cavity. It also is influenced by the technical proficiency of the operator and, in the case of conscious animals, the cooperation of the animal. The total volume collected must be recorded at the time of collection. Certain gross characteristics of body fluids should be recorded at collection, including

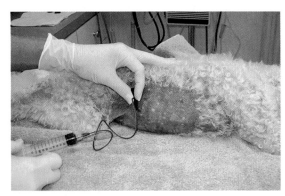

Figure 9-14. Collection of peritoneal fluid by abdominocentesis.

sample color and turbidity. Subsequently, total nucleated cell counts, cell types, and morphologic features are determined.

Color and Turbidity

Color and turbidity are influenced by protein concentration and cell numbers. Gross discoloration, with increased turbidity, may be caused by iatrogenic contamination with peripheral blood, recent or old hemorrhage, inflammation, or a combination of these conditions.

Perforation of superficial vessels during collection may result in contamination with peripheral blood. Such admixture of blood with the sample may be obvious as a streak of blood in otherwise clear fluid at some stage during collection. Blood-tinged fluid also may be the result of recent or old hemorrhage into the body cavity being sampled. Both peripheral blood contamination and recent hemorrhage result in a clear supernatant and red (erythrocyte-rich) sediment after centrifugation. Recent hemolysis imparts a reddish discoloration to the supernatant. Hemorrhage that occurred at least 2 days previously generally causes a yellowish supernatant (because of hemoglobin breakdown products), usually with little erythrocytic sediment (Fig. 9-15).

Cytologic examination of the fluid also may assist in determining the time of hemorrhage. Clumps of platelets may be observed in recent, often iatrogenic (operator-induced), hemorrhage. These clumps are not obvious after approximately 1 hour. Blood must be present in the cavity for

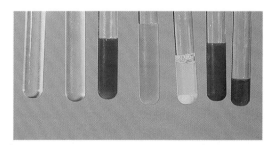

Figure 9-15. Gross appearance of various effusion *(left to right)*: clear and colorless, yellow and slightly turbid, hemolyzed and slightly turbid, orange and turbid, sedimented fluid, bloody and turbid, brown and slightly turbid. (From Raskin RE, Meyer DJ: *Atlas of canine and feline cytology*, St. Louis, 2001, Saunders.)

several hours before macrophage ingestion of erythrocytes becomes evident. If the hemorrhage occurred a day or so before collection, hemoglobin breakdown products, such as hemosiderin, may be seen in the macrophages. Inflammation also may discolor body fluids, with the degree of turbidity reflecting leukocyte numbers. Color may vary from an off-white or cream to a red-cream or dirty brown, depending on the number of erythrocytes also involved and the integrity of the cells present.

Consistent terminology must be used when describing cell types. Specific details on the morphologic features of each cell type also assist the clinician in making the diagnosis. Neutrophils and macrophages should be evaluated for the presence of vacuoles or phagocytized material. Neoplastic cells should be evaluated for malignant changes, such as mitotic figures and basophilic cytoplasm.

Transtracheal/Bronchial Wash

Cytologic evaluation of samples obtained from the trachea, bronchi, or bronchioles may assist with diagnosis of pulmonary disease in animals. Tracheal washes may be performed by passage of a catheter through an endotracheal tube in an anesthetized animal (orotracheal approach), through the nasal passages (nasotracheal approach), or through the skin and trachea (percutaneous approach) in a conscious, sedated animal. The transtracheal route minimizes pharyngeal contamination of the specimen, but it is an invasive procedure and consequently requires aseptic technique. These procedures are commonly used in both small and large animals.

Percutaneous Technique

The percutaneous method requires the use of an 18- to 20-gauge through-the-needle (jugular) catheter. The laryngeal area is clipped of hair and aseptically prepared. A small amount (usually 0.5 to 1.0 ml) of 2% lidocaine is injected into the cricothyroid membrane and surrounding skin. The needle is inserted into the trachea through the cricothyroid membrane (Fig. 9-16). Sterile physiologic saline solution is infused through the catheter at a rate of 0.5 to 1.0 ml/kg body weight.

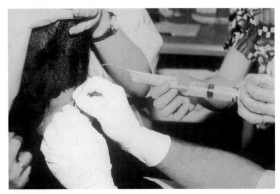

Figure 9-16. Collection of transtracheal wash sample by the percutaneous method. (From McCurnin DM, Bassert JM: *Clinical textbook for veterinary technicians,* ed 6, St Louis, 2006, Saunders.)

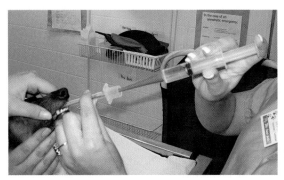

Figure 9-17. Collection of transtracheal wash sample by the orotracheal method.

When the animal coughs, the syringe plunger should be retracted several times and the fluid collected placed into a plain sterile tube. Samples should be processed immediately.

Orotracheal Technique

This technique may be preferred in very small or fractious animals. The patient must be lightly anesthetized and an appropriate-size endotracheal tube placed. A urinary or jugular catheter is then placed through the endotracheal tube and saline is infused as described for the percutaneous method. A red rubber catheter may be used but care must be taken to ensure that the catheter does not collapse upon aspiration as may occur with highly viscous samples (Fig. 9-17). Depending on the level of anesthesia, the animal will often not cough, so the saline should be withdrawn within a few seconds and evaluated. Bronchoalveolar lavage (BAL) is an orotracheal technique used to collect samples specifically from the lower respiratory tract. Bronchoscopy is the preferred method for performing a BAL, but specialized equipment (e.g., bronchoscope) is required.

With either method, only a small amount of the saline infused will be harvested with the initial collection. Subsequent coughing of the animal may also contain cells of interest, so all fluid released during coughing subsequent to the initial collection should be collected once the animal has been returned to its cage. This fluid should be placed in a sterile tube with a notation containing the site of collection. Such fluids are often contaminated but can sometimes be used for evaluation when the initial collection yields insufficient information.

Samples with little mucus (generally corresponding to small numbers of cells) should be centrifuged at low speed and smears prepared from the sediment. Samples containing much mucus (and usually numerous cells) may not need to be centrifuge concentrated before a smear is made. Total nucleated cell counts are usually not performed on tracheal wash fluids. Cell numbers are subjectively recorded from evaluation of the smear. A tracheal wash smear from a normal animal contains few cells, usually with a small amount of mucus. The mucus often appears microscopically as eosinophilic to purple strands that may enmesh the cells. Epithelial cells are the principal cell type.

Cytologic evaluation of samples obtained from the nasal cavity may be useful in investigation of diseases affecting the upper airway. Fluid (normal saline) may be infused into the nasal cavity through the nose with a syringe and tubing, then aspirated. This procedure is referred to as a nasal flush. Such specimens are processed as for a tracheal wash. Various abnormalities may be demonstrated with this procedure, such as inflammation secondary to sepsis, fungi and yeasts, and neoplasia. These should not be confused with glove powder, which may be present in some specimens.

CONCENTRATION TECHNIQUES

When a cytologic smear is to be made of fluid with a cell count less than 500/µl, concentration of cells is mandatory. Such concentration may be helpful even at higher cell counts. Four methods are described.

Low-Speed Centrifugation

To concentrate fluids by centrifugation, the fluid is centrifuged 5 minutes at 165g to 360g using a centrifuge with a radial arm length of 14.6 cm (the arm length of most urine centrifuges) at 1000 to 1500 rpm. After centrifugation, the supernatant is separated from the sediment and analyzed for total protein concentration. The sediment is resuspended in a few drops of supernatant by gently thumping the side of the tube. A drop of the resuspended sediment is placed on a slide, and a smear is made by the blood smear or compression preparation technique. When possible, several smears should be made by each technique. Addition of plasma may help cells adhere to the microscope slide. After air drying, the slide may be stained with a Romanowsky stain.

Gravitational Sedimentation

Gravitational sedimentation is another method used to concentrate cells and is most commonly used for cerebrospinal fluid (CSF) evaluations. One method uses a glass cylinder (which can be made by cutting the end off a test tube) attached to a microscope slide with paraffin wax. (The smooth tube end is dipped in melted wax and placed on a warm slide.) The cells in approximately 1 ml of CSF are allowed about 30 minutes to settle. The supernatant is then carefully removed with a pipette and the tube detached. Excess CSF may be gently removed with absorbent paper. The slide is air dried and residual paraffin carefully scraped off. The slide may be stained with a Romanowsky stain.

Membrane Filtration

Membrane filtration of alcohol-diluted CSF also may be used to concentrate cells. A membrane pore size of five is usually satisfactory. Filter holders that attach to a syringe are available. The CSF is permitted to gravity feed from the syringe barrel, or it is gently injected through the filter at no more than 1 drop/sec. The filter paper must be kept horizontal to distribute the cells evenly. Increased resistance to filtration suggests that the pores are becoming obstructed by cells or protein, and no more CSF should be forced through the filter. Filtration of another, smaller volume of CSF through fresh filter paper results in a less-crowded preparation.

After removal from the syringe holder, the filter is fixed in 95% ethanol for at least 30 minutes. Holders are available for easy handling of the filter paper during fixation and staining. A trichrome-type stain must be used. Romanowsky stains are unsuitable because they stain the filter paper too intensely. A satisfactory staining procedure is as follows.

The filter paper is immersed for 2 minutes in each specific substance in the following order: 80%, 70%, 50%, and 30% ethanol and then distilled water, then 4 minutes in hematoxylin, 5 minutes in running tap water, 4 minutes in Pollak's stain, 1 minute in 0.3% acetic acid, 1 minute in 95% ethanol, 2 minutes in N-propyl-alcohol (propanol), 2 minutes in a 1:1 mixture of propanol and xylene, and finally three rinses of 2 minutes each in xylene. At all stages the filter must be treated gently to avoid dislodging cells. Depending on the size of the filter, it may need to be cut to a suitable size before placement on a microscope slide (cell side up). The filter is then flooded with a mounting medium with a refractive index similar to that of filter paper (approximately 1.5), and a cover slip is applied.

Cytologically, the cells trapped by the membrane filter are rounder than those seen after sedimentation (and therefore may be harder to distinguish) and are in slightly different planes of focus. Furthermore, the filter produces a patterned background that may be distracting. This distraction is minimized by ensuring the sample is not over-stained and by using the appropriate mounting medium. The pore size generally used is far too large to trap free bacteria. Quantitatively, more cells are collected by filtration than by the two sedimentation methods.

Cytocentrifugation

As with any fluid of low cellularity, a cytocentrifuge (e.g., Shandon Cytospin, Thermo Fisher Scientific, Inc., Waltham, MA) can be used for preparation of CSF cytologic smears. Such equipment is generally too expensive for a veterinary practice to justify purchasing. However, it often is used in a referral laboratory. This technique allows cells to be concentrated within a small circular area on the slide.

SMEAR PREPARATION

Preparation of Smears from Solid Masses

Several methods may be used to prepare smears for cytologic evaluation of solid masses including lymph nodes and internal organs. The experience of the person preparing the smears and characteristics of the sample influence the choice of smear preparation technique. A combination of slide preparation techniques is therefore suggested. Some cytologic preparation techniques are described in the following sections.

Compression ("Squash") Preparation

The compression technique, sometimes referred to as the "squash prep," can yield excellent cytologic smears (Procedure 9-8). However, in less experienced hands it often yields unreadable cytologic smears because too many cells are ruptured or the sample is not sufficiently spread. A compression preparation is made by expelling the aspirate onto the middle of one slide and then gently placing a second slide (spreader slide) over the aspirate horizontal with and at right angles to the first slide (prep slide) (Figs. 9-18 and 9-19). The spreader slide is then quickly and smoothly slid across the prep slide. Downward pressure should not be placed on

PROCEDURE 9-8

Preparing a Compression Smear

1. Transfer sample to clean slide near the frosted edge and toward the middle of the slide
2. Add a second slide perpendicular to the first.
   a. Place the second slide on top of the drop of sample with the frosted edge facing down and close to the sample
   b. Allow the sample to spread for a few seconds
3. Using a smooth single motion, pull slide 2 (the top one) evenly across the bottom slide
4. Air dry slide 2 and stain

the spreader slide because this may cause excessive cell rupturing, making the sample unable to be interpreted.

A modification of the compression preparation that has fewer tendencies to rupture cells is to lay the second slide over the aspirate, rotate the second slide 45 degrees, and lift it upward (Procedure 9-9 and Fig. 9-20).

Combination Technique

One combination procedure involves spraying the sample onto the middle of a clean glass microscope slide or prep slide. Place the prep slide on a flat, solid, horizontal surface and pull another slide, called the spreader slide, backward at a 45-degree angle to the first slide until it makes contact with approximately one third of the aspirate. Then the spreader slide is slid smoothly and rapidly forward, as if making a blood smear. Next, the spreader slide is placed horizontally over the back third of the aspirate at a right angle to the prep slide. The weight of the spreader slide (top slide) is usually sufficient to spread the material. Avoid the temptation to compress the slides manually. Keep the spreader slide flat and horizontal, and use a quick, smooth motion to slide the spreader slide across the prep slide (Fig. 9-21).

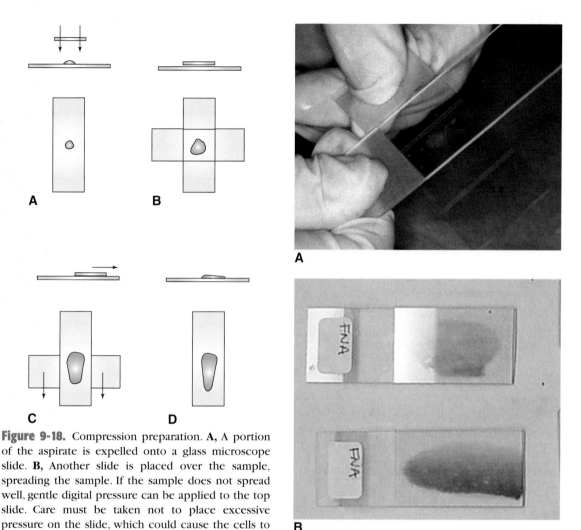

Figure 9-18. Compression preparation. **A,** A portion of the aspirate is expelled onto a glass microscope slide. **B,** Another slide is placed over the sample, spreading the sample. If the sample does not spread well, gentle digital pressure can be applied to the top slide. Care must be taken not to place excessive pressure on the slide, which could cause the cells to rupture. **C,** The slides are smoothly slipped apart, which usually produces well-spread smears (**D**) but may result in excessive cell rupture.

Figure 9-19. A, Preparation of a compression smear. **B,** Completed compression smear.

This procedure makes a compression preparation of the back third of the aspirate. The middle third of the aspirate is left untouched. This procedure leaves the front third of the aspirate gently spread. If the aspirate is of fragile tissue, this area should contain sufficient intact cells to evaluate. The back third of the aspirate has been spread with the shear forces of a compression preparation. If the aspirate contains clumps of cells that are difficult to spread, some clumps should be sufficiently spread in the back third of the preparation. If the aspirate is of low cellularity, the middle third remains more concentrated and is the most efficient area to study.

Starfish Smear
Another technique for spreading aspirates is to drag the aspirate peripherally in several directions

PROCEDURE 9-9

Preparing a Modified Compression Smear

1. Transfer sample to clean slide near the frosted edge and toward the middle of the slide
2. Add a second slide perpendicular to the first.
   a. Place the second slide on top of the drop of sample with the frosted edge facing down and the sample near the middle of the slide
   b. Allow the sample to spread for a few seconds
3. Using a smooth single motion, twist the two slides in opposite directions (like opening an Oreo cookie).
4. Lift the top slide straight up.
5. Air dry slide 2 and stain.

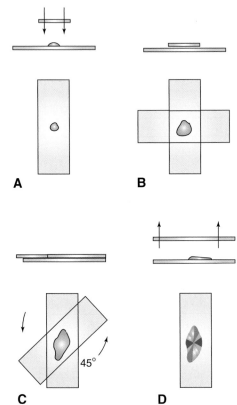

Figure 9-20. Modification of the compression preparation. **A,** A portion of the aspirate is expelled onto a glass microscope slide. **B,** Another slide is placed over the sample, causing the sample to spread. If necessary, gentle digital pressure can be applied to the top slide to spread the sample more. Care must be taken not to place excessive pressure on the slide, which could cause the cells to rupture. **C,** The top slide is rotated approximately 45 degrees and lifted directly upward, producing a squash preparation with subtle ridges and valleys of cells **(D).**

with the point of a syringe needle, producing a starfish shape (Procedure 9-10 and Fig. 9-22). This technique tends not to damage fragile cells but does allow a thick layer of tissue fluid to remain around the cells. Sometimes the thick layer of fluid prevents the cells from spreading well and interferes with evaluation of cell detail. Usually, however, some acceptable areas are present. The starfish smear technique is especially useful for the preparation of highly viscous samples.

Preparation of Smears from Fluid Samples

Cytologic smears should be prepared immediately after fluid collection. When possible, fluid samples for cytologic examination should be collected in EDTA tubes. Smears may be prepared directly from fresh, well-mixed fluid or from the sediment of a centrifuged sample by wedge (blood) smear, line smear, and/or compression preparation techniques. The cellularity, viscosity, and homogeneity of the fluid influence the selection of smear technique.

Line Smear

When the fluid cannot be concentrated by centrifugation or the centrifuged sample is of low cellularity, the line smear technique may be used to concentrate cells in the smear (Procedure 9-11 and Fig. 9-23). A drop of fluid is placed on a clean glass slide and the blood smear technique is used, except the spreading slide is raised directly upward approximately three fourths of the way through the smear, yielding a line containing a much higher concentration of cells than the rest of the slide. Unfortunately, an excessive amount of fluid also

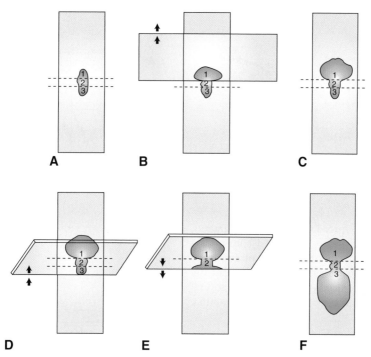

Figure 9-21. Combination cytologic preparation. **A,** A portion of the aspirate is expelled onto a glass microscope slide (prep slide). **B,** Another glass microscope slide is placed over approximately one third of the preparation. If additional spreading of the aspirate is needed, gentle digital pressure can be used. Excessive pressure should be avoided. **C,** The spreader slide is smoothly slid forward. This procedure makes a compression preparation of approximately one third of the aspirate *(area 1)*. The spreader slide also contains a squash preparation (not depicted). Next, the edge of a tilted glass microscope slide (second spreader slide) is slid backward from the end opposite the compression preparation until it makes contact with approximately one third of the expelled aspirate **(D and E). F,** Then the second spreader slide is slid rapidly and smoothly forward. These steps produce an area *(3)* that is spread with mechanical forces like those of a blood smear preparation. The middle area *(2)* is left untouched and contains a high concentration of cells.

PROCEDURE 9-10

Preparing a Starfish Smear

1. Transfer sample to the center of a clean slide
2. Use the tip of a needle to "drag" the sample outward from the center
3. Vary the length and direction of each "drag" through the sample
4. Air dry the slide before staining by gently waving it in the air

may remain in the "line" and prevent the cells from spreading well.

The compression preparation technique often spreads viscous samples and samples with flecks of particulate material better than the blood smear and line smear techniques. The blood smear technique usually produces well-spread smears of sufficient cellularity from homogeneous fluids containing at least 5000 cells/μl but often produces smears of insufficient cellularity from fluids containing less than 5000 cells/μl. The line smear technique may be used to concentrate fluids of low

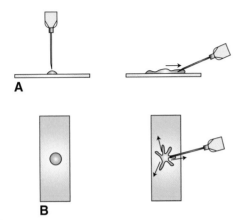

Figure 9-22. Needle spread or "starfish" preparation. **A,** A portion of the aspirate is expelled onto a glass microscope slide. **B,** The tip of a needle is placed in the aspirate and moved peripherally, pulling a tail of the sample with it. This procedure is repeated in several directions, resulting in a preparation with multiple projections.

PROCEDURE 9-11

Preparing a Line Smear

1. Transfer sample to clean slide near the frosted edge.
2. Place a second slide at an angle on the first slide, and back the edge of the second slide into the drop of sample.
3. Allow the sample to spread along the edge of the slide.
4. Use the secone slide to push the sample across the slide.
5. STOP abruptly before the sample makes a feathered edge.
6. Pick the second slide straight up.
7. Air dry slide 1 and stain.

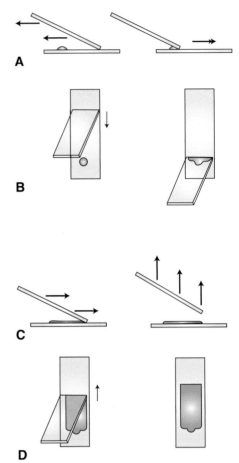

Figure 9-23. Line smear concentration technique. **A,** A drop of fluid sample is placed on a glass microscope slide close to one end, then another slide is slid backward to make contact with the front of the drop **(B).** When the drop is contacted, it rapidly spreads along the juncture between the two slides. **C,** The spreader slide is then smoothly and rapidly slid forward. **D,** After the spreader slide has been advanced approximately two thirds to three fourths the distance required to make a smear with a feathered edge, the spreader slide is raised directly upward. This procedure produces a smear with a line of concentrated cells at its end instead of a feathered edge.

cellularity but often does not sufficiently spread cells from highly cellular fluids. In general, translucent fluids are of low to moderate cellularity, whereas opaque fluids usually have high cellularity. Therefore translucent fluids often require concentration, either by centrifugation or by the line smear technique. When possible, concentration by centrifugation is preferred.

To prepare a smear by the wedge (blood smear) technique, a small drop of the fluid is placed on a glass slide approximately 1.0 to 1.5 cm from the end. Another slide is pulled backward at a 30- to 40-degree angle until it makes contact with the drop. When the fluid flows sideways along the juncture between the slides, the second slide is quickly and smoothly pushed forward until the fluid has all drained away from the second slide. This procedure makes a smear with a feathered edge.

FIXING AND STAINING THE CYTOLOGY SAMPLE

Although many stains incorporate a cellular fixative, accomplishing this as a separate step in the procedure is advantageous to ensure the highest quality preparation. The preferred fixative for cytology specimens is 95% methanol. The methanol must be fresh and not contaminated with stain or cellular debris. Methanol containers must be protected from evaporation and dilution resulting from environmental humidity, which will introduce humidity artifacts onto the slide. The prepared cytology slides should remain in the fixative for 2 to 5 minutes. Longer fixative times will improve the quality of the staining procedure and not harm the samples.

Several types of stains have been used for cytologic preparations. The two general types most commonly used are the Romanowsky-type stains (Wright's, Giemsa, Diff-Quik) and Papanicolaou stain and its derivatives, such as Sano's trichrome. The advantages and disadvantages of both types of stains are discussed. However, because the Romanowsky-type stains are more rewarding, practical, and readily available in practice situations, the remainder of this discussion deals predominantly with Romanowsky-stained preparations.

Romanowsky Stains

Romanowsky stains are inexpensive; readily available; and easy to prepare, maintain, and use. They stain organisms and the cytoplasm of cells excellently. Although nuclear and nucleolar detail cannot be perceived as well with Romanowsky stains as with Papanicolaou stains, nuclear and nucleolar detail usually is sufficient for differen-

tiating neoplasia and inflammation and for evaluating neoplastic cells for cytologic evidence of malignant potential (criteria of malignancy).

Smears to be stained with Romanowsky stains are first air dried. Air drying partially preserves (fixes) the cells and causes them to adhere to the slide so that they do not fall off during the staining procedure.

Many Romanowsky stains are commercially available, including Diff-Quik (Dade Behring, Deerfield, IL.) and other quick Wright's stains (Fig. 9-24). Most, if not all, Romanowsky stains are acceptable for staining cytologic preparations. Diff-Quik stain does not undergo the metachromatic reaction. As a result, granules of some mast cells do not stain. When mast cell granules do not stain, the mast cells may be misclassified as macrophages, which may lead to confusion in examination of some mast cell tumors. Increasing the fixative time to approximately 15 minutes may alleviate this problem. Also, in evaluation of blood smears or bone marrow aspirates, Diff-Quik does not stain polychromatophilic red blood cells well and occasionally does not stain basophils. The variations among different Romanowsky stains

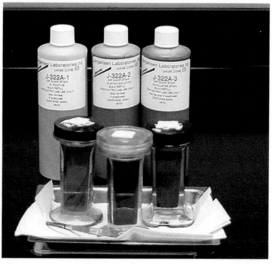

Figure 9-24. A three-step Romanowsky stain suitable for cytology samples.

should not cause a problem once the evaluators become familiar with the stain they routinely use.

Each stain usually has a unique recommended staining procedure. These procedures should be followed in general but should be adapted to the type and thickness of smear being stained and to the evaluator's preference. The thinner the smear and the lower the total protein concentration of the fluid, the less time needed in the stain. The thicker the smear is and the greater the total protein concentration of the fluid, the more time needed in the stain. As a result, fluid smears with low protein and low cellularity, such as abdominal fluid, may stain better in half or less of the recommended time. Thick smears, such as smears of neoplastic lymph nodes, may need to be stained twice the recommended time or longer. Each technician tends to have a different preferred staining technique. By trying variations in the recommended time intervals for stains, the evaluator can establish which times produce the preferred staining characteristics.

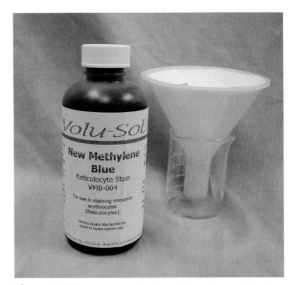

Figure 9-25. New methylene blue is used when critical nuclear detail must be visualized. The stain should be filtered just before use.

New Methylene Blue Stain

New methylene blue (NMB) stain is a useful adjunct to Romanowsky stains (Fig. 9-25). It stains cytoplasm weakly, if at all, but gives excellent nuclear and nucleolar detail. Because NMB stains cytoplasm weakly, the nuclear detail of cells in cell clumps may be better visualized. Generally, red blood cells do not stain with NMB but may develop a pale blue tint. As a result, marked red blood cell contamination of smears does not obscure nucleated cells.

Papanicolaou Stains

The delicate Papanicolaou stains give excellent nuclear detail and delicate cytoplasmic detail. They allow the viewer to see through layers of cells in cell clumps and evaluate nuclear and nucleolar changes well. They do not stain cytoplasm as strongly as Romanowsky stains and therefore do not demonstrate cytoplasmic changes as well. They also do not demonstrate bacteria and other organisms as well as Romanowsky stains do.

Papanicolaou staining requires multiple steps and considerable time. In addition, the reagents often are difficult to locate, prepare, and maintain in practice. Papanicolaou stains and their derivatives require the specimen to be wet fixed (i.e., the smear must be fixed before the cells have dried). Wet fixing requires spraying the smear with a cytologic fixative or placing it in ethanol immediately after preparation. When the smear is to be placed in ethanol, it should be made on a protein-coated slide, which prevents the cells from falling off the slide when it is immersed.

Staining Problems

Poor stain quality often perplexes the novice and experienced cytologist. Most staining problems can be avoided if the following precautions are taken:

- Always use new, clean slides. Even "precleaned" slides should be wiped with alcohol before use to remove residue.
- Fresh, well-filtered (if periodic filtration is required) stain(s) and fresh buffer solution (if a buffer is required) should be used.

- Cytologic preparations should be fixed immediately after air drying unless they are being sent to an outside laboratory. The laboratory should be consulted before fixing slides.
- The surface of the slide or smear should not be touched at any time by human hands.

Occasionally a sample may be contaminated with a foreign substance, such as lubrication jelly, that alters the specimen's staining. Table 9-1 shows some of the problems that can occur with Romanowsky stains and some proposed solutions to these problems.

SUBMISSION OF CYTOLOGIC PREPARATIONS AND SAMPLES FOR INTERPRETATION

When in-house evaluation of a cytologic preparation does not furnish sufficient reliable information for managing a case, the preparation may be submitted to a veterinary clinical pathologist or cytologist for interpretation, or an alternative procedure, such as biopsy and histopathologic evaluation, may be performed. If possible, the person to whom the cytologic preparation is sent should be contacted, and specifics concerning sample handling should be discussed, such as the number of smears to send or whether to fix or stain the smears before mailing.

When possible, two or three air-dried unstained smears, and two or three air-dried Romanowsky-stained smears should be submitted. Pathologists may stain the air-dried unstained smears with the Romanowsky or NMB stains of their choice. The Romanowsky-stained smears are a safety factor. Some tissues stain poorly when air dried but not stained for several days. Also, slides occasionally are shattered during transport and cannot be stained on receipt. Sometimes microscopic examination of shards from the broken prestained smears allows diagnosis. If only a few smears can be prepared from the sample, one should be submitted air dried and unstained and the other submitted air dried, fixed, and stained. Smears should be well labeled with alcohol-resistant ink or another permanent labeling method. If a Papanicolaou stain

is to be used, several wet-fixed smears should be submitted.

Fluid samples should have smears prepared from them immediately. Direct smears and concentrated smears should be submitted. Also, an EDTA (lavender top) and sterile serum tube (red top) fluid sample should be submitted. A total nucleated cell count and total protein concentration can be performed on the EDTA tube sample and, if necessary, chemical analyses can be performed on the serum tube sample.

Slides must be protected when mailed. Simple cardboard mailers do not provide sufficient protection to prevent slide breakage if they are mailed in unpadded envelopes. Marking the envelope with phrases such as "fragile," "glass," "breakable," and "please hand cancel" has little success. Placing a pad of bubble wrap or polystyrene on each side of the slide holder usually prevents slide breakage. Slides may also be mailed in plastic slide holders or innovative holders, such as small pill bottles.

Unfixed slides should not be mailed with formalin-containing samples and should be protected against moisture. Formalin fumes alter the staining characteristics of smears, and water causes cell lysis (Fig. 9-26).

INITIAL MICROSCOPIC EVALUATION

Figure 9-27 summarizes steps in the evaluation of cytology specimens. The initial evaluation of the cytology preparation should be performed on low magnification (100×) to determine if all areas are adequately stained and to detect any localized areas of increased cellularity. To improve resolution by decreasing light refraction, a drop of immersion oil can be placed on the smear and a cover slip added. A consistent approach to examination helps ensure high-quality results. Large objects such as cell clusters, parasites, crystals, and fungal hyphae are normally evident on the low power examination. This initial evaluation should be used to characterize the cellularity and composition of the sample by recording the types of cells present and relative numbers of each type. A high power examination (400× to 450×) should then be performed to

TABLE 9-1

Problems that Can Occur with Romanowsky Stains and Proposed Solutions

Problem	Solution
Excessive Blue Staining (RBCs May Be Blue-Green)	
Prolonged stain contact	Decrease staining time
Inadequate wash	Wash longer
Specimen too thick	Make thinner smears if possible
Stain, diluent, buffer, or wash water too alkaline	Check with pH paper and correct pH
Exposure to formalin vapor	Store and ship cytologic preps separate from formalin containers
Wet fixation in ethanol	Air dry smears before fixation
Delayed fixation	Fix smears sooner if possible
Surface of the slide was alkaline	Use new slides
Excessive Pink Staining	
Insufficient staining time	Increase staining time
Prolonged washing	Decrease duration of wash
Stain or diluent too acidic	Check with pH paper and correct pH; fresh methanol may be needed
Excessive time in red stain solution	Decrease time in red stain solution
Inadequate time in blue stain solution	Increase time in blue stain solution
Mounting cover slip before preparation is dry	Allow preparation to dry completely before mounting cover slip
Weak Staining	
Insufficient contact with one or more of the stain solutions	Increase staining time
Fatigued (old) stains	Change stains
Another slide covered specimen during staining	Keep slides separate
Uneven Staining	
Variation of pH in different areas of slide surface (may be caused by slide surface being touched or slide being poorly cleaned)	Use new slides and avoid touching their surfaces before and after preparation
Water allowed to stand on some areas of the slide after staining and washing	Tilt slides close to vertical to drain water from the surface or dry with a fan
Inadequate mixing of stain and buffer	Mix stain and buffer thoroughly
Precipitate on Preparation	
Inadequate stain filtration	Filter or change the stain(s)
Inadequate washing of slide after staining	Rinse slide well after staining
Dirty slides used	Use clean new slides
Stain solution dries during staining	Use sufficient stain and do not leave it on slide too long

TABLE 9-1

Problems that Can Occur with Romanowsky Stains and Proposed Solutions—cont'd

Problem	Solution
Miscellaneous	
Overstained preparations	Destain with 95% methanol and restain; Diff-Quik-stained smears may have to be destained in the red Diff-Quik stain solution to remove the blue color; however, this damages the red stain solution
Refractile artifact on RBC with Diff-Quik stain (usually result of moisture in fixative)	Change the fixative

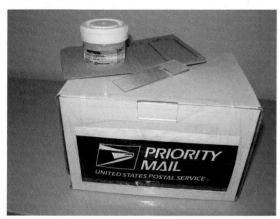

Figure 9-26. Preparing samples for shipment to reference laboratories. Unfixed slides must not be in proximity to formalin containers.

evaluate and compare individual cells and further characterize the types of cells present. Oil immersion must be used to identify specific nuclear criteria of malignancy and cytoplasmic abnormalities indicative of malignancy and various inflammatory reactions. The cytology report should indicate the cell types present, their appearance, and relative proportions.

Inflammation

Inflammation is a normal physiologic response to tissue damage or invasion by microorganisms. This damage releases substances that have a chemo-tactic effect on certain white blood cells. These chemotactic factors are therefore involved in attracting white blood cells to the site of inflammation. The first white blood cells to arrive are the neutrophils. Neutrophils phagocytize dead tissue and microorganisms. The process of phagocytosis creates pH changes both within the neutrophils and in the site. As the pH changes, neutrophils become unable to phagocytize any further and the cells quickly die. At this point, macrophages move in to the site and pick up the phagocytic activity. Cytology samples from inflammatory sites are therefore characterized by the presence of white blood cells, particularly neutrophils and macrophages. Occasionally eosinophils or lymphocytes may also be present. In fluid samples, total nucleated cell counts of greater than 5000/µl is a common finding with inflammation. The fluid is often turbid and may be white or pale yellow. Total protein is often greater than 3 g/dl

Inflammation can be categorized as suppurative (purulent), granulomatous, pyogranulomatous, or eosinophilic based on the relative numbers of the various cell types present.

Suppurative (purulent) inflammation (Fig. 9-28) is characterized by the presence of large numbers of neutrophils, usually greater than 85% of the total nucleated cell count. When significant numbers of macrophages are present (greater than 15%), the sample is classified as granulomatous or pyogranulomatous (Fig. 9-29). Fungal and parasitic infections often manifest with this presentation. The

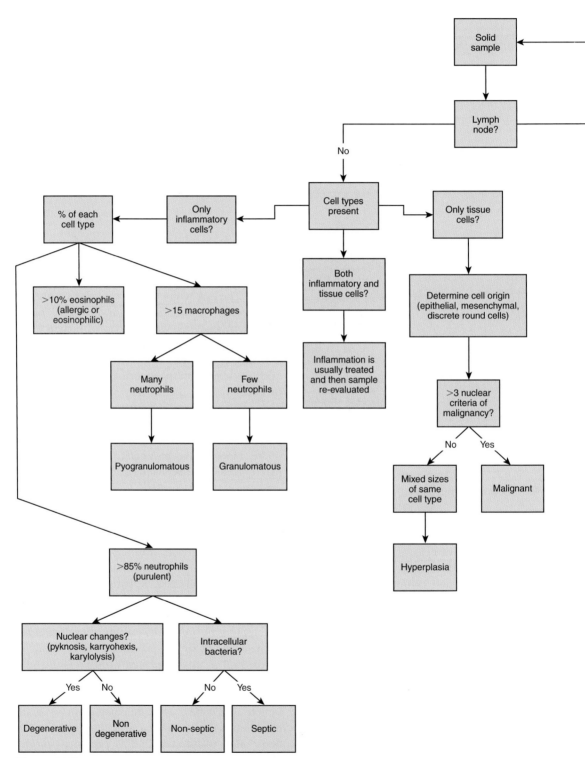

Figure 9-27. Flow chart for the examination of cytology specimens.

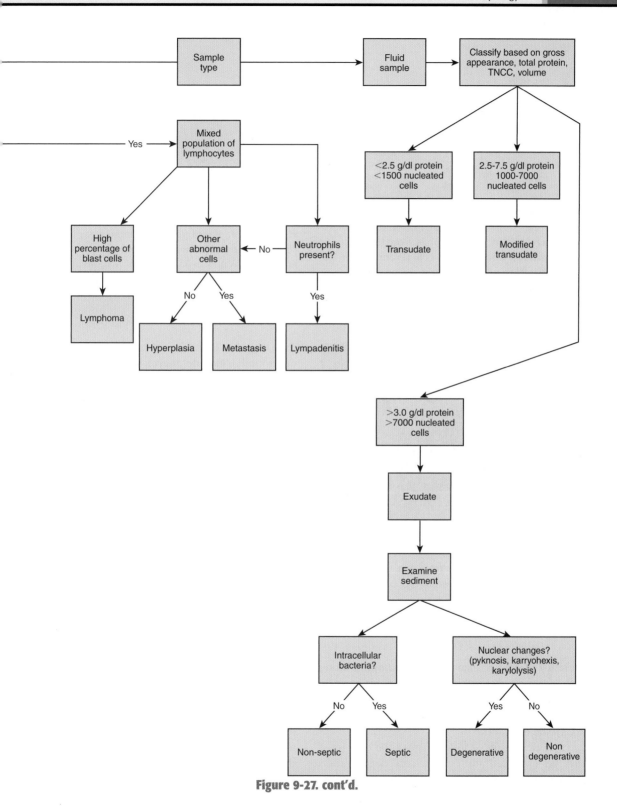

Figure 9-27. cont'd.

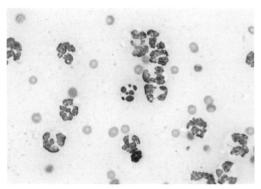

Figure 9-28. Suppurative inflammation as evidenced by the large number of neutrophils. Note the presence of karyorrhexis in the center cell. (From Raskin RE, Meyer DJ: *Atlas of canine and feline cytology*, St Louis, 2001, Saunders.)

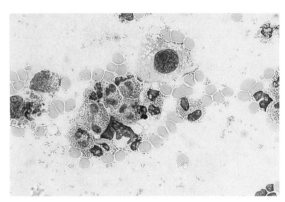

Figure 9-30. Eosinophilic inflammation. Note the single macrophage and numerous free eosinophilic granules. (From Cowell RL, Tyler RD, Meinkoth JH: *Diagnostic cytology and hematology of the dog and cat*, ed 2, St Louis, 1999, Mosby.)

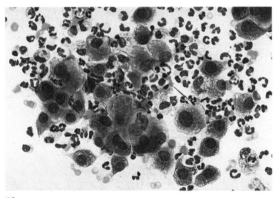

Figure 9-29. Pyogranulomatous inflammation. Macrophages represent more than 15% of the cells present. (From Cowell RL, Tyler RD, Meinkoth JH: *Diagnostic cytology and hematology of the dog and cat*, ed 2, St Louis, 1999, Mosby.)

presence of greater than 10% of eosinophils along with increased neutrophils indicates an eosinophilic inflammation (Fig. 9-30). This is usually found with parasitic infection but may also be present in some neoplastic disorders.

Once designated as inflammatory, the cells must also be evaluated for evidence of degeneration and presence of microorganisms. Nuclear changes that may be found in inflammatory cells (e.g., neutrophils) include karyolysis, karyorrhexis, and pyknosis, with karyolysis having the greatest significance. Pyknosis represents slow cell death (aging) and refers to a small, condensed, dark nucleus that may fragment (karyorrhexis). Karyolysis represents rapid cell death, as in some septic (bacterial) inflammatory reactions, and appears as a swollen, ragged nucleus without an intact nuclear membrane and with reduced staining intensity. Cells should also be evaluated for the presence of bacteria. Inflammatory cells that contain phagocytized microorganisms are referred to as septic (Fig. 9-31). Additional phagocytized material may include erythrocytes, parasites, and fungal organisms (Fig. 9-32).

Neoplasia

Unlike inflammation, neoplastic specimens normally contain rather homogeneous populations of a single cell type. Although mixed cells populations are sometimes seen, these usually involve a neoplastic area with a concurrent inflammation. Neoplasia is indicated when the cells present are of the same tissue origin. Once identified as neoplastic, the technician should identify the tissue origin and evaluate the cells for the presence of malignant characteristics (Table 9-2).

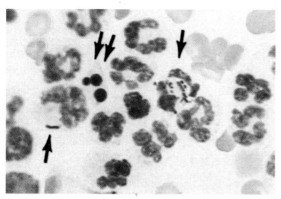

Figure 9-31. Septic inflammation. Degenerated neutrophils with phagocytized bacterial rods. A pyknotic cell *(double arrow)* is also present. (From Cowell RL, Tyler RD, Meinkoth JH: *Diagnostic cytology and hematology of the dog and cat,* ed 2, St Louis, 1999, Mosby.)

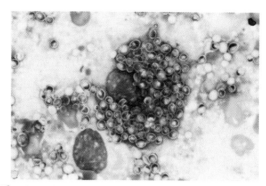

Figure 9-32. A macrophage with phagocytized *Histoplasma capsulatum* organisms. Numerous organisms are also free in the sample. (From Raskin RE, Meyer DJ: *Atlas of canine and feline cytology,* St Louis, 2001, Saunders.)

Neoplasia must first be differentiated as either benign or malignant. Benign neoplasia is represented by hyperplasia with no criteria of malignancy present in the nucleus of the cells. The cells are of the same type and are relatively uniform in appearance. Cells that display at least three abnormal nuclear configurations are identified as malignant. Nuclear criteria of malignancy can include any of the following:

- Anisokaryosis: Any unusual variation in overall cell size.
- Pleomorphism: Variability in the size and shape of same cell type.
- High or variable nucleus/cytoplasm ratio
- Increased mitotic activity: Mitosis is rare in normal tissue, and cells usually divide evenly in two Any increase in the present of mitotic figures or cells that are not dividing equally is considered a malignant criteria.
- Coarse chromatin pattern: The chromatin pattern is coarser than normal and may appear ropy or cordlike.
- Nuclear molding: A deformation of nuclei by other nuclei within the same cell or adjacent cells.
- Multinucleation: Multiple nuclei within a cell.

- Nucleoli that vary in size (anisonucleoliosis), shape (angular nucleoli), and number (multiple nucleoli).

In general, if three or more nuclear criteria of malignancy are present, the specimen is identified as malignant. Exceptions to this general rule are indicated if inflammation is also present or only a few cells display malignant characteristics. Histopathologic verification of cytologic findings is important for most tumors (whether cytologically benign or malignant). Also, cytologically benign cells may be obtained from malignant tumors. Histopathologic examination offers the advantage of enabling assessment of factors such as local tissue infiltration and vessel or lymphatic invasion by tumor cells. These characteristics of malignant tumors are not evident cytologically.

Specimens that have been classified as malignant should be further evaluated to determine the cell type involved. The primary types of tumors encountered in veterinary medicine are categorized as epithelial cell tumors, mesenchymal cell tumors, and discrete round cell tumors. The overall characteristics of samples from each of these cell types are summarized in Table 9-3. A variety of terminology is used to describe these various tumor types, and some references may differ in their classifications of specific types of tumors.

TABLE 9-2

Nuclear Criteria of Malignancy

Criteria	Description	Schematic Representation
Nuclear Criteria		
Macrokaryosis	Increased nuclear size. Cells with nuclei larger than 10 μ in diameter suggest malignancy.	RBC
Increased nucleus: cytoplasm ratio (N:C)	Normal nonlymphoid cells usually have an N:C of 1:3 to 1:8; depending on the tissue. Ratios ≥ 1:2 suggest malignancy.	See *"Macrokaryosis"*
Anisokaryosis	Variation in nuclear size. This is especially important if the nuclei of multinucleated cells vary in size.	
Multinucleation	Multiple nucleation in a cell. This is especially important if the nuclei vary in size.	
Increased mitotic figures	Mitosis is rare in normal tissue.	Normal Abnormal
Abnormal mitosis	Chromosomes are improperly aligned.	See *Increased mitotic figures*
Coarse chromatin pattern	The chromatin pattern is coarser than normal. It may appear ropy or cordlike.	
Nuclear molding	Nuclei are deformed by other nuclei within the same cell or adjacent cells.	
Macronucleoli	Nucleoli are increased in size. Nucleoli ≥5 μ strongly suggest malignancy. For reference, RBCs are 5 to 6 μ in cats and 7 to 8 μ in dogs.	RBC
Angular nucleoli	Nucleoli are fusiform or have other angular shapes; instead of their normal round to slightly oval shape.	
Anisonucleoliosis	Nucleolar shape or size varies. This is especially important if the variation is within the same nucleus.	See *"Angular nucleoli"*

RBC, Red blood cell.

TABLE 9-3

Characteristics of Tumor Types

Tumor Type	Cell Size	Cell Shape	Cellularity	Clumps or Clusters
Epithelial	Large	Round to caudate	Usually high	Common
Mesenchymal	Small to medium	Spindle to stellate	Usually low	Uncommon
Discrete round cell	Small to medium	Round	Usually high (except histiocytoma)	Uncommon

Epithelial cell tumors are also referred to as carcinoma or adenocarcinoma. The samples tend to be highly cellular and often exfoliate in clumps or sheets (Fig. 9-33). Mesenchymal cell tumors are also referred to as sarcoma and are usually less cellular. The cells tend to exfoliate singly or in wispy spindles (Fig. 9-34). Discrete round cell tumors exfoliate very well but are usually not in clumps or clusters. Round cell tumors include histiocytoma, lymphoma, mast cell tumors, plasma cell tumors, transmissible venereal tumors, and melanoma. Histiocytoma and transmissible venereal tumors appear somewhat similar except that histiocytoma is not usually highly cellular (Fig. 9-35). Plasma cell tumors can be recognized by the presence of large numbers of cells with an eccentrically located nucleus and prominent perinuclear clear zone (Fig. 9-36). Mast cells can be recognized

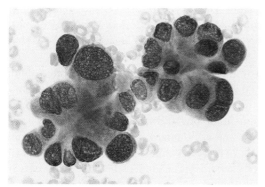

Figure 9-33. Lung carcinoma. Clusters of cells with anisokaryosis, binucleation, and high and variable nucleus/cytoplasm ratios. (From Raskin RE, Meyer DJ: *Atlas of canine and feline cytology,* St Louis, 2001, Saunders.)

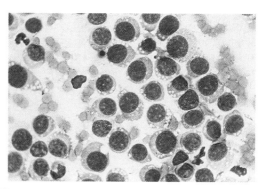

Figure 9-35. Large numbers of round cells from an imprint of a transmissible venereal tumor. (From Raskin RE, Meyer DJ: *Atlas of canine and feline cytology,* St Louis, 2001, Saunders.)

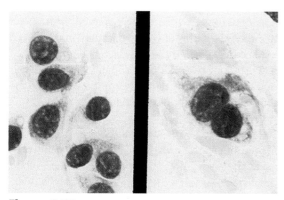

Figure 9-34. Sarcoma. Aspirate from a malignant spindle cell tumor with cells showing anisokaryosis; anisonucleiosis; and large, prominent, and occasionally angular nucleoli. (From Cowell RL, Tyler RD, Meinkoth JH: *Diagnostic cytology and hematology of the dog and cat,* ed 2, St Louis, 1999, Mosby.)

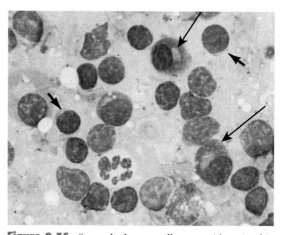

Figure 9-36. Several plasma cells are evident in this sample *(long arrows)* from a hyperplastic lymph node. Small lymphocytes are also present *(short arrows).* (From Cowell RL, Tyler RD, Meinkoth JH: *Diagnostic cytology and hematology of the dog and cat,* ed 2, St Louis, 1999, Mosby.)

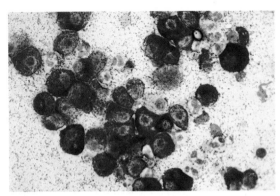

Figure 9-37. Aspirate from a highly granular mast cell tumor. Several eosinophils are also present. (From Cowell RL, Tyler RD, Meinkoth JH: *Diagnostic cytology and hematology of the dog and cat,* ed 2, St Louis, 1999, Mosby.)

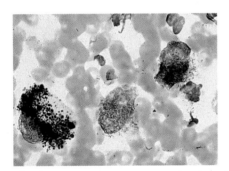

Figure 9-38. A melanophage *(lower left cell)* and two melanocytes. (From Cowell RL, Tyler RD, Meinkoth JH: *Diagnostic cytology and hematology of the dog and cat,* ed 2, St Louis, 1999, Mosby.)

by their prominent purple/black granules (Fig. 9-37). Melanoma is characterized by cells with prominent dark black granules (Fig. 9-38). Occasionally, cells from poorly differentiated tumors may contain few or no granules (amelanotic melanoma).

CYTOLOGY OF SPECIFIC SITES

Peritoneal and Pleural Fluid

Under normal circumstances, the peritoneal and thoracic cavities contain only enough fluid to ade-

quately lubricate the surfaces of the organs and the cavity walls. Fluid is collected in EDTA tubes for total nucleated cell counts, cytologic examination, and refractometric protein measurements and in a plain tube for determination of the total protein concentration. Other clinical chemistry determinations are performed infrequently on peritoneal and pleural fluid.

Color, Turbidity, and Odor

Normal peritoneal and pleural fluids are colorless to straw yellow and transparent to slightly turbid. Both fluids should be odorless. Gross discoloration and increased turbidity may be the result of increased cell numbers and/or protein concentration. Collection of malodorous peritoneal fluid at abdominocentesis may indicate a necrotic segment of bowel within the peritoneal cavity, a ruptured segment of bowel with free gut contents in the cavity, or accidental enterocentesis. These conditions may be distinguishable cytologically and by reference to other clinical findings. Although not commonly seen, chylothorax may be evident as a "milky" fluid, especially if the animal has recently eaten, because of the chylous effusion's high fat content and large number of mature lymphocytes. In fasted animals, the fluid may be tan. Unlike fluids with high leukocyte counts (which also may have a whitish color), chylous fluid does not have a clear supernatant after centrifugation. The fat in chylous fluid is present as small droplets (chylomicrons), which can be stained with Sudan III or IV. The fat in chylous fluid may be dissolved with ether after the fluid has been alkalinized with sodium hydroxide or sodium bicarbonate. If significant numbers of erythrocytes are present, the fluid may have a reddish color.

Total Nucleated Cell Count

A total nucleated cell count (TNCC) is performed using the same methods as for a complete blood count (see Chapter 2). As a cross-species generalization, normal peritoneal and pleural fluids have less than 10,000 nucleated cells/µl, usually 2000 to 6000/µl. Mononuclear cells may be visible as clusters of cells, which can make counting individual cells difficult.

A differential count of at least 100 nucleated cells should be performed, noting cell type and morphologic characteristics. Nucleated cells are categorized as neutrophils, large mononuclear cells (a collective grouping of mesothelial cells and macrophages), lymphocytes, eosinophils, and any other nucleated cells. Notes on cell morphologic characteristics should include comments on nuclear and cytoplasmic appearance. If bacteria are present, their morphologic features (bacilli, coccobacilli, cocci) and location (free or intracellular; i.e., phagocytosed) must be recorded. In such cases, another smear can be stained with Gram stain and the fluid cultured.

Cellular Elements

Normal peritoneal and pleural fluids contain few erythrocytes. The number present on a smear should be estimated. Suitable categories include rare, few, many, and large numbers. The number present varies with the method of sample preparation. Iatrogenic contamination and acute and chronic hemorrhage are distinguished grossly, as previously outlined. If erythrocytes have been present in the fluid for several hours, they may be

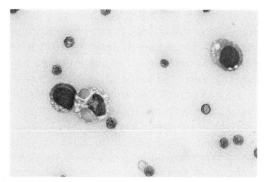

Figure 9-39. Fluid aspirate with macrophages. One cell is exhibiting erythrophagia. (From Raskin RE, Meyer DJ: *Atlas of canine and feline cytology*, St Louis, 2001, Saunders.)

phagocytosed by macrophages (erythrophagocytosis) (Fig. 9-39).

Peritoneal and pleural fluid samples should also be evaluated for cellularity. The TNCC and total protein values for the sample allow it to be classified as transudate, modified transudate, or exudate (Table 9-4). Published normal values for peritoneal and pleural fluid cytology of dogs and

TABLE 9-4

Characteristics of Fluid Samples

	Transudate	Exudate	Normal	Modified Transudate
Origin	Noninflammatory hypoalbuminemia Vascular stasis Neoplasia	Inflammatory Infection Necrosis		Feline infectious peritonitis Chylous effusion Lymphatic fluid
Amount of fluid	Large	Variable	Small	Variable
Color	Clear, colorless, or red tinged	Turbid, white, slightly yellow	Clear, colorless	Variable, usually clear
Protein	<3.0 g/dL	>3.0 g/dL	<2.5 g/dL	2.5-7.5 g/dL
TNCC	<1500/μL	>5000/μL	<3000/μL	1000-7000/μL
Cell types	Mixture of monocytes, macrophages, lymphocytes, and mesothelial cells* (normal and/or reactive)	Inflammatory: neutrophils, macrophages, lymphocytes,* and eosinophils*	Same as transudate	Lymphocytes, nondegenerate neutrophils, mesothelial cells, macrophages, and neoplastic cells

*Variable numbers.

cats are scarce. Normal horses generally have an average of approximately 55% to 60% neutrophils, 25% to 30% large mononuclear cells, 10% to 20% lymphocytes, and an occasional eosinophil (less than 1%). Values for cattle are somewhat similar, but normal animals often have comparable numbers of neutrophils and lymphocytes.

Exudates are fluids with increased cellularity and protein concentration because of inflammation. The following cross-species generalization can be made. Suppurative inflammatory reactions increase the total cell count, the percentage, and the absolute numbers of neutrophils to greater than 85% of the nucleated cells. Suppurative inflammatory reactions usually cause high-normal to elevated total nucleated cell counts, with elevated neutrophil percentages and numerous mesothelial cells and/or macrophages. Mesothelial cells line the body cavities. In the presence of increased fluid within the cavities, these cells may become reactive (i.e., multinucleate, with anisocytosis and anisokaryosis, prominent nucleoli, and basophilic cytoplasm) (Fig. 9-40). Reactive mesothelial cells may be difficult to distinguish from some neoplastic cells. Some mesothelial cells may be present as clusters or rafts of cells. These clusters result from proliferation and exfoliation of cells from the peritoneal lining, or mesothelium, in response to a decrease in contact inhibition

between cells on opposing surfaces of the peritoneum, because of the effusion. Macrophages may phagocytize degenerate cells or cellular debris. Migrating parasite larvae can cause increased neutrophil and eosinophil percentages, with or without an elevated total nucleated cell count.

Cellular morphologic features depend on microorganism(s) present and may vary from cytoplasmic vacuolation with few nuclear changes evident to marked cytoplasmic vacuolation, marked nuclear swelling and disruption (karyolysis), and general cellular degeneration or fragmentation. Bacteria may be evident within the cytoplasm of neutrophils and/or macrophages (Fig. 9-41). Cases of simple peritonitis may have a single type of bacterium evident or the bacterial population may be mixed as a result of devitalization or rupture of the bowel. Accidental penetration of the bowel during abdominocentesis may also result in a mixed pop-

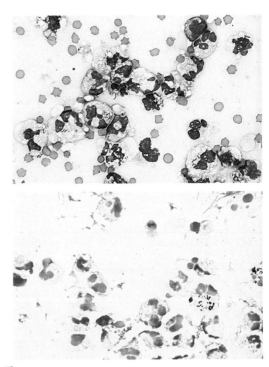

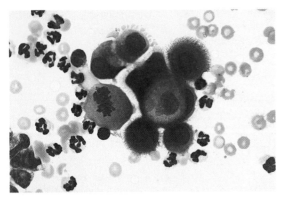

Figure 9-40. A cluster of reactive mesothelial cells. Note the mitotic figure. (From Cowell RL, Tyler RD, and Meinkoth JH: *Diagnostic cytology and hematology of the dog and cat,* ed 2, St Louis, 1999, Mosby.)

Figure 9-41. Septic exudates. Note the presence of intracellular bacterial rods. (From Raskin RE, Meyer DJ: *Atlas of canine and feline cytology,* St Louis, 2001, Saunders.)

ulation of bacteria in the smear. However, in the latter case, leukocyte numbers and morphologic characteristics are usually normal, and the bacteria are frequently not phagocytosed. Large ciliated organisms also may be noted in large-bowel enterocentesis in horses.

Transudates (ascitic effusions) typically have low protein concentrations and low total nucleated cell counts (less than 1500/μl), with fairly normal differential counts or possibly an increase in the percentage of large mononuclear cells (Fig. 9-42). The mononuclear cells are principally mesothelial cells, which may be in clusters or rafts and may be quite reactive in appearance. Transudates are frequently secondary to congestive heart failure or may occur in animals with low blood albumin concentration.

Modified transudates are characterized by relatively low to moderate total cell counts, predominantly resulting from leakage of lymphatics. This leakage is responsible for the high total protein concentration of modified transudates. Cells present include low numbers of inflammatory cells (nondegenerate), mostly small mature lymphocytes; few macrophages; and some mesothelial cells (Fig. 9-43).

Intraabdominal tumors may exfoliate cells into the peritoneal fluid. Cytologic diagnosis of such neoplasia may be difficult and is often a task for

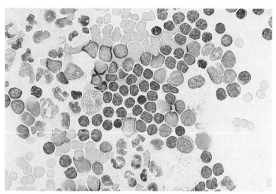

Figure 9-43. Smear from a chylous effusion. A mixture of mature lymphocytes, neutrophils, and an eosinophil are present. This is characteristic of a modified transudate. (From Cowell RL, Tyler RD, Meinkoth JH: *Diagnostic cytology and hematology of the dog and cat,* ed 2, St Louis, 1999, Mosby.)

a specialist cytologist. However, the technician should be able to recognize abnormal lymphocytes by using the criteria of malignancy previously outlined and should be suspicious of clusters of pleomorphic, secretory-type cells. The presence of unexpected cells, such as mast cells, must also be noted.

Lymph Nodes

Cytologic evaluation of lymph node tissue is performed to diagnose causes of lymph node enlargement and differentiate hyperplasia, inflammation, primary neoplasia (lymphoma), and metastatic neoplasia. Lymph nodes may show evidence of inflammation (lymphadenitis), hyperplasia (benign neoplasia), mixed (both inflammatory and neoplastic cells present), neoplasia (lymph node cells with abnormal nuclear features), and metastasis (neoplastic cells from other body tissues that spread to lymph nodes). Each of these has specific cell types associated with the abnormality.

Lymph node tissue is normally collected from the periphery of an enlarged lymph node by fine-needle biopsy. In patients with generalized lymphadenopathy, samples should be obtained from two lymph nodes. Because lymph nodes that drain

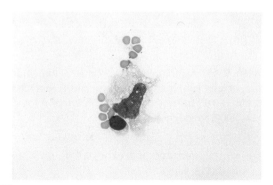

Figure 9-42. Macrophage, small lymphocyte, and several red blood cells. This sample is characteristic of normal fluid and transudates. (From Raskin RE, Meyer DJ: *Atlas of canine and feline cytology,* St Louis, 2001, Saunders.)

TABLE 9-5

Cell Types Found in Lymph Node Aspirates

Cell Type	Characteristics
Lymphocytes, small	Similar in appearance to the small lymphocyte seen on a peripheral blood film. Slightly larger than a Scanty cytoplasm, dense nucleus.
Lymphocytes, intermediate	Nucleus approximately twice as large as an RBC. Abundant cytoplasm.
Lymphoblasts	Two to four times as large as an RBC. Usually contain a nucleolus. Diffuse nuclear chromatin.
Plasma cells	Eccentrically located nucleus, trailing basophilic cytoplasm, perinuclear clear zone. Vacuoles and/or Russell bodies may be present.
Plasmablasts	Similar to lymphoblasts with more abundant, basophilic cytoplasm. May contain vacuoles.
Neutrophils	May appear similar to neutrophils in peripheral blood or show degenerative changes.
Macrophages	Large phagocytic cell. May contain phagocytized debris, microorganisms, etc. Abundant cytoplasm.
Mast cells	Round cells that are usually slightly larger than lymphoblasts. Distinctive purple-staining granules may not stain adequately with Diff-Quik.
Carcinoma cells	Epithelial tissue origin. Usually found in clusters; pleomorphic.
Sarcoma cells	Connective tissue origin. Usually occur singly with spindle-shaped cytoplasm.
Histiocytes	Large, pleomorphic, single or multinuclear; nuclei are round to oval.

the oral cavity and gastrointestinal tract are antigenically stimulated under normal conditions, these should be avoided. Samples are then prepared by the compression technique and stained with standard Romanowsky-type stains.

A variety of cell types may be found in lymph node aspirates. These include lymphocytes, plasma cells, white blood cells, and neoplastic cells. Microorganisms, lymphoglandular bodies, and bacteria may also be present. Lymphoglandular bodies are small cytoplasmic fragments that may be seen between cells and are not a pathologic feature. Table 9-5 contains a summary of the cell types that may be found in lymph node aspirates.

In a normal lymph node, the predominant cell type is the small, mature lymphocyte. These tend to comprise more than three fourths of the total cells present. Smaller numbers of intermediate lymphocytes and lymphoblasts as well as macrophages are also present. Plasma cells may occasionally be seen (Fig. 9-44). Mast cells are usually rare in cytologic preparations of lymph node tissue. Lymph nodes with evidence of inflammation (lymphadenitis) will

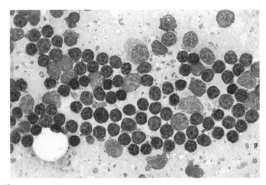

Figure 9-44. Aspirate from a normal lymph node. Small, mature lymphocytes predominate. (From Raskin RE, Meyer DJ: *Atlas of canine and feline cytology*, St Louis, 2001, Saunders.)

have a predominance of leukocytes, as previously described (Fig. 9-45).

Reactive Lymph Node

Lymph nodes that are responding to antigenic stimulation also contain predominantly small, mature lymphocytes. However, plasma cells, lym-

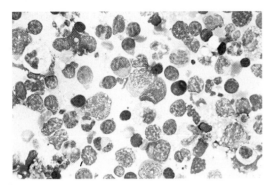

Figure 9-45. Pyogranulomatous lymphadenitis. Numerous macrophages and neutrophils are evident along with a mixture of lymphocyte types. (From Raskin RE, Meyer DJ: *Atlas of canine and feline cytology*, St Louis, 2001, Saunders.)

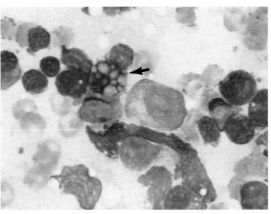

Figure 9-47. The plasma cell that appears vacuolated *(arrow)* is a Mott cell containing Russell bodies. Small lymphocytes and lymphoblasts are also present. (From Cowell RL, Tyler RD, Meinkoth JH: *Diagnostic cytology and hematology of the dog and cat*, ed 2, St Louis, 1999, Mosby.)

phoblasts, and intermediate lymphocytes are more abundant than in a normal lymph node (Fig. 9-46). Occasional Mott cells (plasma cells containing secretory vesicles of immunoglobulin) may also be seen (Fig. 9-47). Antigenic stimulation can also cause an inflammatory response and would be characterized by the presence of neutrophils and/or macrophages.

Malignant Neoplasia

Primary lymphoid neoplasia, or lymphoma, is characterized by a predominance of lymphoblasts,

and mitotic figures are common. Macrophages are also present, and plasma cells are scarce. Other neoplastic cells that may be present in lymph node aspirates include mast cells, carcinoma cells, sarcoma cells, and histiocytes. Cells that display at least three abnormal nuclear configurations usually are identified as malignant (Fig. 9-48). Lymph node

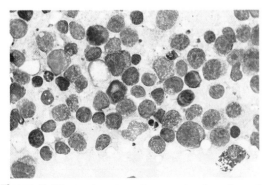

Figure 9-46. An imprint of a reactive lymph node. Note the mixed population of small, medium, and large lymphocytes, plasma cells, and a mast cell *(lower right)*. (From Raskin RE, Meyer DJ: *Atlas of canine and feline cytology*, St Louis, 2001, Saunders.)

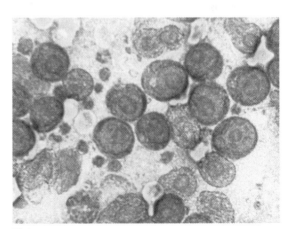

Figure 9-48. Immature, neoplastic lymphocytes are present in this sample from a dog with malignant lymphoma. (From Cowell RL, Tyler RD, Meinkoth JH: *Diagnostic cytology and hematology of the dog and cat*, ed 2, St Louis, 1999, Mosby.)

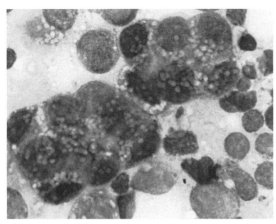

Figure 9-49. An epithelial cell cluster from a transitional cell carcinoma that metastasized to a local lymph node. (From Cowell RL, Tyler RD, Meinkoth JH: *Diagnostic cytology and hematology of the dog and cat,* ed 2, St Louis, 1999, Mosby.)

samples may also contain metastatic cells from other body parts (Fig. 9-49).

Cerebrospinal Fluid

As a cross-species generalization, normal CSF contains no erythrocytes and less than 25 nucleated cells per milliliter (usually 0 to 10/L) (Fig. 9-50). Pleocytosis is an elevated CSF nucleated cell count.

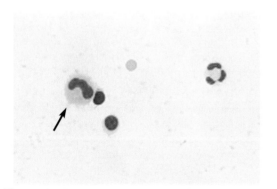

Figure 9-50. Cell types found in CSF. Two small lymphocytes, one large mononuclear cell *(arrow),* one neutrophil, and one erythrocyte are present. (From Raskin RE, Meyer DJ: *Atlas of canine and feline cytology,* St Louis, 2001, Saunders.)

Normal CSF contains 95% to 100% mononuclear cells, almost all of which are lymphocytes. Bacterial infections involving CSF generally cause marked pleocytosis, mostly because of neutrophils. Inflammation associated with viruses, fungi, neoplasia, or degenerative conditions generally causes less dramatic pleocytosis, with a significant proportion of mononuclear cells (often lymphocytes). Eosinophils sometimes are seen, especially in parasitic inflammatory responses. In general, the causative agent often is not cytologically apparent. Neoplastic cells are seldom observed in CSF.

Normal CSF contains virtually no erythrocytes. Erythrocytes may be counted by charging a hemacytometer with a well-mixed sample of undiluted and unstained CSF. All cells in the entire boxed area of one side are counted. With this method both erythrocytes and nucleated cells are observed. Distinguishing between these two groups of cells is usually possible, but not to subcategorize the nucleated cells. Cell counts for undiluted CSF are multiplied by 1.1 to give the total number of cells per milliliter. (If ethanol-diluted CSF is used, the cell counts are multiplied by 2.2.) If distinguishing erythrocytes from nucleated cells in unstained CSF is difficult, the total number of cells counted by the latter method can be subtracted from the number of nucleated cells counted to calculate the erythrocyte count.

Use of various correction factors has been advocated to adjust CSF nucleated cell counts (NCC) for any peripheral blood leukocytic contamination. Because normal CSF contains no erythrocytes, the observed nucleated cell count may be corrected if the number of erythrocytes per milliliter of CSF is known. The simplest approach is to consider that each 500 to 1000 erythrocytes would be accompanied by one leukocyte. A more complicated method is to use the following equation:

$$\text{Corrected NCC} = \frac{\text{observed NCC}}{\text{blood WBC} \times \dfrac{\text{CSF RBC}}{\text{blood RBC}}}$$

This equation requires values for blood leukocyte (white blood cells) and erythrocyte (red blood cell) counts and a CSF erythrocyte count.

Despite its complexity, it is no more accurate than the preceding approximation. Ideally CSF samples should be free of iatrogenic peripheral blood contamination. Use of the previous correction factor is, at best, a rough guide to the uncontaminated CSF nucleated cell count.

In addition to the cytology evaluation, a variety of chemical and immunologic tests are performed on CSF samples. These include the Pandy test, Nonne-Apelt test, sulfosalicylic acid test, trichloroacetic acid test, fibrinogen concentration, glucose concentration, lactate concentration, electrolyte concentrations, and creatine kinase concentration. These tests are discussed further in Chapter 3.

Aqueous and Vitreous Humor

Fluid from the eye is similar to CSF in that it has low cellularity, being composed of mostly small mononuclear cells, essentially no erythrocytes, and a low protein concentration. Interpretation of changes in aqueous humor is similar to that for CSF.

Synovial Fluid Analysis

If only one or two drops can be obtained, as in some normal joints of cats and dogs, gross assessment of fluid color and turbidity and cytologic examination of a direct smear, possibly with concurrent subjective assessment of viscosity, may be all that is practical. If 0.5 to 1 ml is collected, a total nucleated cell count and refractometric protein measurement (on EDTA-preserved fluid) may be added to the list of tests. Collection of larger volumes permits additional tests, such as the mucin clot test.

Color and Turbidity

Normal synovial fluid is clear to straw yellow and nonturbid. Yellow synovial fluid is common in large animals, especially horses. Turbidity, when present, is caused by cells, protein (or fibrin), or cartilage.

Normal synovial fluid contains few erythrocytes. Iatrogenic contamination at arthrocentesis is common. Differentiation of contamination and recent or old hemorrhage is as previously described.

Viscosity

Viscosity reflects the quality and concentration of hyaluronic acid, which is part of the synovial fluid mucin complex. The function of mucin is joint lubrication. Viscosity may be quantitated with a viscometer; however, subjective assessment is most often used.

Normal synovial fluid is sticky. If a drop is placed between the thumb and forefinger, as the digits are separated it forms a 1- to 2-inch strand before breaking. Similarly, when gently expressed through a needle on a horizontally held syringe, it hangs in a 1- to 2-inch strand before separating from the needle tip.

In general, viscosity is not decreased in normal joints and those with degenerative problems. It frequently is decreased in joints with bacterial inflammation as a result of mucin degradation by bacterial hyaluronidase and in joints with a significant effusion (including hydrarthrosis) as a result of dilution of mucin (and hyaluronic acid).

Because EDTA may degrade hyaluronic acid, both viscosity and mucin clot formation usually are assessed on fluid to which no anticoagulant has been added. If anticoagulation is necessary because of a high fluid fibrinogen concentration, heparin is the preferred anticoagulant.

Cytologic Examination (Cell Counts)

Slides for cytologic examination may be prepared on EDTA-preserved fluid or fluid without anticoagulant, the latter especially if only a few drops are obtained and the smear is made immediately. Thin smears are made by slowly advancing the spreader slide. Because of the high viscosity of normal synovial fluid, cells usually do not accumulate at the feathered edge of the smear. Margination of cells increases as viscosity of the fluid decreases. At low cell counts, especially less than 500/μl, concentration of cells by centrifugal sedimentation and subsequent resuspension of cells in a small volume of supernatant fluid produces a more cellular smear. Slides usually are stained with a Romanowsky stain. Table 9-6 summarizes classification of synovial fluid.

Normal synovial fluid generally contains at least 90% mononuclear cells and less than 10%

TABLE 9-6

Classification of Synovial Fluid

	Normal	Hemarthrosis	Degenerative Arthropathy	Inflammatory Arthropathy
Appearance	Clear to straw colored	Red, cloudy, or xanthochromic	Clear	Cloudy
Protein	<2.5 g/dL	Increased	Normal to decreased	Normal to increased
Viscosity	High	Decreased	Normal to decreased	Normal to decreased
Mucin clot	Good	Normal to poor	Normal to poor	Fair to poor
Cell count (/μL)	<3000	Increased RBCs	1000 to 10,000	5000 to >100,000
PMN	<5%	Relative to blood	<10%	>10 to 100%
Mononuclear	>95%	Relative to blood	>90%	10 to <90%
Comments	Only a small amount should be present (<0.5ml in most joints)	Erythrophagia helps confirm previous hemorrhage	Cells are typically macrophages or found in thick sheets (synoviocytes)	Septic and nonseptic etiologies. Bacteria are rarely observed in infected joints

From Raskin RE, Meyer DJ: *Atlas of canine and feline cytology,* St Louis, 2001, Saunders.

neutrophils (Fig. 9-51). Eosinophils are rarely observed. Mononuclear cells comprise about equal numbers of lymphocytes and monocytic/macrophage-type cells, which are nonvacuolated and nonphagocytic. Large vacuolated or phagocytic mononuclear cells comprise less than 10% of the differential count of normal synovial fluid.

Macrophages become vacuolated in normal synovial fluid that is not processed soon after collection; therefore prompt preparation of smears is important to prevent this artificial finding.

Cells in synovial fluid with good viscosity tend to align in a linear fashion in the direction of the smear, giving a "windrow" appearance (Fig. 9-52).

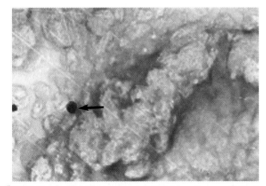

Figure 9-51. Normal synovial fluid has low cellularity with primarily mononuclear cells *(arrow)*. The background material is related to the mucin content and may appear granular to ropy. (From Raskin RE, Meyer DJ: *Atlas of canine and feline cytology,* St Louis, 2001, Saunders.)

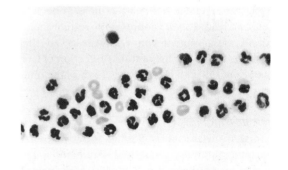

Figure 9-52. Synovial fluid from a patient with inflammatory joint disease. These neutrophils are in the typical "windrow" arrangement commonly seen in synovial fluid. (From Raskin RE, Meyer DJ: *Atlas of canine and feline cytology,* St Louis, 2001, Saunders.)

Mucin precipitation produces an eosinophilic granular background in Romanowsky-stained smears, the density of which reflects smear thickness. Cells in smears from viscous fluid may not spread out well on the slide, which can make their identification difficult. Such fluid may be diluted 1:1 with saline-reconstituted hyaluronidase (150 U/ml). This decreases sample viscosity after a few minutes, allowing more accurate cell morphology when smeared.

As a generalization, mononuclear cells predominate in traumatic and degenerative arthropathies, usually with increased numbers of large vacuolated or phagocytic cells.

Occasionally when joint erosion has progressed through to subchondral bone, osteoclasts may be observed. In contrast, neutrophils predominate in infectious arthropathies (because of bacteria, viruses, and mycoplasmas, for example) and many noninfectious conditions, such as rheumatoid arthritis and systemic lupus erythematosus. When cells are clumped together in a smear, NMB stain may demonstrate interlocking fibrin strands. Rarely the causative organism in septic joint fluid may be observed cytologically, especially when phagocytosed. Culture is recommended when an infectious process is suspected. A granulomatous type of arthropathy is suggested when neutrophils and vacuolated/phagocytic macrophages are both increased in number. Lupus erythematosus cells, which are neutrophils or macrophages containing phagocytosed nuclear chromatin, are seen occasionally in the synovial fluid of animals with systemic lupus erythematosus.

Tracheal Wash

Total nucleated cell counts are usually not performed on tracheal wash fluids. Cell numbers are subjectively recorded from evaluation of the smear. A tracheal wash smear from a normal animal contains few cells, usually with a small amount of mucus. The mucus often appears microscopically as eosinophilic to purple strands that may enmesh the cells. Epithelial cells are the principal cell type. If the sample is collected from the level of the trachea, ciliated epithelial cells predominate.

These cells are columnar to cuboidal, with a polar nucleus on the border opposite the cilia (Fig. 9-53). If the specimen is collected from the bronchi, bronchoalveolar epithelial cells are also fairly common. They are round, nonciliated cells with basophilic cytoplasm and may occur in clumps. A few goblet cells (secretory epithelial cells) also may be observed (Fig. 9-54).

If the sample is a bronchoalveolar wash, alveolar macrophages may predominate. These are large individual cells with a large round to oval nucleus

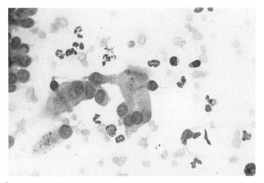

Figure 9-53. Normal ciliated columnar epithelial cells in a normal tracheal wash sample. (From Raskin RE, Meyer DJ: *Atlas of canine and feline cytology,* St Louis, 2001, Saunders.)

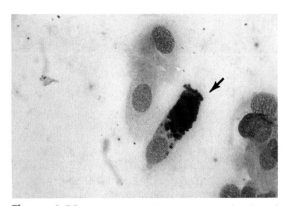

Figure 9-54. A goblet cell *(arrow)* and ciliated columnar cells in a tracheal wash sample. (From Cowell RL, Tyler RD, and Meinkoth JH: *Diagnostic cytology and hematology of the dog and cat,* ed 2, St Louis, 1999, Mosby.)

and a moderate amount of basophilic cytoplasm. If they become reactive or activated, the cytoplasm increases in volume and becomes more granular and vacuolated. Neutrophils, lymphocytes, eosinophils, plasma cells, mast cells, and erythrocytes are seen rarely in specimens from normal animals.

Abnormal tracheal washes are generally exudates. These samples contain numerous mucus strands and are cellular. Eosinophilic, spiral casts from small bronchioles (Curschmann's spirals) suggest a chronic bronchiolar problem (Fig. 9-55). Cell morphology is highly variable among and within samples. Many cells may be unidentifiable. Neutrophils and macrophages are numerous. In acute inflammation, neutrophils are the predominant cell type and may represent more than 95% of nucleated cells (Fig. 9-56). As the process becomes more chronic, mononuclear macrophages increase in number. The causative agent, possibly bacterial or fungal, may be noted, free and/or phagocytosed, in the smear. Tracheal wash samples can be cultured by routine microbiologic procedures.

The presence of bacteria or fungi in a tracheal wash does not necessarily mean the organism is pathogenic. Plant or fungal spores sometimes contaminate tracheal washes from herbivores

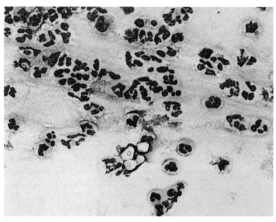

Figure 9-56. High numbers of neutrophils, an alveolar macrophage, and a cluster of four granules of cornstarch from glove powder in a tracheal wash sample. (From Cowell RL, Tyler RD, Meinkoth JH: *Diagnostic cytology and hematology of the dog and cat,* ed 2, St Louis, 1999, Mosby.)

(inhaled from feed) and may be phagocytosed by macrophages. Oral or pharyngeal contamination of the collection apparatus, or increased inspiratory effort with contamination of the upper tracheal mucosa by pharyngeal microflora, may cause inclusion of bacteria in a tracheal wash specimen. Such bacteria frequently are associated with or are adherent to squamous epithelial cells of the pharyngeal mucosa.

Eosinophils are prominent (possibly more than 10% of nucleated cells) in inflammatory reactions with an allergic or parasitic component. Because cell preservation is often only fair, free eosinophil granules rather than intact eosinophils may be noted. Rarely parasite eggs or larvae may be noted in the smear.

Erythrocytes rarely are seen in normal tracheal wash specimens. Recent hemorrhage may be evidenced by numerous intact erythrocytes in the smear. In contrast, with old hemorrhage few erythrocytes may be noted, and many of the macrophages may contain hemosiderin granules (dark-blue or red cytoplasmic granules).

Neoplastic cells may be detected in tracheal wash specimens. Criteria for malignancy are as previously described. Neoplastic cells are fre-

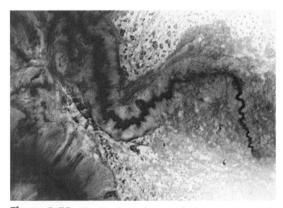

Figure 9-55. Tracheal wash sample from a dog with chronic bronchial disease. A large Curschmann's spiral and several macrophages are present. The eosinophilic background represents mucus. (From Cowell RL, Tyler RD, Meinkoth JH: *Diagnostic cytology and hematology of the dog and cat,* ed 2, St Louis, 1999, Mosby.)

quently in clusters, generally epithelial in origin, and frequently secretory in appearance (i.e., their cytoplasm is basophilic and vacuolated).

Nasal Flush

A nasal flush from a normal animal contains cornified and noncornified squamous epithelial cells, often with adherent bacteria, and negligible evidence of hemorrhage or inflammation. Various abnormalities may be demonstrated with this procedure, such as inflammation secondary to sepsis, fungi and yeasts, and neoplasia (Fig. 9-57). These should not be confused with glove powder, which may be present in some specimens (see Fig. 9-56).

Ear Swabs

"Normal" specimens contain cornified squamous epithelial cells, with negligible evidence of inflammation and few microorganisms. Common abnormal findings are bacteria and yeasts, with or without inflammation. The organism *Malassezia,* a potential cause of chronic skin lesions and ear infections, will stain with Gram stain, Diff-Quik, or even NMB for a quick "wet prep." Look for the characteristic peanut-shaped organisms (Fig. 9-58). Some controversy exists among specialists regard-

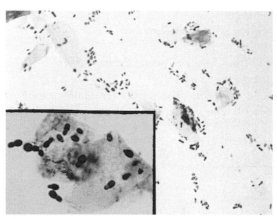

Figure 9-58. Sample from an ear swab containing *Malassezia* organisms. (From Cowell RL, Tyler RD, Meinkoth JH: *Diagnostic cytology and hematology of the dog and cat,* ed 2, St Louis, 1999, Mosby.)

ing whether the presence of *Malassezia* in small numbers is significant. Some believe that any organisms found are grounds for treatment, whereas others claim that low numbers may be found in normal ears.

Vaginal Cytology

Exfoliative vaginal cytology is a useful adjunct to the history and clinical examination in determining the stage of the estrous cycle in bitches and queens. It assists with optimal timing of mating or artificial insemination in small animals but is not of practical value for these purposes in mares, cows, does, ewes, or sows. Cytologic findings must be interpreted in conjunction with the history and clinical signs. The findings at each stage of the canine estrous cycle are detailed subsequently. These stages are convenient divisions in a continuum of change, brought about by variations in blood estrogen and progesterone concentrations. Because determination of the stage of the estrous cycle may be difficult on the basis of a single examination, repeat examinations every few days may be necessary. Unlike the bitch, the queen (female cat) ovulates after coital stimulation. Cytologic findings at different stages of the estrous cycle are similar to those of the bitch for epithelial cells and

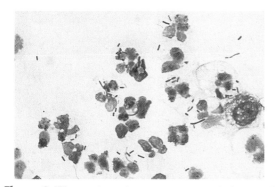

Figure 9-57. Nasal wash in a patient with bacterial rhinitis. Note the large number of degenerate neutrophils and bacteria present both intracellularly and extracellularly. (Reprinted from Raskin RE, Meyer DJ: *Atlas of canine and feline cytology,* St Louis, 2001, Saunders.)

neutrophils; however, erythrocytes are usually not present at any stage.

Cell Types Seen on Vaginal Cytology Sample Preparations

Some variation exists in the terminology used to describe the cell types commonly seen in vaginal cytology preparations. In addition to neutrophils and erythrocytes, a variety of squamous epithelial cells are also seen in vaginal cytology preparations (Fig. 9-59). These cells are further categorized on the basis of their size and degree of cornification. The epithelial cells present may include the small basal cells; the slightly larger parabasal epithelial

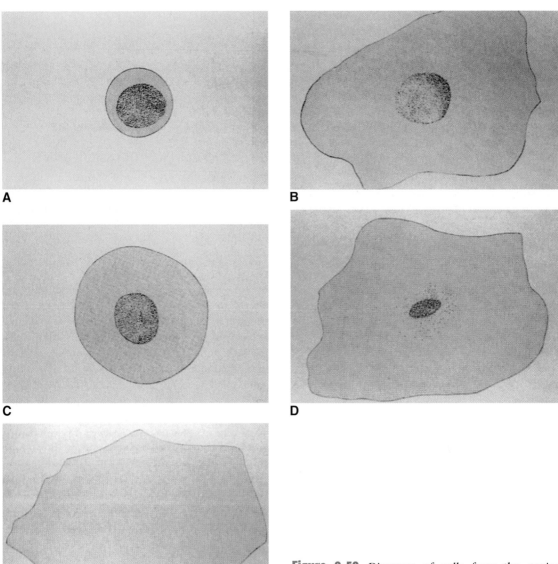

Figure 9-59. Diagrams of cells from the canine vagina. **A,** Parabasal epithelial cell. **B,** Small intermediate cell. **C,** Large intermediate cell. **D,** Superficial cell with pyknotic nucleus. **E,** Anuclear superficial cell. (Courtesy of Kal Kan Forum.)

cells (Fig. 9-60); and the largest sized noncornified squamous epithelial cells, sometimes referred to as intermediate (Fig. 9-61). At some stages of the estrous cycle, these intermediate cells may contain pyknotic nuclei (Fig. 9-62). Cornified epithelial cells are angular in appearance and usually have no nuclei (Fig. 9-63) or contain a pyknotic nuclei. Bacteria may be present in vaginal smears at any stage of the estrous cycle (but especially during estrus) and usually have no pathologic significance (i.e., they are part of the normal vaginal microflora).

Anestrus

The anestrual bitch has no vulvar swelling and does not attract male dogs. A vaginal smear reveals predominantly noncornified squamous epithelial cells (large cells with a rounded border; abundant basophilic cytoplasm; and a large, round nucleus) (Fig. 9-64). On the basis of size, these cells may be categorized as intermediate, parabasal, or basal epithelial cells. The smear also may contain some neutrophils but no erythrocytes. Anestrus is variable in length but generally lasts less than 4.5 months.

Proestrus

A bitch in proestrus has a swollen vulva, with a reddish vulvar discharge. The bitch attracts but does not accept male dogs attempting to breed.

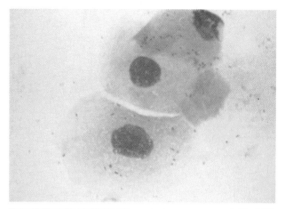

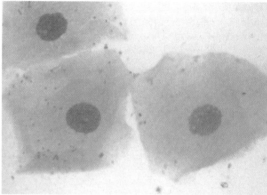

Figure 9-61. Small and large intermediate vaginal epithelial cells from a dog. (From Cowell RL, Tyler RD, Meinkoth JH: *Diagnostic cytology and hematology of the dog and cat,* ed 2, St Louis, 1999, Mosby.)

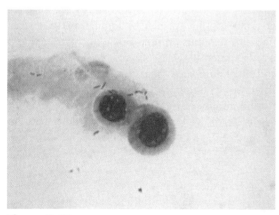

Figure 9-60. Parabasal vaginal epithelial cells from a dog. (From Cowell RL, Tyler RD, Meinkoth JH: *Diagnostic cytology and hematology of the dog and cat,* ed 2, St Louis, 1999, Mosby.)

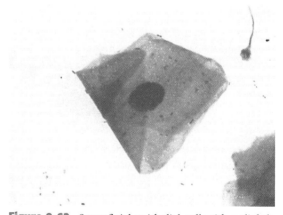

Figure 9-62. Superficial epithelial cell with a slightly pyknotic nucleus and folded angular cytoplasm. (From Cowell RL, Tyler RD, Meinkoth JH: *Diagnostic cytology and hematology of the dog and cat,* ed 2, St Louis, 1999, Mosby.)

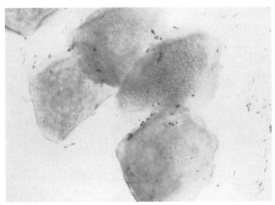

Figure 9-63. Anuclear superficial (cornified) vaginal epithelial cells from a dog. (From Cowell RL, Tyler RD, Meinkoth JH: *Diagnostic cytology and hematology of the dog and cat,* ed 2, St Louis, 1999, Mosby.)

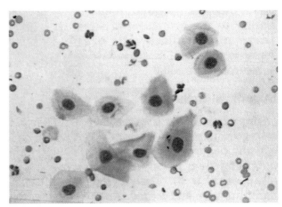

Figure 9-65. Vaginal smear from a dog in proestrus. Intermediate epithelial cells predominate. Red blood cells and a few neutrophils are also present. (From Cowell RL, Tyler RD, Meinkoth JH: *Diagnostic cytology and hematology of the dog and cat,* ed 2, St Louis, 1999, Mosby.)

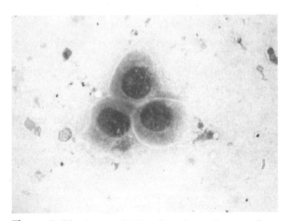

Figure 9-64. A superficial cell and two intermediate cells. Abundant bacteria are also present. (From Cowell RL, Tyler RD, Meinkoth JH: *Diagnostic cytology and hematology of the dog and cat,* ed 2, St Louis, 1999, Mosby.)

Proestrus may last 4 to 13 days, with an average of 9 days. Proestrus is often further subdivided into early proestrus and late proestrus. Gradual changes in physiology and cellular morphology are seen as the stages progress. In early proestrus, high numbers of erythrocytes are present along with basal and parabasal epithelial cells (Fig. 9-65). As proestrus continues, the numbers of erythrocytes gradually decrease and the epithelial cells begin to show signs of cornification, such as pyknotic nuclei. In late proestrus, nearly all epithelial cells present are intermediate cells with pyknotic nuclei. Small numbers of neutrophils are sometimes seen in proestrus samples, especially in the earlier stage.

Estrus

The estrual bitch has a history of recent proestrus and a swollen vulva, with possibly a pinkish to straw-colored discharge, becoming whiter as diestrus approaches. Bitches in estrus accept male dogs attempting to mate. A vaginal smear reveals that all squamous epithelial cells are cornified and usually anuclear (Fig. 9-66), neutrophils are absent, and small numbers of erythrocytes may be present. Erythrocyte numbers decrease further and neutrophil numbers increase rapidly at the end of estrus. Estrus generally lasts 4 to 13 days, with an average of 9 days.

Diestrus

A bitch in diestrus has a history of recent estrus. The vulvar swelling and discharge have decreased, and she no longer attracts or is receptive to male dogs. Cornified squamous epithelial cells are replaced by noncornified squamous epithelial cells

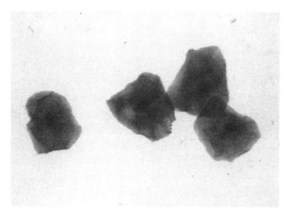

Figure 9-66. Superficial epithelial cell with a pyknotic nuclei and folded angular cytoplasm from a dog in estrus. (From Cowell RL, Tyler RD, Meinkoth JH: *Diagnostic cytology and hematology of the dog and cat,* ed 2, St Louis, 1999, Mosby.)

and abundant cytologic debris. By approximately the tenth day after estrus, all epithelial cells are noncornified. Neutrophils increase in number until approximately the third day of diestrus and then decrease to few by about the tenth day. Erythrocytes are generally absent throughout diestrus (Fig. 9-67). Diestrus may last 2 to 3 months. Cytologically, diestrus and anestrus are often

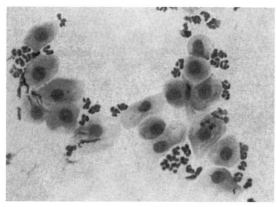

Figure 9-67. Numerous neutrophils and intermediate cells from a vaginal smear of a dog in diestrus. (From Cowell RL, Tyler RD, Meinkoth JH: *Diagnostic cytology and hematology of the dog and cat,* ed 2, St Louis, 1999, Mosby.)

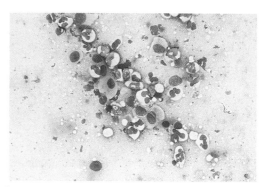

Figure 9-68. Degenerate neutrophils in an imprint of a tissue scraping of vaginal papules. A few parabasal and intermediate epithelial cells are also present. (From Raskin RE, Meyer DJ: *Atlas of canine and feline cytology,* St Louis, 2001, Saunders.)

difficult to differentiate. Pregnancy is not cytologically distinguishable from diestrus or anestrus. Some references may refer to diestrus as metestrus.

Vaginitis and Metritis

Inflammation of the vagina or uterus results in a pinkish-white vulvar discharge, usually without vulvar swelling or clinical signs of proestrus or estrus. A vaginal swab reveals noncornified squamous epithelial cells and massive numbers of neutrophils, possibly with free and/or phagocytosed bacteria (Fig. 9-68).

SEMEN EVALUATION

The American Society of Theriogenologists has published some guidelines for examination of male animals for breeding soundness. Evaluation of semen is an important part of such an assessment. Techniques for semen collection in common domestic animals are described in standard theriogenology texts.

Avoid exposing semen samples to marked changes in temperature (especially cold), water, disinfectants, or variations in pH. All laboratory equipment used in semen collection and examination should be clean and dry and warmed to approximately 37° C (98.6° F). This equipment includes microscope slides, cover slips, and pipettes. Stains and diluents also should be warmed to approximately 37° C. Samples should be processed in a warm room as soon as possible after collection.

The following characteristics are readily determined in the laboratory: volume of ejaculate, gross appearance, wave motion, microscopic motility, spermatozoal concentration, ratio of live/dead spermatozoa, assessment of morphologic features, and presence of foreign cells or material. Recording the animal's species, breed, age, brief history with salient clinical findings, suspected abnormalities, and the method of semen collection (e.g., artificial vagina, electroejaculation, massage) is important.

Volume of Ejaculate

The volume of ejaculate is measured with a volumetric flask, which may be incorporated into the collection receptacle. Marked species variations occur, and the method of collection greatly influences the volume obtained, its gross appearance, and spermatozoal concentration. As a generalization, ejaculate volume is larger but spermatozoal concentration lower (and the specimen apparently more dilute) when collected by electroejaculation than when collected by artificial vagina. Further, repeated ejaculation, whether associated with semen collection or sexual activity, decreases the volume and concentration of semen obtained at subsequent collections. Semen volume tends to be greater if collection is preceded by a period of sexual arousal ("teasing").

The ejaculate is composed of three portions: a sperm-free watery secretion, a sperm-rich fraction, and a sperm-poor fraction. The first and third fractions are derived from accessory sex glands. In bucks, bulls, rams, and toms, all three fractions are collected together. However, with boars, dogs, and stallions, the third fraction conveniently may be collected separately, which is advisable because the third fraction is voluminous in these three animals and is therefore an unnecessary encumbrance in subsequent evaluation of the semen sample. In these three species, the first two fractions (collected together) are used in the other procedures that follow.

Approximate average total ejaculate volumes (all three fractions) are as follows: boar, 250 ml; buck and ram, 1 ml; bull, 5 ml; dog, 10 ml; stallion, 65 ml; and tom, 0.04 ml. Ejaculate volume does not necessarily correlate with fertility. In general, spermatozoal number, motility, and morphologic characteristics are better guides to fertility. However, small ejaculates may be of concern in species that should have voluminous ejaculates. Knowledge of the ejaculate volume is necessary to determine total spermatozoal numbers if the sample is to be divided (and possibly diluted) for artificial insemination procedures.

Gross Appearance of Ejaculate

The opacity and color of the sample should be recorded. Opacity subjectively reflects the concentration of spermatozoa. Categories used include thick, creamy, opaque; milky opaque; opalescent milky; and watery white. This rule of thumb works best for semen from bucks, bulls, and rams, which normally have opaque, creamy-white semen because of high spermatozoal concentration. As the density of spermatozoa decreases, the specimen becomes more translucent and milkier in appearance. Semen from boars, dogs, and stallions is normally fairly translucent and white to gray. Contaminants, especially intact or degenerate erythrocytes, cause discoloration of semen.

Sperm Motility

Sperm motility (movement) is subjectively assessed and depends on careful handling of the sample for meaningful results. Variations in temperature and exposure to nonisotonic fluids or destructive chemicals (including detergents) must be avoided. Motility is correlated with fertility; however, improper specimen handling adversely affects its assessment. If other tests, especially sperm morphology, suggest the semen is normal but sperm motility is poor, another sample should be examined to ensure that technical errors were not responsible for the poor motility. Motility may be conveniently assessed in two ways.

Wave Motion

Wave motion is a subjective assessment of the gross motility of sperm. Four general classifications are used—very good, good, fair, and poor—on the basis of the amount of swirling activity observed in a drop of semen on a microscope slide at low power (40×) magnification. These categories respectively correspond to distinct vigorous swirling, moderate slow swirling, barely discernible swirling, and lack of actual swirling but with motile sperm present, which may cause the sample to have an irregular oscillating appearance. Wave motion depends on high sperm density and is therefore best in samples from bucks, bulls, and rams, which normally have high sperm concentrations. Wave motion decreases as sperm concentration decreases. Consequently, normal boars, dogs, stallions, and toms may have fair or poor wave motion. As a guide, if wave motion is very good or good, the sample should be diluted for evaluation of the percentage of motile sperm and their rate of motility.

Motility

Progressive motility of individual spermatozoa is determined on a relatively dilute drop of semen under a cover slip examined at 100× magnification. Because the motility of individual spermatozoa is difficult to appreciate in dense samples, such concentrated samples should be diluted before examination. Warm physiologic saline or fresh, buffered 2.9% sodium citrate solutions are suitable diluents.

A drop of semen is placed on a slide and diluted until a satisfactory concentration of spermatozoa is observed. A cover slip is placed on top to produce a monolayer of cells. Excessive dilution of the sample makes evaluation of motility difficult. The rate of motility is generally subjectively classified as very good, good, fair, or poor, corresponding to rapid linear activity, moderate linear activity, slow linear or erratic activity, and very slow erratic activity, respectively. The percentage of motile spermatozoa is broadly categorized as very good, good, fair, or poor, corresponding to approximately 80% to 100%, 60% to 80%, 40% to 60%, and 20% to 40% motile cells, respectively. As a generalization, to be considered satisfactory a sample should have at least 60% moderately active spermatozoa.

Sperm Concentration

Several solutions are satisfactory for semen dilution before counting sperm numbers, including 5 g of sodium bicarbonate or 9 g of sodium chloride with 1 ml of formalin in 1 L of distilled water; 3% chlorazene; or 12.5 g of sodium sulfate with 33.3 ml of glacial acetic acid in 200 ml of distilled water (Gower's solution). The sample is diluted to a 1:200 dilution and thoroughly mixed. A Neubauer hemacytometer is charged with fluid. The sample is allowed to settle for a few minutes and is then checked for homogeneous distribution of spermatozoa. If this is not present, the sample should be thoroughly mixed again and the cleaned hemacytometer recharged.

The number of spermatozoa in the central grid area of one side of the chamber is counted at 400× magnification. The number of spermatozoa per milliliter of semen is calculated by multiplying the number observed by 2 million. If spermatozoal concentration is high (e.g., in bucks, bulls, and toms), fewer squares may be counted and the multiplication factor adjusted accordingly. Spermatozoal concentration also may be determined by colorimetric and electronic particle counter techniques.

As previously outlined, sperm concentration varies with the method of collection. As a generalization, average sperm concentrations (in millions per milliliter) are approximately 150 for boars and stallions, 3000 for bucks and rams, 1200 for bulls, 300 for dogs, and 1700 for toms.

Live/Dead Sperm Ratio

Staining with a vital dye permits discrimination between live and dead spermatozoa. An eosin/nigrosin mixture is popular for this purpose and also permits examination of sperm morphologic features. The stain is prepared by adding 1 g of eosin B and 5 g of nigrosin to a 3% solution of sodium citrate dihydrate. This solution is stable for at least 1 year.

A small drop of warm stain is gently mixed with a small drop of semen on a warm microscope slide. After several seconds of contact between specimen and dye, the mixture is smeared, as when making a blood smear, and then rapidly dried. Once the smear is dried, microscopic examination may be delayed. Live sperm resist staining and appear white (clear) against the blue-black nigrosin background. In contrast, dead sperm passively take up the eosin and are stained a pinkish red. The ratio of live/dead sperm, expressed as a percentage, is determined by examination at 400× or 1000× magnification, preferably by observation of 200 cells.

Unfortunately, this procedure is susceptible to technical problems. Conditions that kill sperm, especially temperature changes, produce misleading results. Findings should always be interpreted with regard to other results, such as sperm concentration, motility, and morphology.

Sperm Morphology

Sperm morphology is readily assessed on a nigrosin and eosin stained smear, prepared as outlined previously. Other stains, such as India ink, hematoxylin and eosin, Wright's stain, Giemsa stain, and Cavarett's stain (a mixture of eosin B and phenol), have been used but offer no distinct advantages over nigrosin and eosin.

Species differences exist regarding the fine points of sperm morphology, but all sperm have the same basic structure (Fig. 9-69). The percentage of abnormal spermatozoa and their types are recorded after observing 100 to 500 cells. Counting the lower number of cells (100) is usually adequate once the technician has become proficient. Abnormalities are conveniently divided into head, midpiece, and

tail problems. Abnormalities often are categorized as primary or secondary.

Primary defects occur during spermatozoal production and include heads that are double, too large, too small, or ⌐ᵈˡy shaped (e.g., pearlike, round, twisted, knobby) (Fig. 9-70); midpieces that are swollen, kinked, twisted, double, or eccentrically attached to the head (abaxial); and tails that are coiled (Fig. 9-71). Primary abnormalities generally are considered more serious than sec-

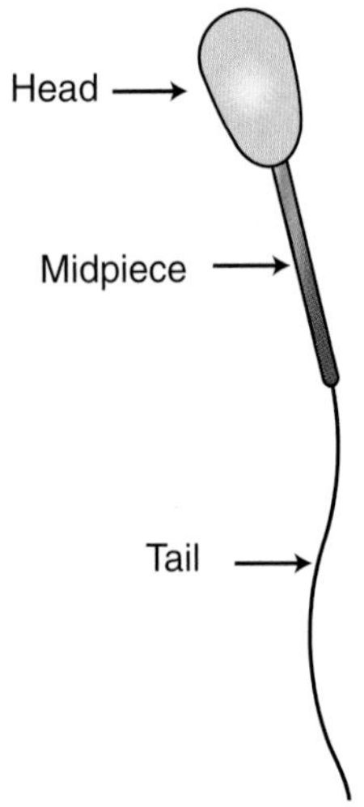

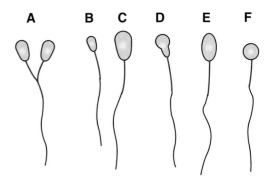

Figure 9-70. Diagrammatic representation of primary spermatozoal abnormalities involving the head. Abnormalities depicted are double head (bicephaly) **(A)**, small head (microcephaly) **(B)**, large head (macrocephaly) **(C)**, pear-shaped head (pyriform) **(D)**, elongated head **(E)**, and round head **(F)**.

Head →
Midpiece →
Tail →

Figure 9-69. Diagram of normal spermatozoa.

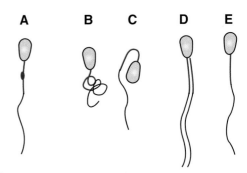

Figure 9-71. Diagrammatic representation of primary spermatozoal abnormalities involving the midpiece and tail. Abnormalities depicted are swollen midpiece **(A)**, coiled midpiece and coiled tail **(B)**, bent midpiece **(C)**, double midpiece **(D)**, and abaxial midpiece **(E)**.

ondary ones. Their percentage is fairly consistent if another semen sample is collected within several days. Slightly abaxial midpiece attachment in boars is probably not as significant as in other species because it may be found in numerous spermatozoa of apparently normal boars.

Secondary defects may occur at any time from storage in the epididymis until the smear is made. Therefore, because secondary abnormalities may be artifactual, careful specimen handling is mandatory. Minimization of technique-induced secondary abnormalities permits easier sample interpretation. Secondary defects include tailless heads, protoplasmic droplets on the midpiece, and bent or broken tails (Fig. 9-72). Obviously, for every tailless head is a headless tail, so the latter need not be counted. Protoplasmic droplets are distinct from swollen midpieces. Protoplasmic droplets are normally present while spermatozoa are in the epididymis. The droplets migrate caudally along the midpiece while the sperm cells mature in the epididymis. The droplets usually are shed before the spermatozoa leave the epididymis.

As a broad generalization, less than 20%—and usually less than 10%—of spermatozoa are abnormal in a normal animal. Higher percentages of abnormal spermatozoa may compromise fertility. Obviously, however, the total number of normal spermatozoa is important, not the percentage of abnormal sperm.

Other Cells in Semen

Normal semen contains few (if any) leukocytes, erythrocytes, or epithelial cells and no bacteria or fungi. If present, their approximate quantity should be noted. If bacteria or fungi are observed without an inflammatory response, sample contamination by the normal preputial microflora should be suspected. Attention to preputial sanitation before sample collection should remedy the problem. If indicated, a semen sample may be submitted for microbiologic examination.

Cells from the germinal layers of the testes are an unusual finding in semen and represent severe testicular damage. Such cells include spermatids, spermatocytes, and large ciliated cells (often called medusa heads). Precise categorization is unimportant as long as these cells are classified as immature sperm cells.

EVALUATION OF PROSTATIC SECRETIONS

Disorders of the prostate are not uncommon in dogs but are rare in other domestic animals. Cells of prostatic origin may be collected by urethral catheterization combined with prostatic massage (or penile massage) performed per rectum to stimulate prostatic secretion. Prostatic tissue may be aspirated by transcutaneous needle biopsy. Cytologic smears are prepared as previously described.

An enlarged prostate may be the result of prostatic hypertrophy, hyperplasia, metaplasia, neoplasia, or inflammation. Prostatic cells may occur singly or in clusters. Spermatozoa may be present in some fluid samples, especially those collected by penile massage.

Normal prostatic cells have a uniform size and shape, with a fairly high nucleus/cytoplasm ratio, transparent to gray cytoplasm, homogeneous nuclear chromatin, and no obvious nucleoli. Normal prostatic fluid or tissue contains few leukocytes. Prostatic hypertrophy is gland enlargement because of increased size of individual cells, without

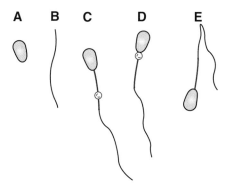

Figure 9-72. Diagrammatic representation of secondary spermatozoal abnormalities involving the midpiece and tail. Abnormalities depicted are tailless head **(A)**, Headless tail **(B)**, distal protoplasmic droplets **(C)**, proximal protoplasmic droplets **(D)**, and bent tail **(E)**.

increased cell numbers. A hypertrophic prostate is not cytologically distinguishable from a normal prostate. The distinction is made on the basis of gland size at palpation or radiography. Prostatic hyperplasia is gland enlargement because of increased numbers of cells. The cells are uniform in size and appearance and have a high nucleus/cytoplasm ratio; basophilic cytoplasm that is often vacuolated; and a nucleus with a "roughened" chromatin pattern and a uniform, small, single nucleolus. Few leukocytes are present. Metaplasia is a change (from normal) in the population of prostatic cells. Exfoliated or biopsied cells have the appearance of noncornified squamous epithelial cells. Consequently, they have a low nucleus/cytoplasm ratio and a somewhat pyknotic nucleus. Prostatic neoplasia is characterized by a pleomorphic population of cells with a high nucleus/cytoplasm ratio and very basophilic cytoplasm. Nuclear size varies among cells and contain variable numbers of large, irregular (angular), and pleomorphic nucleoli. A cytologic diagnosis of prostatic abcessation is based on finding large numbers of neutrophils in the fluid or tissue sample. Macrophages and lymphocytes also may be present in variable numbers.

EXAMINATION OF MILK

Subclinical and clinical bovine mastitis (mammary gland infection) is an important economic concern for dairy farmers. Mastitis may be detected by several laboratory procedures. Those most frequently used indirectly or directly reflect milk nucleated cell counts and/or bacterial counts. Tests are performed on milk samples from individual quarters, all four quarters pooled together, or bulk milk (several cows together, usually the whole herd).

When individual animals are being screened, foremilk (sample obtained before milking begins) is generally used. It has more cells than a sample obtained in the middle of milking but fewer cells than one collected at the end of milking. Cell counts also vary with the stage of lactation. Milk samples from normal cows within the first week and at the end of lactation have higher cell counts than throughout the interim.

Nucleated cell counts of normal milk are generally less than 300,000 to 500,000 cells/ml. Counts greater than 500,000 cells/ml indicate mastitis.

Differential cell counts sometimes are performed. Nucleated cells are categorized as neutrophils or mononuclear cells. Normal milk in midlactation generally has less than 10% neutrophils, whereas in severe acute mastitis the milk may have up to 95% neutrophils.

Recommended Reading

Anthony A, Sirois M: Microbiology, cytology and urinalysis. In Sirois M: *Principles and practice of veterinary technology,* ed 2, St Louis, 2004, Mosby.

Cowell R, Tyler R, Meinkoth J: *Diagnostic cytology and hematology of the dog and cat,* ed 2, St Louis, 1999, Mosby.

Latimer KS, Prasse KW, Mahaffey EA: *Duncan and Prasse's veterinary laboratory medicine: clinical pathology,* Ames, IA, 2003, Blackwell.

Raskin R, Meyer D: *Atlas of canine and feline cytology,* St Louis, 2001, WB Saunders.

Appendix A

Reference Ranges

The data on the following pages was compiled from a variety of sources, including personal notes, workshops, conference presentations, and references listed at the end of each chapter. These values can be affected by a large number of factors such as the test methods used, type of equipment used, and the characteristics of the patient. Each laboratory should establish its own reference ranges for the methods used in that laboratory.

Hematology Reference Ranges

	Canine	Feline	Equine	Bovine	Ovine	Caprine	Porcine
RBC × 10^6/μl	5.0-8.5	5.0-10.0	5.5-12.5	5.0-10.0	9.0-15.0	8.0-17.0	5.0 -7.0
WBC × 10^3/μl	6.0-15.0	5.5-19.5	5.5-12.5	4.0-12.0	4.0-12.0	4.0-13.0	10.5-22.0
PCV (%)	37-55	30-45	32-57	24-42	25-45	21-38	32-43
Hgb (g/dl)	12-18	8-15	10.5-18	8-14	8-16	8-13	9-16
MCV (fl)	60-77	39-55	34-58	40-60	23-40	16-25	50-67
MCH (pg)	14-25	13-20	13-19	11-17	8-12	5-8	17-21
MCHC (g/dl)	31-36	30-36	31-37	28-36	30-35	28-36	29-34
RDW (%)	14-19	14-17	18-21	15-20			
Neutrophils (segmented) %	60-70	35-75	30-75	15-45	10-50	10-50	20-70
× 10^3/μl	3.0-11.3	2.5-12.5	3-6	0.6-4.0	3.0-10.0	0.7-6.0	2-15
Neutrophils (bands) %	0-4	0-3	0-1	0-2	0-0.2	0-0.15	0-4.0
× 10^3/μl	0-0.4	0-0.3	0-0.1	0-0.12	0-0.01	0-0.01	0-0.8
Lymphocytes %	12-30	20-55	25-60	45-75	40-75	40-75	35-75
× 10^3/μl	1-4.8	1.5-7.0	1.5-5.0	2.5-7.5	2-9	2-9	2-16
Monocytes %	3-9	1-4	0-10	2-7	0-6	0-4	0-10
× 10^3/μl	0.2-1.3	0-0.9	0-0.7	0.02-0.85	0-0.75	0-0.55	0.2-2.2
Eosinophils %	2-10	2-10	1-10	2-20	0-10	1-8	0-15
× 10^3/μl	0.1-0.75	0-0.8	0-0.7	0-2.4	0.1-0.75	0.05-0.65	0.2-2.0
Basophils %	0-0.3	0-0.3	0-3	0-2	0-3	0-1	0-3
× 10^3/μl	0-0.03	0-0.03	0-0.5	0-0.2	0-0.3	0-0.12	0-0.5
Reticulocytes (%)	0-1.5	0-10 0.4 (aggregate) 1.5-10 (punctuate)	0	0	0	0	0-2
ESR	5-25 mm/hour	7-23 mm/hour	15-38 mm/ 20 minutes	2-4 mm/day	3-8 mm/day	2-2.5 mm/day	1-14 mm/hour

Coagulation Reference Ranges

	Canine	Feline	Equine	Bovine	Ovine	Caprine	Porcine
Platelets x $10^3/\mu l$	160-625	160-700	100-350	100-600	100-800		120-720
Mean platelet volume (fl)	6.1-13.1	12-18	6.0-11.1	3.5-7.4			
Thrombin time (seconds)	4-10	10-21	9-10.5	7.8-9.5			
Prothrombin time (seconds)	6-14	8.6-20	9.8-12	18-28			
PTT (seconds)	15-30	10-25	50-65	37-57			
APTT (seconds)	13-17	12-20	37-56				
Fibrinogen (mg/dl)	200-400	100-300	112-372	300-700	300-700		100-500
Bleeding time (minutes)	1.4-5	1.4-5	2.2-3.4	1-5			
ACT (seconds)	60-100	10-65	120-190	90-120			

Clinical Chemistry Reference Ranges

	Canine	Feline	Equine	Bovine	Ovine	Caprine	Porcine
Albumin (g/dl)	2.3-4.3	2.8-3.4	2.6-4.1	3.4-4.3	2.4-3.9	2.7-3.9	1.8-3.9
ALT (U/L)	8.2-109	25-97	2.7-21	5-35	10-44	15-52	9-47
AST (U/L)	9-49	7-40	160-595	46-176	49-90	43-230	8-55
ALP (U/L)	22-114	16-65	30-227	18-153	27-156	61-283	41-176
Amylase (U/L)	220-1400	280-1200	47-188	41-98	140-260	—	—
Bicarbonate (mEq/L)	17-25	17-25	22-30	20-30	20-27	—	18-27
Bile acids-fasting (µmol/L)	0-9	0-5	0-20	—	—	—	—
Bile acids-2 hour postprandial (µmol/L)	0-30	0-7	11-60	—	—	—	—
Bilirubin, total (mg/dl)	0.07-0.6	0-0.5	0.3-3.5	0.01-0.8	0-0.4	0-0.1	0-0.6
Bilirubin, direct (mg/dl)	0.06-0.15	0-0.1	0-0.4	0.01-0.4	0-0.27	0-0.01	0-0.3
Calcium (mg/dl)	8.7-12	7.9-11.9	10.2-13.4	8.0-11.4	9.8-12	9.8-12	9.5-11.5
Chloride (mEq/L)	95-120	105-130	97-110	94-111	101-110	99-112	90-106
Cholesterol (mg/dl)	116-330	50-156	71-142	80-120	76-102	100-112	97-106
Creatine kinase (U/L)	40-368	59-362	60-333	44-350	—	—	0-800
Creatinine (mg/dl)	0.5-1.7	0.7-2.2	0.4-1.9	0.7-1.4	1.0-2.7	—	1.0-3.0
Glucose (mg/dl)	76-120	58-120	62-127	37-79	45-80	45-75	65-150
Lipase (U/L)	60-200	0-83	—	—	—	—	—
Magnesium (mg/dl)	1.2-2.7	1.5-3.5	1.4-3.5	1.4-3.0	2.0-2.7	2.1-2.9	2.3-3.5
Phosphorus (mg/dl)	2.5-6.2	2.5-7.3	1.5-5.4	4.6-8.0	4.0-7.3	3.7-8.5	5.0-9.3
Potassium (mEq/L)	3.9-6.1	3.5-6.1	2.5-5.4	3.5-5.3	4.5-5.1	3.5-6.7	3.5-7.1
Protein, total serum (g/dl)	5.4-7.5	5.7-7.6	5.4-7.9	6.0-7.5	6.0-7.9	6.4-7.9	6.0-8.9
SDH (U/L)	2.9-8.2	2.4-7.7	1.0-7.9	4.0-18.0	4.0-28.0	9.0-21.0	0.5-6.0
Sodium (mEq/L)	141-155	140-159	128-146	136-148	132-154	137-152	135-153
Urea nitrogen (mg/dl)	9.0-27.0	18.0-34.0	10.0-27.0	10.0-26.0	8.0-30.0	10.0-30.0	8.0-30.0

Bacterial Pathogens of Veterinary Importance

The following table is a summary of characteristics of and diseases produced by microbial pathogens seen in mammals and birds. A comprehensive bacteriology text should be consulted for additional characteristics used to identify these species definitively and for additional information on less-common species.

Organism	Primary Species Affected	Disease or Lesion	Characteristics
***Actinobacillus* Species**			
A. arthritidis	Horses	Arthritis and septicemia	• Gram-negative bacilli and coccobacilli
A. equuli equuli	Foals, pigs, calves	"Sleepy foal" disease; diarrhea, meningitis, pneumonia, purulent nephritis, or septic polyarthritis	• Facultative anaerobe; require carbon dioxide • Pus may contain club-shaped structures representing bacterial colonies surrounded by spicules of calcium phosphate <1 mm in diameter
A. equuli haemolyticus	Horses	Endocarditis, meningitis, metritis, abortion	

A. lignieresii	Cattle, sheep	Granulomatous/pyogranulomatous lesions. Commonly affects tongue (wooden tongue); may also cause pyogranulomatous lesions in soft tissues of the head, neck, limbs, lungs, pleura, udder, and subcutaneous tissue.	• Identification/differentiation
			  • Growth on MacConkey agar
			  • CAMP test
			  • Esculin hydrolysis
			  • Acid production in carbohydrate substrates
			  • Oxalase test
			  • Catalase test
			  • Urease test

A. pleuropneumoniae	Pigs	Pleuropneumonia; pleuritis, pulmonary abscess in pigs <5 months	
A. rossii	Pigs	Abortion, metritis	

Continued

Organism	Primary Species Affected	Disease or Lesion	Characteristics
***Actinobacillus* Species–cont'd**			
A. seminis	Sheep	Epididymitis in rams; purulent polyarthritis in lambs	
A. salpingitidis	Chickens	Salpingitis and peritonitis in chickens of layer type	
A. suis	Young pigs, foals	Fatal septicemia in animals <6 weeks, arthritis, pneumonia, pericarditis, abscesses in older animals	
***Actinomyces* Species**			
A. bovis	Cattle, horses	Lumpy jaw and lung abscesses in cattle, chronic fistulous withers and chronic poll evil in horses	• Gram-positive, non-acid-fast bacilli • Non–spore-forming • Poor growth on Sabouraud dextrose agar
A. hordeovulneris	Dogs	Localized abscesses, pleuritis, peritonitis, visceral abscesses, septic arthritis	• Facultative anaerobe; require carbon dioxide • Usually filamentous • Often contain yellowish granules
A. hyovaginalis	Pigs	Vaginitis, abortion	• Identification/differentiation
A. suis	Pigs	Pyogranulomatous mastitis	• Colony characteristics • Hemolysis pattern

A. viscosus	Dogs, hamsters	Chronic pneumonia, pyothorax, localized subcutaneous abscesses	• Esculin hydrolysis test
			  • Acid production in carbohydrate substrates
			  • Nitrate reduction test
			  • Catalase test
			  • Urease test

***Anaplasma* Species**			
A. bovis	Cattle	Anemia, weight loss	• Gram-negative coccoid to ellipsoid forms
A. caudatum	Ruminants	Anemia, icterus, splenomegaly, erythrophagocytosis	• Located within cytoplasmic vacuoles of myeloid cells, neutrophils, erythrocytes, or thrombocytes
A. centrale	Ruminants	Fever, anemia	• Identification/differentiation
A. marginale	Ruminants	Fever, anorexia, weight loss, lethargy	• Demonstration of organisms on blood film • Immunology
A. ovis	Sheep, goats	Anemia, depression, fever, anorexia	

Organism	Primary Species Affected	Disease or Lesion	Characteristics
***Anaplasma* Species—cont'd**			
A. phagocytophilum	Horses, small ruminants	Granulocytic ehrlichiosis	
A. platys	Dogs	Infectious thrombocytopenia	
***Arcobacter* Species**			
A. cryaerophilus	Cattle, horses, pigs, sheep, dogs	Abortion, mastitis	• Gram-negative curved or spiral bacilli • Microaerophilic • Identification/differentiation
A. butzleri	Horses, cattle, pigs, nonhuman primates	Diarrhea	• Colony characteristics • Nitrate reduction test • Catalase test • Growth on MacConkey agar
A. skirrowii	Cattle, pigs	Abortion, diarrhea (lambs and calves)	• Hydrogen sulfide production
***Arcanobacterium* Species**			

A. pyogenes	Cattle, goats, sheep, pigs	Liver abscess, endocarditis, abortion, endometriosis, suppurative mastitis, pneumonia, septic arthritis, umbilical infections, seminal vesiculitis	• Gram-positive, nonmotile, coccoid bacilli
			• Identification/differentiation
			  • Colony characteristics
			  • Hemolysis pattern

A. hippocoleae	Horses	Vaginitis	
***Bacillus* Species**			
B. anthracis	Ruminants, dogs, cats, horses	Septicemia, pharyngitis (dogs and cats)	• Gram-positive spore-forming bacilli • Identification/differentiation
B. cereus	Cattle, sheep, horses	Gangrenous mastitis, abortion	• Colony characteristics • Hemolysis pattern • Motility test
B. licheniformis	Cattle	Abortion	• Nitrate reduction test • PCR testing
***Bacteroides* Species**			
B. asaccharolyticus	Dogs, cats, horses, cattle	Osteomyelitis	• Gram-negative, non-spore-forming bacilli • Anaerobic

B. fragilis	Cattle, sheep, goats, horses, pigs, dogs, cats	Neonatal diarrhea, abortion, mastitis, soft tissue abscess (dogs and cats)	• Identification/differentiation
			  • Cellular morphology
			  • Colony characteristics
			  • Bile sensitivity test

Continued

Organism	Primary Species Affected	Disease or Lesion	Characteristics
***Bacteroides* Species—cont'd**			
B. levii	Cattle	Mastitis	• Esculin hydrolysis test • Indole production test • Fermentation of sugars
***Bordetella* Species**			

B. bronchiseptica	Dogs, cats, horses, pigs, nonhuman primates, rodents, rabbits	Sinusitis, pneumonia, rhinitis, tracheobronchitis, conjunctivitis, endocarditis, meningitis, peritonitis	• Gram-negative bacilli
			• Identification/differentiation
			  • Colony characteristics
			  • Growth on MacConkey and blood agar
			  • Slide agglutination test
			  • Urease test

B. avium	Birds	Turkey coryza	• Oxidase test • Nitrate reduction test • Citrate utilization test • Motility test
***Borrelia* Species**			
B. anserina	Birds	Fatal septicemia	• Coiled spirochetes • Microaerophilic or anaerobic
B. burgdorferi	Dogs, cats, horses, cattle	Lyme disease	• Identification/differentiation • Demonstration of organisms on blood films, smears of spleen or liver tissue
B. coriaceae	Cattle	Abortion	• Immunologic testing
B. theileri	Cattle, sheep, horses	Relapsing fever, anemia	
***Brachyspira* Species**			
B. aalborgi	Nonhuman primates	Colonic spirochetosis	• Gram-negative, slender spirochetes • Identification/differentiation
B. alvinipulli	Poultry	Colonic spirochetosis	• Cellular morphology • Colony characteristics
B. hyodysenteriae	Pigs	Dysentery	• Hemolysis pattern • Indole production test
B. intermedia	Poultry	Colonic spirochetosis	
B. pilosicoli	Pigs, chickens	Colonic spirochetosis	

Organism	Primary Species Affected	Disease or Lesion	Characteristics
***Brucella* Species**			
B. abortus	Cattle, pigs, sheep, goats, dogs	Abortion, orchitis, epididymitis, chronic bursitis, fistulous withers	• Gram-negative bacilli and coccobacilli • Nonmotile • Facultative intracellular parasites

B. canis	Dogs	Abortion, epididymitis, osteomyelitis, meningitis, glomerulonephritis	• Identification/differentiation
			  • Hemolysis pattern
			  • Indole production test

B. melitensis	Sheep, goats	Abortion, mastitis, orchitis, lameness	• Oxidase test
			  • Catalase test
			  • Nitrate reduction test

B. ovis	Sheep	Epididymitis, orchitis, infertility, nephritis, abortion, vaginitis	• Urease test
B. suis	Pigs	Abortion, arthritis, infertility, orchitis, posterior paralysis	
***Burkholderia* Species**			
B. mallei	Horses	Glanders	• Gram-negative bacilli • Identification/differentiation

B. pseudomallei	Dogs, carnivores	Pseudoglanders, fever, myalgia, dermal abscess, epididymitis	• Cellular morphology
			  • Colony characteristics
			  • Growth on MacConkey agar
			  • Motility
			  • Oxidase test
			  • Catalase test
			  • Nitrate reduction test
			  • Carbohydrate metabolism

***Campylobacter* Species**			
C. fetus fetus	Cattle, sheep	Abortion	• Gram-negative slender spiral or curved bacilli
C. fetus venerealis	Cattle	Abortion, infertility	• Microaerophilic • Motile

C. jejuni jejuni	Dogs, cats, pigs, cows, sheep	Diarrhea in young animals, abortion	• Identification/differentiation
			  • Colony characteristics
			  • Hydrogen sulfide production
			  • Oxidase test
			  • Catalase test
			  • Nitrate reduction test
			  • Carbohydrate metabolism

Continued

Organism	Primary Species Affected	Disease or Lesion	Characteristics
Chlamydia Species			
C. muridarum	Mice, hamsters	Pneumonitis	• Gram-negative intracellular bodies
C. psittaci	Birds	See _Chlamydiophila psittaci_	• Identification/differentiation
C. suis	Pigs	Conjunctivitis, pneumonia, pericarditis, enteritis, rhinitis, pneumonia	• Cytology impression smears • Immunology (fluorescent antibody test, PCR) • Cell culture
Chlamydiophila Species			
C. abortus	Ruminants, pigs	Abortion	• Gram-negative intracellular bodies
C. caviae	Guinea pigs	Conjunctivitis	• Identification/differentiation
C. felis	Cats	Conjunctivitis, rhinitis, pneumonitis	• Cytology impression smears • Immunology (fluorescent antibody test, PCR)
C. pecorum	Ruminants, pigs	Abortion, infertility, arthritis, conjunctivitis, cystitis, encephalitis, enteritis, pneumonia	• Cell culture
C. psittaci	Birds	Conjunctivitis, encephalitis, enteritis, pneumonia, hepatitis	
Citrobacter Species			

C. rodentium	Mice, gerbils, guinea pigs	Transmissible murine colonic hyperplasia	• Identification/differentiation
			  • Colony characteristics
			  • Hydrogen sulfide production
			  • Motility
			  • Acid production in carbohydrate substrates

Clostridium Species			
C. botulinum	Ruminants, horses, swine, carnivores	Botulism	• Gram-positive spore-forming bacilli
C. chauvoei	Cattle, sheep	Blackleg	• Oxygen tolerant or anaerobic • Produce toxins

C. colinum	Chickens, quail, turkeys	Quail disease	• Identification/differentiation
			  • Colony characteristics
			  • Hemolysis pattern
			  • Immunology (ELISA)

C. difficile	Horses, dogs, rodents, pigs	Diarrhea, colitis	• Histology • Cytology

Organism	Primary Species Affected	Disease or Lesion	Characteristics
***Clostridium* Species—cont'd**			
C. novyi	Sheep, goats	Infectious hepatitis, myonecrosis	
C. perfringens	Warm-blooded animals	Myonecrosis, gas gangrene	
C. piliforme	Mammals	Tyzzer's disease	
C. septicum	Sheep, cattle	Myonecrosis, malignant edema, gangrenous dermatitis, enteritis, braxy	
C. sordelli	Sheep, cattle	Myonecrosis, enteritis	
C. spiroforme	Rabbits, rodents	Enterotoxemia	
C. tetani	Horses, cattle, pigs, carnivores	Tetanus	
***Corynebacterium* Species**			
C. auriscanis	Dogs	Otitis, dermatitis, vaginitis	• Gram-positive, non-spore-forming pleomorphic bacilli
C. cystitidis	Cattle	Bladder and kidney infection	• Aerobic or facultative anaerobes
C. diphtheriae	Cattle, horses	Mastitis, dermatitis, wound infection (equine)	• Most are nonmotile • Non–acid-fast
C. equi	Horses, pigs	See *Rhodococcus equi*	• Identification/differentiation • Colony characteristics • Catalase test
C. kutscheri	Rats, mice	Abscesses of lung, liver, lymph node, kidney	• Hemolysis pattern • Nitrate reduction test • Esculin hydrolysis test
C. pilosum	Cattle	Bladder and kidney infection	• Acid production in carbohydrate substrates
C. pseudotuberculosis	Cattle, sheep, goats	Abscesses, lymphadenitis, abortion, arthritis	• Urease test
C. renale	Cattle, sheep, pigs	Bladder and kidney infection	
C. ulcerans	Cattle, rodents	Mastitis, abscesses, gangrenous dermatitis (rodents)	

Continued

Organism	Primary Species Affected	Disease or Lesion	Characteristics
Dermatophilus Species			

D. congolensis	Cattle, horses, goats, sheep, pigs, dogs, cats	Exudative dermatis, alopecia	• Gram-positive filamentous bacilli
			• Aerobic
			• Motile zoospores
			• Non–acid-fast
			• Identification/differentiation
			  • Cellular morphology
			  • Colony characteristics
			  • Catalase test
			  • Hemolysis pattern
			  • Acid production from glucose
			  • Nitrate reduction test

Dichelobacter Species			

D. nodosus	Sheep, cattle, pigs, goats	Foot rot	• Gram-negative, pleomorphic, slightly curved bacilli
			• Anaerobic
			• Identification/differentiation
			  • Cellular morphology
			  • Colony characteristics
			  • Esculin hydrolysis test
			  • Acid production in carbohydrate substrates
			  • Indole production test

Ehrlichia Species			

E. bovis	Cattle	See Anaplasma bovis	• Gram-negative coccoid to ellipsoid forms
			• Located within cytoplasmic vacuoles of endothelium, myeloid cells, granulocytes, or thrombocytes
			• Identification/differentiation
			  • Demonstration of organisms on blood film
			  • Immunology

E. canis	Dogs, other canids	Monocytic ehrlichiosis	
E. chaffeensis	Dogs	Monocytic ehrlichiosis	
E. ewingii	Dogs	Granulocytic ehrlichiosis	
E. muris	Mice	Ehrlichiosis	
E. platys	Dogs	See Anaplasma platys	
E. ruminantium	Ruminants	Heartwater	
Enterobacter Species			
E. aerogenes	Most mammals	Mastitis, neonatal septicemia, metritis, urinary tract infection, wound infection	• Gram-negative, motile bacilli • Identification/differentiation • Colony characteristics
E. cloacae	Birds		

Organism	Primary Species Affected	Disease or Lesion	Characteristics
***Enterobacter* Species–cont'd**			• Cellular morphology • Citrate utilization test • Hydrogen sulfide production • Acid and gas production from lactose
***Eperythrozoon* Species** See *Mycoplasma*			

***Erysipelothrix* Species**
E. rhusiopathiae
	Cattle, pigs, sheep, turkeys	Diamond skin disease, arthritis, endocarditis	• Gram-positive non-spore-forming bacilli
			• Facultative anaerobes
			• Nonmotile
			• Identification/differentiation
			  • Cellular morphology
			  • Colony characteristics
			  • Hemolysis pattern
			  • Catalase test
			  • Esculin hydrolysis test
			  • Acid production from carbohydrates
			  • Hydrogen sulfide production
			  • CAMP test
			  • Immunology (agglutination)

***Escherichia* Species**
E. coli
(numerous pathotypes)
	Most vertebrates	Enteritis, septicemia, ruminant mastitis, canine pyometra, cystitis, calf scours	• Gram-negative bacilli
			• Most are motile
			• Identification/differentiation
			  • Cellular morphology
			  • Colony characteristics
			  • Hemolysis pattern
			  • Growth on MacConkey agar
			  • Catalase test
			  • Oxidase test
			  • Acid and gas production from glucose
			  • Hydrogen sulfide production
			  • Immunology (agglutination, ELISA, PCR)
			  • Histology

Continued

Organism	Primary Species Affected	Disease or Lesion	Characteristics
Francisella Species			

F. tularensis	Rabbits, most other mammals	Pneumonia, fever, lymphadenitis, ulcerative dermatitis	• Gram-negative coccobacilli
			• Identification/differentiation
			  • Cellular morphology with fluorescent antibody stain
			  • Immunology (agglutination, ELISA, antibody titer)
			  • Histology

Fusobacterium Species			
F. equinum	Horses	Lower respiratory tract disease	• Gram-negative, non-spore-forming fusiform bacilli • Identification/differentiation
F. necrophorum	Cattle, sheep, horses, pigs, rabbits	Foot rot, mastitis, liver abscess, metritis, calf diphtheria, thrush (equine), abortion, ulcerative stomatitis, "bull nose"	• Cellular morphology • Colony characteristics • Hemolysis pattern • Catalase test • Nitrate reduction test • Esculin hydrolysis test • Fermentation of glucose • Indole production test
F. nucleatum	Cattle, sheep	Abortion	
Haemobartonella Species			
H. canis	Dogs	See Mycoplasma haemocanis	
H. felis	Cats	See Mycoplasma haemofelis	
Haemophilus Species			
H. felis	Cats	Rhinitis, conjunctivitis	• Gram-negative, pleomorphic bacilli or coccobacilli • May form filaments • Nonmotile • Facultative anaerobes • Growth on chocolate agar • Identification/differentiation
H. haemoglobinophilus	Dogs	Vaginitis, cystitis	
H. influenzaemurium	Rodents	Respiratory, ocular disease	
H. paragallinarium	Chickens	Infectious coryza	
H. parasuis	Pigs	Glasser's disease, meningitis, myositis, pneumonia, septicemia	• Catalase test • Indole production test • CAMP test • Acid production in carbohydrate substrates • Urease test • Immunology (immunohistochemistry, PCR)
Helicobacter Species			
H. bilis	Mice	Hepatitis	• Gram-negative helical, curved, or unbranched bacilli

Organism	Primary Species Affected	Disease or Lesion	Characteristics
Helicobacter Species—cont'd			
H. canis	Dogs	Gastroenteritis	• Motile • Microaerophilic
H. cholecystus	Hamsters	Cholecystitis, pancreatitis	• Identification/differentiation
H. felis	Cats, dogs	Gastritis	• Colony characteristics • Catalase test
H. hepaticus	Mice, rats	Hepatitis	• Oxidase test • Urease test
H. muridarum	Mice, rats	Gastritis	
H. mustelae	Ferrets	Gastritis	
H. nemestrinae	Macaques	Gastritis	
H. pillorum	Poultry	Gastroenteritis, hepatitis	
H. pylori	Monkeys, cats	Gastritis	
H. rappini	Mice, rats, dogs, sheep	Abortion	
Histophilus Species			

H. somni	Cattle	Bronchopneumonia, "honker syndrome," myocarditis, otitis, conjunctivitis, myelitis, vaginitis, orchitis, thromboembolic meningoencephalitis	• Gram-negative, nonmotile pleomorphic bacilli
			• Capnophilic
			• Identification/differentiation
			  • Colony characteristics
			  • Hemolysis pattern
			  • Catalase test
			  • Oxidase test
			  • Nitrate reduction test
			  • Immunology

Klebsiella Species			

K. pneumoniae ssp. pneumoniae	Cattle, horses, sheep, dogs, birds	Metritis, mastitis, neonatal septicemia	• Gram-negative, nonmotile encapsulated bacilli
			• Identification/differentiation
			  • Colony characteristics
			  • Cellular morphology

K. oxytoca	Horses	Vaginitis, metritis, abortion, infertility	• Citrate utilization test
			  • Hydrogen sulfide production
			  • Acid and gas production from Lactose
			  • Urease test
			  • Indole production test

Continued

Organism	Primary Species Affected	Disease or Lesion	Characteristics
Lawsonia Species			

L. intracellularis	Pigs, hamsters, cats, dogs, horses, ferrets	Proliferative enteritis, "wet tail," ileitis	• Gram-negative curved intracellular body
			• Motile
			• Identification/differentiation
			  • Cellular morphology with silver staining
			  • Immunology (ELISA, immunofluorescence)

Leptospira Species			

L. bratislava	Horses, pigs	Abortion	• Spiral bacteria
			• Aerobic
			• Motile
			• Identification/differentiation
			  • Cellular morphology with darkfield microscopy
			  • Immunology (agglutination, PCR, fluorescent antibody stain)

L. canicola	Cattle, pigs, dogs	Uremia, abortion	
L. grippotyphosa	Cattle, pigs, horses	Fever, jaundice uremia	
L. hardjo	Cattle	Abortion, infertility	
L. icterohaemorrhagiae	Dogs, cattle, rats	Septicemia, abortion	
L. kennewicki	Horses	Abortion	
L. pomona	Pigs, cattle, horses	Abortion	
Listeria Species			

L. monocytogenes	Cattle, sheep, goats, horses, birds, dogs, rodents, pigs	Central nervous system infection, abortion, mastitis, septicemia	• Gram-positive, non-spore-forming bacilli
			• Facultative anaerobes
			• Motile
			• Identification/differentiation
			  • Cellular morphology
			  • Colony characteristics
			  • Hemolysis pattern
			  • Catalase test
			  • Esculin hydrolysis test
			  • Acid production from carbohydrates
			  • Hydrogen sulfide production
			  • CAMP test

Organism	Primary Species Affected	Disease or Lesion	Characteristics
Mannheimia Species			
M. haemolytica	Cattle, sheep	Pneumonia, septicemia, mastitis	• Gram-negative bacilli and coccobacilli • Nonmotile
M. granulomatis	Cattle	Panniculitis	• Facultative anaerobes • Identification/differentiation

M. varigena	Cattle	Pneumonia, septicemia, mastitis	• Colony characteristics
			  • Hemolysis pattern
			  • Oxidase test
			  • Acid production from glucose
			  • Nitrate reduction test

Moraxella Species			
M. bovis	Cattle	Infectious keratoconjunctivitis	• Gram-negative coccobacilli • Nonmotile
M. canis	Dogs	Bite wound infections	• Identification/differentiation • Colony characteristics

M. ovis	Small ruminants	Pinkeye	• Growth on MacConkey agar
			  • Hemolysis pattern
			  • Oxidase test
			  • Catalase test
			  • Nitrate reduction test
			  • Immunology (fluorescent antibody stain, ELISA)

Morganella Species			

M. morganii	Dogs	Otitis externa, cystitis	• Gram-negative bacilli
			• Identification/differentiation
			  • Colony characteristics
			  • Oxidase test
			  • Indole production test

Mycobacterium Species			
M. avium ssp. avium	Birds	Tuberculosis	• Gram-positive non-spore-forming bacilli
M. avium ssp. paratuberculosis	Ruminants	Johne's disease	• Nonmotile • Aerobic • Acid fast

M. bovis	Ruminants, dogs, cats, pigs, goats, nonhuman primates	Tuberculosis	• Identification/differentiation
			  • Colony characteristics
			  • Cellular morphology
			  • Intradermal skin test
			  • Carbohydrate utilization test

Continued

Organism	Primary Species Affected	Disease or Lesion	Characteristics
***Mycobacterium* Species—cont'd**			
M. fortuitum	Cattle, cats, dogs, pigs	Mastitis; joint, lung, and skin disease	
M. intracellularae	Pigs, cattle, nonhuman primates	Tuberculosis, granulomatous enteritis	
M. lepraemurium	Cats, Rats	Leprosy	
M. porcinum	Pigs	Lymphadenitis	
M. smegmatis	Cattle, cats	Mastitis, ulcerative skin disease	
M. vaccae	Cattle	Skin disease	
M. xenopi	Cats, pigs	Nodular skin lesions, lymphadenitis	
***Mycoplasma* Species**			
Nonhemotropic mycoplasmas			

M. agalactiae	Goats, sheep	Contagious agalactia	• Identification/differentiation
			  • Colony characteristics
			  • Colony stain with Diene stain
			  • Urease test
			  • Immunology (immunodiffusion, immunofluorescent assay, agglutination, ELISA)

M. alkalescens	Cattle	Arthritis, mastitis	
M. bovigenitalum	Cattle	Infertility, mastitis	
M. bovis	Cattle	Arthritis, mastitis, pneumonia, abortion, abscesses, otitis media, genital infections	
M. bovoculi	Cattle	Conjunctivitis	
M. californicum	Cattle	Mastitis	
M. canadense	Cattle	Abortion, mastitis	
M. capricolum	Goats	Abortion, mastitis, septicemia, polyarthritis, pneumonia	
M. conjunctivae	Sheep	Infectious keratoconjunctivitis	
M. cynos	Dogs	Pneumonia	

Organism	Primary Species Affected	Disease or Lesion	Characteristics
***Mycoplasma* Species–cont'd**			
Nonhemotropic mycoplasmas			
M. dispar	Cattle	Respiratory disease	
M. felis	Cats, horses	Conjunctivitis, pneumonia	
M. gallisepticum	Chickens, turkeys	Airsacculitis, sinusitis	
M. gatae	Cats	Arthritis	
M. hyopneumoniae	Pigs	Pneumonia	
M. hyorhinis	Pigs	Polyarthritis	
M. meleagridis	Turkeys	Airsacculitis, skeletal abnormalities	
M. mycoides ssp. *capri*	Goats	Arthritis, mastitis, pleuropneumonia, septicemia	
M. mycoides ssp. *mycoides*	Cattle, goats, sheep	Pleuropneumonia, mastitis, septicemia, polyarthritis, pneumonia	
M. ovipneumoniae	Goats, sheep	Pleuropneumonia	
M. pulmonis	Rats, mice	Murine respiratory mycoplasmosis	
M. synovale	Chickens, turkeys	Infectious synovitis	
Hemotropic Mycoplasmas			
M. haemocanis	Dogs	Haemobartonellosis	• Coccoid organisms
M. haemofelis	Cats	Haemobartonellosis, feline infectious anemia	• Obligate intracellular parasites • Attached to red blood cell surface
M. haemomuris	Rats, mice	Haemobartonellosis	• Identification/differentiation
M. ovis	Sheep, goats	Eperythrozoonosis	• Cellular morphology
M. suis	Pigs	Eperythrozoonosis	• Immunology (PCR)
M. wenyonii	Cattle	Eperythrozoonosis	

Continued

Organism	Primary Species Affected	Disease or Lesion	Characteristics
Neisseria Species			
N. canis	Dogs	Bite wound infections	• Gram-negative coccobacilli • Nonmotile

N. weaveri	Dogs	Bite wound infections	• Identification/differentiation
			  • Colony characteristics
			  • Hemolysis pattern
			  • Oxidase test
			  • Catalase test
			  • Acid production from carbohydrates

Neorickettsia Species			
N. helminthoeca	Dogs, other canids	"Salmon poisoning"	• Gram-negative coccoid to ellipsoid forms

N. risticii	Horses	Potomac horse fever, monocytic ehrlichiosis	• Located within cytoplasmic vacuoles of myeloid cells or enterocytes
			• Identification/differentiation
			  • Demonstration of organisms on blood film
			  • Immunology

Nocardia Species			
N. asteroids	Dogs, cats, cattle, horses, pigs	Lymphadenitis, subcutaneous abscess, stomatitis, mastitis, pleuritis, peritonitis, abortion	• Gram-positive, pleomorphic, non-spore-forming bacilli • Nonmotile • Aerobic • Acid-fast
N. brasiliensis	Horses	Pneumonia, pleuritis	• Identification/differentiation • Colony characteristics

N. otitidis-caviarum	Cattle, guinea pigs	Ear infections, mastitis	• Cellular morphology
			  • Nitrate reduction test
			  • Esculin hydrolysis test
			  • Urease test

Pasteurella Species			
P. caballi	Horse	Respiratory infection, metritis	• Gram-negative bacilli and coccobacilli
P. canis	Dogs	Puppy septicemia	• Nonmotile • Aerobes
P. gallinarum	Chickens, turkeys	Fowl cholera, salpingitis	• Identification/differentiation • Colony characteristics
P. haemolytica	Cattle, sheep	See _Mannheimia haemolytica_	• Hemolysis pattern • Growth on chocolate agar and MacConkey agar
P. lymphangitidis	Cattle	Lymphangitis	• Catalase test

Organism	Primary Species Affected	Disease or Lesion	Characteristics
Pasteurella Species—cont'd			
P. mairii	Pigs	Abortion, septicemia	• Urease test
P. multocida	Ruminants, pigs, rodents, dogs, cats, cattle	Pneumonia, fowl cholera, rhinitis, mastitis, hemorrhagic septicemia, bite wound infections	• Indole production test • Oxidase test • Acid and gas production from carbohydrates • Nitrate reduction test
P. pneumotropica	Rodents, rabbits	Pneumonia	
P. trehalosi	Sheep	Septicemia, pneumonia	
Porphyromonas Species			
P. levii	Cattle, most mammals	Bovine summer mastitis, pleuritis	• Non-spore-forming, pleomorphic bacilli • Nonmotile

P. gingivalis	Numerous	Periodontitis, gingivitis	• Obligate anaerobes
			• Identification/differentiation
			  • Colony characteristics
			  • Hemolysis pattern
			  • Acid production on carbohydrate substrates
			  • Indole production test

Prevotella Species			
P. melaninogenica	Cattle	Foot rot	• Non-spore-forming, pleomorphic bacilli

P. heparinolytica	Horses	Lower respiratory tract disease	• Nonmotile
			• Obligate anaerobes
			• Identification/differentiation
			  • Colony characteristics
			  • Hemolysis pattern
			  • Acid production on carbohydrate substrates
			  • Indole production test

Proteus Species			

P. mirabilis
P. vulgaris
	Dogs, horses, calves	Cystitis, pyelonephritis, prostatitis, otitis externa	• Gram-negative bacilli
			• Motile
			• Identification/differentiation
			  • Colony characteristics
			  • Oxidase test
			  • Hydrogen sulfide production
			  • Indole production test

Continued

Organism	Primary Species Affected	Disease or Lesion	Characteristics
Pseudomonas Species			

P. aeruginosa	Cattle, dogs, horses, sheep	Mastitis, otitis externa, metritis, corneal ulcer, fleece rot	• Gram-negative, non-spore-forming bacilli
			• Aerobic
			• Identification/differentiation
			  • Colony characteristics
			  • Oxidase test
			  • Growth on MacConkey agar

P. fluorescens	Cattle	Mastitis	
P. mallei		See Burkholderia mallei	
Rhodococcus Species			

R. equi	Horses, pigs	Bronchopneumonia, cervical lymphadenitis	• Gram-positive, pleomorphic coccobacillus
			• Aerobic
			• Partially acid-fast
			• Identification/differentiation
			  • Colony characteristics
			  • Catalase test
			  • Hemolysis pattern
			  • CAMP test
			  • Immunology (immunodiffusion, ELISA)

Rickettsia Species			
R. felis	Cats	Flea typhus	• Intracellular coccobacilli • Located in endothelial cells and smooth muscle cells • Identification/differentiation • Immunology (fluorescent antibody tests, PCR)
R. rickettsii	Dogs	Rocky Mountain spotted fever	
R. typhi	Rats	Murine typhus	
Salmonella Species			

S. ser. abortus-ovis	Sheep	Abortion	• Gram-negative, non-spore-forming bacilli
			• Most are motile
			• Nearly 2500 serovars
			• Organisms are referred to by the genus name and serovar
			• Identification/differentiation
			  • Colony characteristics
			  • Growth on MacConkey agar
			  • Growth on Simmons citrate
			  • Urease test
			  • Indole production test
			  • Hydrogen sulfide production

S. ser. anatum	Sheep, goats, horses	Peracute septicemia; acute, subacute, or chronic enteritis	
S. ser. choleraesuis	Pigs		
S. ser. dublin	Cattle, sheep, goats		
S. ser. enteritidis	Horses		
S. ser. newport	Cattle		
S. ser. pullorum	Poultry		

Organism	Primary Species Affected	Disease or Lesion	Characteristics
***Salmonella* Species–cont'd**			
S. ser. typhimurium	Cattle, sheep, goats, horses, pigs		
***Staphylococcus* Species**			
S. aureus	Mammals	Wound infections, mastitis, skin infections, vaginitis	• Gram-positive cocci • Aerobic • Identification/differentiation
S. epidermidis	Cattle, other mammals	Mastitis, skin abscess	• Colony characteristics • Hemolysis pattern • Catalase test
S. felis	Cats	Otitis externa, cystitis, abscesses, wound infections	• Coagulase test • Fermentation of sugars
S. intermedius	Dogs, cattle	Skin and ear infections, mastitis	
***Streptococcus* Species**			
S. agalactiae	Cattle, horses	Mastitis	• Gram-positive non-spore-forming cocci
S. canis	Dogs, cats	Genital, skin, and wound infections; metritis, mastitis, kitten septicemia	• Facultative anaerobes • Identification/differentiation • Colony characteristics • Hemolysis pattern
S. dysgalactiae ssp. *dysgalactiae*	Cattle, dogs	Mastitis, dermatitis, abortion, septicemia	• Catalase test • Esculin hydrolysis test • CAMP test
S. equi ssp. *equi*	Horses	Strangles, genital infection, mastitis	• Fermentation of sugars
S. zooepidemicus ssp. *equi*	Rats, cattle, goats, sheep, chickens	Mastitis, lymphadenitis, wound infections, pneumonia, septicemia	
S. porcinus	Pigs	Abscesses, lymphadenitis	
S. suis	Pigs	Encephalitis, meningitis, arthritis, septicemia, abortion, endocarditis	
***Taylorella* Species**			
T. equigenitalis	Horses	Contagious equine metritis	• Gram-negative coccobacilli • Identification/differentiation • Colony characteristics • Growth on chocolate agar

Continued

Organism	Primary Species Affected	Disease or Lesion	Characteristics
Taylorella Species–cont'd			• Indole production test • Oxidase test • Catalase test • Esculin hydrolysis test • Immunology (PCR)
Treponema Species			
T. brennaborense	Cattle, horses	Digital dermatitis, "hairy foot warts"	• Tight spiral bacteria • Motile • Identification/differentiation
T. paraluis-cuniculi	Rabbits	Rabbit syphilis	• Cellular morphology with silver staining
Ureaplasma Species			

U. diversum	Cattle	Abortion, vulvitis, pneumonia	• Small mycoplasmas
			• Identification/differentiation
			  • Colony characteristics
			  • Urea hydrolysis
			  • Immunology (PCR, immunofluorescence assay)

Yersinia Species			
Y. enterocolitica	Rabbits, dogs, pigs, horses	Ileitis, gastroenteritis	• Gram-negative bacilli • Facultative anaerobes • Identification/differentiation
Y. pestis	Dogs, cats, goats	Plague	• Cellular morphology • Colony characteristics

Y. pseudotuberculosis	Rodents, guinea pigs, cats, cattle, goats	Pseudotuberculosis, abortion, epididymitis, orchitis	• Oxidase test
			  • Catalase test
			  • Fermentation of sugars

Appendix C

Professional Associations Related to Veterinary Clinical Laboratory Diagnostics

American Association of Veterinary Laboratory Diagnosticians
http://www.aavld.org/mc/page.do

American Association of Veterinary Parasitologists
http://www.aavp.org/

American Board of Veterinary Toxicology
http://www.abvt.org/

American College of Veterinary Microbiologists
http://www.vetmed.iastate.edu/acvm/about.htm

American Society for Veterinary Clinical Pathology
http://www.asvcp.org/

Association of Veterinary Hematology and Transfusion Medicine
http://www.vetmed.wsu.edu/org-AVHTM/index.asp

Veterinary Laboratory Association
http://www.vetlabassoc.com/

Glossary

Abdominocentesis Removal of fluid from the abdominal cavity

Absolute value Number of each type of leukocyte in peripheral blood; calculated by multiplying the relative percentage from the differential count by the total white blood cell count

Acanthocyte An erythrocyte with spiny projections of varying lengths distributed irregularly over its surface

Acariasis Infestation with mites

Accuracy The closeness with which test results agree with the true quantitative value of the constituent

Acid-fast A staining procedure for demonstrating presence of microorganisms that are not readily decolorized by acid after staining; a characteristic of certain bacteria, particularly *Mycobacterium* and *Nocardia*

Acidosis Pathologic decrease in pH of blood or body tissues caused by accumulation of acids or a decrease in bicarbonate

ACTH stimulation Test designed to test the response of the hormone that stimulates adrenocortical growth and secretion (adrenocorticotropic hormone)

Activated clotting time Test of the intrinsic and common pathways of blood coagulation that uses a diatomaceous earth tube to initiate clotting

Active immunity Refers to an animal's production of antibody as a result of infection with an antigen or immunization

Adaptive immunity Component of the immune system that responds to specific antigens

Adipocytes Fat cells

Aerobic In the presence of oxygen

Agar A seaweed extract used to solidify culture media

Agar diffusion Type of test that uses an agar gel plate to allow test substances to disperse in the gel

Agglutination Clumping of particles

Agranulocyte White blood cell group that has no visible cytoplasmic granules

Albumin A group of plasma proteins that comprises the majority of protein in plasma

Alkaline phosphatase A group of enzymes that functions at alkaline pH and catalyzes reactions of organic phosphates

Alpha hemolysis Characterized by partial destruction of blood cells on a blood agar; evident as a greenish zone around the bacterial colony

ALT Alanine aminotransferase; cytoplasmic enzyme of hepatocytes released when hepatocytes are damaged

Ammonium biurate Brownish crystal seen in the urine of animals with severe liver disease

Amorphous crystals Granular precipitate material seen on urine sediment examination

Amylase Enzyme derived primarily from the pancreas that functions in the breakdown of starch

Amyloclastic Method of measuring serum amylase by evaluating the disappearance of starch substrate

Anaerobic In the absence of oxygen

Anemia Reduction in the oxygen-carrying capacity of blood because of a reduced number of circulating red blood cells or a reduced concentration of hemoglobin

Anion Negatively charged ion

Anisocytosis   Variation in the size of cells in a sample

Anisokaryosis   Variation in the size of the nuclei in cells of a sample

Anisonucleosis   Variation in size of nucleoli

Anticoagulant   Any substance that inhibits or prevents clotting

Antigen   Any substance capable of eliciting an immune response

Anulocyte   Bowl-shaped erythrocyte

Anuria   Absence of urine

Arthrocentesis   Removal of fluid from a joint

Arthropod   Ectoparasite belonging to the phylum Arthropoda (insects)

AST   Aspartate aminotransferase; enzyme of hepatocytes found free in the cytoplasm and attached to the mitochondrial membrane that is released when hepatocytes are damaged

Autoimmunity   Any condition that results in production of antibody against a body's own tissues

Azotemia   Increased retention of urea in the blood

Bacilli   Rod-shaped bacteria

Bacteriology   Study of bacteria

Baermann technique   Parasitology test used to recover larvae

Band cell   Immature granulocyte characterized by a nucleus with parallel sides and no nuclear lobes or indentations

Basophilia   Increase in numbers of basophils in a cell; bluish-gray appearance of cells or components of cells that have high affinity for stains with alkaline pH (e.g., methylene blue)

Basophilic stippling   Erythrocytes characterized by small, blue-staining granules; represents residual RNA

Beer's law   Describes the relation between light absorbance, transmission, and concentration of a substance in solution

Bence Jones proteins   Light chain proteins of immunoglobulin molecules that readily pass through the glomerulus into urine

Benign   A tumor or growth that is not malignant; can refer to any condition that is not life threatening

Beta hemolysis   Complete destruction of red blood cells on a blood agar that creates a clear zone around the bacterial colony

Bile acids   Group of compounds synthesized by hepatocytes from cholesterol that aid in fat absorption

Bilirubin   Insoluble pigment derived from the breakdown of hemoglobin, which is processed by hepatocytes

Bilirubinuria   Abnormal increase in concentration of bilirubin in the urine

Biopsy   Removal of cells or tissues for microscopic or chemical examination

Bladderworm   Fluid-filled larval stage of some cestodes

Blast cell   Any immature cell representing a precursor in the development of a particular cell line

Blood agar   An enriched medium that supports the growth of most bacterial pathogens; usually composed of sheep blood

Blood groups   Describes the antigens present on the surface of erythrocytes and antibodies that may be present in serum

Broth   Liquid media used for culture of microorganisms

Buffy coat   Layer of material above the packed erythrocytes after centrifugation; consists primarily of leukocytes and thrombocytes

Calcium carbonate   Type of crystal commonly seen in the urine of rabbits and horses

Calcium oxalate   Crystal found in acidic and neutral urine; commonly seen in small numbers in dogs and horses

Capnophilic   An organism requiring high levels of carbon dioxide for growth or for enhancement of growth

Carboxyhemoglobin   Molecule formed from the irreversible reaction of hemoglobin binding to carbon monoxide

Carcinoma   Describes tumors of epithelial cell origin

Cast   Structure formed from protein precipitate of degenerating kidney tubule cells; may contain embedded materials

Catalase   An enzyme that catalyzes the breakdown of hydrogen peroxide to oxygen and water

Cation   Positively charged ion

Cell-mediated immunity Immune system mechanism involving actions of the cells of the immune system rather than antibodies

Centesis Act of puncturing a body cavity or organ with a hollow needle to draw out fluid

Centrifuge Used to separate substances of different densities that are in a solution

Cercaria Life cycle stage of trematodes that develops in the intermediate host

Cestode Organism in the order Cestoda; tapeworms

Chédiak-Higashi Syndrome Characterized by the presence of large, eosinophilic granules in the cytoplasm of granulocytes and monocytes

Cholestasis Any condition in which bile excretion from the liver is blocked

Cholesterol Plasma lipoprotein produced primarily in the liver as well as ingested in food; used in the synthesis of bile acids

Chylomicron A small fat globule composed of protein and lipid

Chylous Describes fluid that appears milky; results from the presence of emulsified fats

Clearance studies Type of test designed to measure the movement of a specific substance through a specific organ

Coagulase Molecule produced by some bacteria that allows adhesion of fibrinogen to the cell surface

Cocci Describes a bacteria with a round shape

Codocytes Erythrocyte characterized by an increased membrane surface area relative to the cell volume

Colloidal gold assay A type of immunochromatographic test that uses a colloidal gold/antibody conjugate in the test system

Colorimeter A type of photometer that uses a filter to select the wavelength

Complement A group of plasma proteins that function to enhance the activities of the immune system

Control A biologic solution of known values used for verification of accuracy and precision of test results

Coombs test Immunologic test designed to detect antibodies on the surface of erythrocytes (direct Coombs test) or antibodies in plasma against erythrocytes (indirect Coombs test)

Cortisol Steroid hormone produced by the adrenal glands

Creatine kinase An enzyme found predominantly in cells of the heart, brain, and skeletal muscle; released when cells are damaged

Creatinine Waste product formed during normal muscle cell metabolism

Crenation An erythrocyte with multiple small projections evenly spaced over the cell circumference; an artifact from immersion in hypertonic fluid

Cuvette Optical-quality glass or plastic container used to contain reacted samples in photometric assays

Cysticercus A larval form of tapeworm consisting of a single scolex enclosed in a bladderlike cyst

Cytokines Soluble molecules that serve as mediators of cell responses

Dacryocyte An abnormal erythrocyte shaped like a teardrop

d-dimer A protein fragment formed from the breakdown of fibrin

Definitive host The host that harbors the adult, mature, or sexual stages of a parasite

Dermatophyte A group of cutaneous mycotic organisms commonly known as ringworm fungi

DIC Disseminated intravascular coagulation; acquired secondary coagulation disorder characterized by depletion of thrombocytes and coagulation factors; also referred to as consumption coagulopathy and defibrination syndrome

Differential cell count Procedure for classifying cells to determine relative percentages of each cell type present in a peripheral blood or bone marrow sample

Differential media Bacterial culture method that allows bacteria to be differentiated into groups on the basis of their biochemical reactions on the medium

Dipteran An insect of the taxonomic order Diptera (flies); most adults contain a single pair of wings

Döhle bodies   Small, gray-blue areas representing ribosomes seen in the cytoplasm of some immature and toxic granulocytes

Dye excretion   Type of test utilizing biological dyes; evaluates movement of a specific dye through a specific organ

Echinocytes   An erythrocyte with multiple small projections evenly spaced over the cell circumference

Ectoparasite   A parasite that resides on the surface of its host

Effector cell   Collective term for the lymphocytes that function in the immune system to enhance the functions of other cells

Effusion   Excess fluid in a tissue or body cavity

Electrical impedance   Method for counting particles by detection of alterations in electrical current in a solution as particles are passed through the solution

Electrolyte   Any substance that dissociates into ions when in solution

ELISA   Enzyme-linked-immunosorbent assay; an immunologic test

Elliptocyte   An abnormal oval-shaped erythrocyte

Endoparasite   A parasite that resides within a host's tissues

Endospore   Dormant form of a bacterium; intracellular refractile bodies resistant to heat, desiccation, chemicals, and radiation; formed by some bacteria when environmental conditions are poor

Enrichment media   A type of culture media formulated to meet the requirements of the most fastidious pathogens

Enteric bacteria   Bacteria inhabiting the intestinal tract

Enzyme   A protein molecule that catalyzes chemical reactions without being altered or destroyed after the reaction has occurred

Eosinophil   A granulocyte with granules that have an affinity for the acidic components of stains

Eosinophilia   An increase in circulating eosinophils; reddish appearance of cells or components of cells that have high affinity for stains with acid pH

ERPF   Effective renal plasma flow; a clearance study to evaluate kidney function; uses test substances eliminated both by glomerular filtration and renal secretion

Erythrocyte indices   Calculated values that provide the average volume and hemoglobin concentrations of erythrocytes in a peripheral blood sample

Erythroid   Of or relating to a red blood cell or one of its developmental precursors

Erythropoiesis   Production of erythrocytes

Erythropoietin   Hormone that stimulates erythropoietic activity in bone marrow

Exfoliative cytology   Study of cells shed from body surfaces

Exudate   Fluid accumulation resulting from inflammatory processes; characterized by increased cellularity and protein concentration

Facultative anaerobe   Describes a bacteria that does not require oxygen for metabolism but can survive in the presence of oxygen

Fastidious   Describes a bacterial species with complex growth or nutritional requirements

Fibrin   Insoluble plasma protein formed from fibrinogen during blood coagulation

Fibrin split products   A protein fragment formed from the breakdown of fibrin

Flagella   Long, thin, helical structures that function in cell motility

Fractional clearance of electrolytes   Mathematic manipulation that describes the excretion of specific electrolytes relative to the glomerular filtration rate

Fructosamine   Molecule formed as a result of the irreversible reaction of glucose bound to protein

GD   Glutamate dehydrogenase; a mitochondrial-bound enzyme found in high concentrations in the hepatocytes of cattle, sheep, and goats

Generation time   Time required for bacterial colonies to double in size

GFR   Glomerular filtration rate; rate at which substances are filtered through the glomerulus and excreted in urine

Ghost cell   A dead cell in which the cell outline remains visible; an erythrocyte that may be seen in a urine sample that has its cytoplasmic contents removed by cell lysis so that only its outer cytoplasmic membrane remains

Globulin   Complex group of plasma proteins designated as alpha, beta, or gamma; includes immunoglobulins, complement, and transferrin

Glucose   Monosaccharide that represents the end product of carbohydrate metabolism

Glucosuria   Presence of excess glucose in urine

Granular cast   Structure formed from protein precipitate of degenerating kidney tubule cells containing granular material

Granulocyte   Any cell with distinct cytoplasmic granules

Granulomatous   Inflammatory condition characterized by high numbers (more than 70%) of macrophages

Heinz body   Round structure of erythrocytes representing denatured hemoglobin that appear as a pale area with Wright's stain

Helminth   Worm

Hemacytometer   Counting chamber

Hematopoiesis   Production of blood cells and platelets

Hematuria   Presence of intact erythrocytes in urine

Hemoglobinuria   Presence of free hemoglobin in urine

Hemolysis   Destruction of erythrocytes

Hemoprotozoa   Parasites located in peripheral blood

Hemostasis   Blood coagulation

Heterophil   Leukocyte of avian, reptile, and some fish species containing prominent eosinophilic granules; functionally equivalent to the mammalian neutrophil

Hexacanth   Infective stage of some cestodes

Histopathology   Microscopic study of diseased tissues

Howell Jolly body   Basophilic inclusions of young erythrocytes representing nuclear remnants

Humoral immunity   Immune response involving production of specific antibody

Hyaline cast   Structure formed from protein precipitate of degenerating kidney tubule cells with no imbedded materials

Hydatid cyst   Larval cyst stage of the tapeworms *Echinococcus granulosus* and *E. multilocularis,* which contains daughter cysts, each of which contains many scolexes

Hypercalcemia   Increased plasma calcium

Hyperchromatophilic   Cell appearing darker than normal on a peripheral blood sample

Hyperkalemia   Increased plasma potassium

Hypernatremia   Increased plasma sodium

Hyperplasia   Increase in the number of the cells of an organ or tissue

Hypersegmented   Denotes a neutrophil with more than five nuclear lobes

Hypersensitivity   Immune system reactions that damage a body's own tissues

Hyphae   Body of a fungus created as a result of the linear arrangements of cells that form multicellular or multinucleate growth

Hypocalcemia   Decreased plasma calcium

Hypochromic   Erythrocytes with decreased staining intensity from decrease in hemoglobin concentration

Hypoglycemia   Decreased plasma glucose

Hypokalemia   Decreased plasma potassium

Hyponatremia   Decreased plasma sodium

Icterus   Abnormal yellowish discoloration of skin, mucous membranes, or plasma as a result of increased concentration of bile pigments

Immunodiffusion   Immunologic test performed by placing reactants in an agar plate and allowing them to migrate through the gel toward each other

Immunoglobulin   Antibody; plasma proteins produced against specific antigens

Immunologic tolerance   A state of nonresponsiveness to antigens, whether self or foreign

Inflammation   Defensive response of body tissues initiated by release of histamine from damaged cells

Innate immunity   The nonspecific components of the immune system that function the same way regardless of which antigen is present

Interferons   Small soluble proteins that enhance the function of the immune system

Intermediate host   The host that harbors the larval, immature, or asexual stages of a parasite

International unit   Système Internationale (SI) set of basic units, which is based on the metric system

Isoenzymes   Group of enzymes with similar catalytic activities but different physical properties

Isosthenuria   A condition in which urine specific gravity approaches that of the glomerular filtrate

Karyolysis   Degeneration or dissolution of a cell nucleus

Karyorrhexis   Fragmentation of a cell nucleus

Katal   Basic unit of enzyme activity; the amount of activity that converts 1 mole of substrate per second

Keratocyte   In hematology, an abnormally shaped erythrocyte that appears to have horns

Ketoacidosis   Accumulation of ketone bodies in the body tissues and fluids

Ketonuria   Presence of detectable ketone bodies in urine

Kinetic assay   A chemical test that measures the rate of change of a substance in the test system

Left shift   Presence of increased numbers of immature cells in a peripheral blood sample

Leptocyte   Erythrocyte characterized by an increased membrane surface area relative to the cell volume

Leukopenia   Decreased number of leukocytes in blood

Leukemia   Neoplastic cells in the blood or bone marrow

Leukocytosis   Increased numbers of leukocytes in the blood

Leukopoiesis   Production of leukocytes

Lipase   Pancreatic enzyme that functions in the breakdown of fats

Lipemia   Presence of fatty material in plasma or serum

Lymphadenitis   Inflammation of one or more lymph nodes

Lymphopenia   Decreased numbers of leukocytes in a peripheral blood sample

Macrocyte   Cell that appears to have a larger than normal diameter

Macrophage   Phagocytic cell derived from the monocyte

Mast cell   Tissue cell characterized by abundant, small, metachromatic cytoplasmic granules that functions in the immune system

MCH   Mean corpuscular hemoglobin; the mean weight of hemoglobin contained in the average erythrocyte

MCHC   Mean corpuscular hemoglobin concentration; the ratio of weight of hemoglobin in the average erythrocyte to the volume in which it is contained

MCV   Mean corpuscular volume; average size of the erythrocytes in peripheral blood

Megakaryocyte   Bone marrow cell from which blood platelets arise

M/E ratio   Relative percentages of myeloid and erythroid cells in bone marrow

Merozoite   Life cycle stage of a protozoal parasite that results from asexual reproduction

Mesenchymal   Cells or tissues derived from the embryonic mesoderm

Mesophiles   Organisms with an optimal growth temperature between 25° C and 40° C

Mesothelial   Cells that line body cavities; derived from the embryonic mesoderm

Metastasis   Neoplastic cells present in areas other than the location where they originated

Methemoglobin   Form of hemoglobin containing oxidized iron; inefficient at oxygen transport

Microaerophilic   An organism requiring oxygen for growth at a level below that found in air

Microalbuminuria   Abnormal presence of small concentrations of albumin in urine

Microcyte   Cell that appears to have a smaller than normal diameter

Microfilaria   Larval offspring of the group of filarial worms in the phylum Nematoda

Miracidium   Ciliated larval stage of a digenic trematode

Mott cell   Plasma cells containing multiple globular cytoplasmic inclusions composed of immunoglobulin (Russell bodies)

Mueller Hinton media   Standard culture media used to evaluate susceptibility of microorganisms to antimicrobial agents

Mycology   Study of fungi

Myeloid cells   Bone marrow stem cell that gives rise to erythrocyte precursors, megakaryocytes, and nonlymphocytic leukocytes

Myiasis   Infestation with larvae (maggots) of dipterans

Myoglobinuria   Presence of myoglobin (muscle protein) in urine

Natural killer (NK) cell   A subpopulation of lymphocytes capable of direct lysis of cells infected with antigen

N/C ratio   Relative percentage of nuclear and cytoplasmic material in a cell

Neoplasia   Generic term to describe any growth; often used to describe a tumor, which may be malignant or benign

Neutropenia   Abnormal decrease in neutrophils in a peripheral blood sample

Neutrophilia   Abnormal increase in neutrophils in a peripheral blood sample

Nit   The egg stage of lice bound to hair or feather shaft of the host

Normochromic   Cells that stain with their characteristic color

Normocytic   Cells that appear with their characteristic morphology

Nuclear molding   A deformation of nuclei by other nuclei within the same cell or adjacent cells

Reticle   Ocular micrometer disks that impose a calibrated image over the microscope viewing area

Oliguria   Decrease in the volume of urine produced

Oocyst   Resistant spore phase of some parasitic protozoans

Operculum   A lid or flap covering an opening; common structure on the eggs of some trematodes

Opportunistic   Organism that is not normally harmful but can be pathogenic under certain circumstances

Opsonization   Complement-mediated adherence of phagocytes to antigens that enhances phagocytosis of the antigen

Oxidase   Enzyme present in some groups of bacteria that is involved with the reduction of oxygen during normal bacteria metabolism

Oxyhemoglobin   Form of hemoglobin containing a full complement of oxygen molecules for dispersal to tissues

Packed cell volume   Ratio of red blood cells to total plasma volume

Palisade   Parallel arrangement of some species of bacteria; often described as looking like a picket fence

Pancytopenia   Decreased numbers of all blood cells and platelets in a peripheral blood or bone marrow sample

Paracentesis   Removal of fluid from a body cavity

Parthenogenic   Condition in which female organisms produce eggs that develop without fertilization

Passive immunity   Receiving antibodies from colostrum or synthesized antibodies

Pediculosis   Infestation with lice

Pelger-Huët anomaly   An inherited anomaly characterized by the appearance of bi-lobed neutrophils in a peripheral blood sample

Perinuclear   Situated around the nucleus

Periodic parasite   Describes a parasite that lives part of its life cycle on its host and part off the host

pH   Measure of hydrogen ion concentration of a solution

Plasma   Fluid portion of the blood

Plasma cell   A leukocyte that has differentiated to an antibody-secreting cell

Pleomorphic   Taking a variety of shapes and forms

Pleomorphism   Taking a variety of shapes and forms; multiple morphologies

Poikilocytosis   Any abnormal cell shape

Pollakiuria   Increase in the frequency of urination

Polychromasia   Variable staining pattern; basophilia

Polymerase chain reaction   Method used to replicate and amplify DNA molecules in a sample

Polyuria   Increase in the total volume of urine produced

Potentiometers   Type of electrochemical analyzer used to evaluate ionic concentration in a solution

Precision   The magnitude of random errors and the reproducibility of measurements

Prepatent period   The time interval between infection with a parasite and demonstration of the infection

Proglottid   Segments that comprise the body of a cestode

Proteinuria   Abnormal presence of protein in the urine

Psychrophiles   Organisms with optimal growth at cold temperatures (between 15° C and 20° C)

Purulent   Containing, discharging, or causing the production of pus; cytology sample characterized by the presence of neutrophils representing more than 85% of total nucleated cells in the sample

Pyknosis   Condensed nuclear chromatin in a degenerating cell

Pyogranulomatous   Cytology sample characterized by the presence of macrophages representing more than 15% of total nucleated cells in the sample

Redia   A secondary larval form of some digenic trematodes that develops within a mollusk intermediate host

Refractive index   Measure of the degree of light bending as it passes from one media to another, relative to air; function of the dissolved material in the sample

Refractometer   Used to measure the refractive index of a solution

Reliability   The ability of a method to be accurate and precise

Resolving power   Indicator of image quality; numerical aperture

Reticulocyte   An anuclear, immature erythrocyte

Right shift   Presence of an increased number of hypersegmented neutrophils in a peripheral blood sample

Rouleaux   Arrangement of erythrocytes in a column or stack

Russell bodies   Cytoplasmic inclusions in plasma cells representing packets of immunoglobulins

Sarcoma   Generic term to describe any cancer arising from cells of the connective tissues

Schistocyte   Fragmented erythrocytes usually formed as a result of shearing of the red cell by intravascular trauma

Schizont   Life cycle stage of some protozoal organisms; arises from multiple asexual fission

Scolex   The head of a cestode by which it attaches to its host

Selective media   A type of culture media that contains antibacterial substances that inhibit or kill all but a few types of bacteria

Sensitivity testing   Method used to determine the resistance or susceptibility of a microorganism to specific antimicrobials

Serum   The fluid portion of blood after it has clotted; does not contain cells or coagulation proteins

Smudge cell   A leukocyte that has ruptured

Specific gravity   The weight (density) of a quantity of liquid compared with that of an equal amount of distilled water

Specificity   Ability of a test to evaluate a given parameter correctly

Spectrophotometers   Designed to measure the amount of light transmitted through a solution

Spherocyte   Intensely stained erythrocyte having reduced or no central pallor

Sporocyst   Larval stage of a digenic trematode that develops in a mollusk intermediate host

Sporozoite   Infective stage of some protozoal parasites

Stage micrometer   Microscope slide etched with a 2-mm line marked in 0.01-mm divisions; 1 micron equals 0.001 mm

Standard   A nonbiologic solution of an analyte, usually in distilled water, with a known concentration

Stomatocyte   Erythrocyte with a linear area of central pallor

Struvite   Common crystal seen in alkaline to slightly acidic urine; sometimes referred to as triple phosphate crystals or magnesium ammonium phosphate crystals

Substrate   Any substance acted upon by an enzyme

Suppurative   Purulent

Target cells   Leptocyte with a peripheral ring of cytoplasm surrounded by a clear area and a dense, central, rounded area of pigment

Thermophiles   Organisms with optimal growth at elevated temperatures

Thoracocentesis   Removal of fluid from the thoracic cavity

Thrombocyte   Platelet; cytoplasmic fragment of bone marrow megakaryocyte

Thrombocytopenia Decrease in circulating platelets

Thrombopoiesis Production of platelets

Tick paralysis Condition resulting from introduction of a neurotoxin into the body during attachment of and feeding by the female of several tick species

Titer The greatest dilution at which a patient sample no longer yields a positive result for the presence of a specific antibody

Toxic neutrophil A neutrophil characterized by the presence of cytoplasmic basophilia, Döhle bodies, vacuoles, heavy granulation, and/or giantism

Toxicology Study of hazardous substances and their effects on health

Transudate An effusion characterized by low protein concentration and low total nucleated cell counts

Trematode Organism in the phylum Trematoda; commonly referred to as a fluke

Trophozoite The motile form of a protozoal parasite

Urea The principal end product of amino acid breakdown in mammals

Uric acid Metabolic byproduct of nitrogen catabolism

Urochromes Pigments that impart color to a urine sample

Urolithiasis Presence of calculi (stones) in the urinary tract

Vector Any organism that transmits a disease-causing organism to new hosts

Veterinary technician A dedicated, tireless, and vital member of the veterinary health care team; individual with a minimum of 2 years of college education who performs myriad diagnostic and nursing procedures in the veterinary facility; saint

Virology Study of viruses

Warble Common name for the larva of some species of flies; often in swollen, cystlike subcutaneous sites, with a fistula or pore communicating to the outside environment

Zone of inhibition Area of no bacterial growth around a an antimicrobial disk, indicates some sensitivity of the organism to the particular antimicrobial

Zoonotic infection A disease that is transmitted from a nonhuman animal to a human being

Index

Page numbers followed by *f* indicate figures; *t*, tables; *b*, boxes; *p*, procedure boxes.